Multidisciplinary Management of Urinary Stone Disease

Editor

OJAS SHAH

UROLOGIC CLINICS OF NORTH AMERICA

www.urologic.theclinics.com

Consulting Editor

SAMIR S. TANEJA

February 2013 • Volume 40 • Number 1

ELSEVIER

1600 John F. Kennedy Blvd. • Suite 1800 • Philadelphia, PA 19103-2899

http://www.theclinics.com

UROLOGIC CLINICS OF NORTH AMERICA Volume 40, Number 1
February 2013 ISSN 0094-0143, ISBN-13: 978-1-4557-7344-2

Editor: Stephanie Donley

Urologic Clinics of North America (ISSN 0094-0143) is published quarterly by Elsevier Inc., 360 Park Avenue South, New York, NY 10010-1710. Months of issue are February, May, August, and November. Business and Editorial Offices: 1600 John F. Kennedy Blvd., Suite 1800, Philadelphia, PA 19103-2899. Periodicals postage paid at New York, NY and additional mailing offices. Subscription prices are $339.00 per year (US individuals), $561.00 per year (US institutions), $396.00 per year (Canadian individuals), $687.00 per year (Canadian institutions), $492.00 per year (foreign individuals), and $687.00 per year (foreign institutions). Foreign air speed delivery is included in all *Clinics* subscription prices. All prices are subject to change without notice. **POSTMASTER:** Send address changes to *Urologic Clinics of North America*, Elsevier Health Sciences Division, Subscription Customer Service, 3251 Riverport Lane, Maryland Heights, MO 63043. Customer Service: 1-800-654-2452 (US). From outside the United States, call 1-314-447-8871. Fax: 1-314-447-8029. E-mail: JournalsCustomerServiceusa@elsevier.com (for print support) and JournalsOnlineSupport-usa@elsevier.com (for online support).

Reprints. For copies of 100 or more, of articles in this publication, please contact the Commercial Reprints Department, Elsevier Inc., 360 Park Avenue South, New York, New York 10010-1710. Tel.: 212-633-3813; Fax: 212-462-1935; E-mail: reprints@elsevier.com.

Urologic Clinics of North America is covered in MEDLINE/PubMed (*Index Medicus*), *Excerpta Medica, Current Contents/Clinical Medicine, Science Citation Index,* and *ISI/BIOMED*.

Printed and bound by CPI Group (UK) Ltd, Croydon, CR0 4YY

Transferred to digital print 2013

Contributors

CONSULTING EDITOR

SAMIR S. TANEJA, MD
The James M. Neissa and Janet Riha Neissa Professor of Urologic Oncology; Professor of Urology and Radiology; Director, Division of Urologic Oncology; Co-Director, Smilow Comprehensive Prostate Cancer Center, Department of Urology, NYU Langone Medical Center, New York, New York

GUEST EDITOR

OJAS SHAH, MD
Assistant Professor of Urology; Director, Endourology and Stone Disease; Chief of Urology, Bellevue Hospital; Residency Program Director, NYU Langone Medical Center, New York University School of Medicine, New York, New York

AUTHORS

JODI A. ANTONELLI, MD
Fellow, Department of Urology, University of Texas Southwestern Medical Center, Dallas, Texas

OMOTAYO AROWOJOLU, BS
New York University School of Medicine, New York, New York

HERMAN SINGH BAGGA, MD
Department of Urology, University of California San Francisco, San Francisco, California

NAEEM BHOJANI, MD
Endourology Fellow, Department of Urology, Indiana University School of Medicine, Indianapolis, Indiana

MICHAEL S. BOROFSKY, MD
Resident in Urology, Department of Urology, NYU Langone Medical Center, New York University School of Medicine, New York

JUAN C. CALLE, MD
Department of Nephrology, Glickman Urological & Kidney Institute, The Cleveland Clinic, Cleveland, Ohio

DOH YOON CHA, MD
Department of Urology, Columbia University Medical Center, New York, New York

THOMAS CHI, MD
Department of Urology, University of California San Francisco, San Francisco, California

BRIAN H. EISNER, MD
Department of Urology, Harvard Medical School, Massachusetts General Hospital, Boston, Massachusetts

DAVID S. GOLDFARB, MD
Chief, Nephrology Section, New York Harbor Healthcare System; Director, Kidney Stone Prevention Program, Lenox Hill Hospital; Professor of Medicine and Physiology, New York University School of Medicine, New York, New York

MANTU GUPTA, MD
Department of Urology, Columbia University Medical Center, New York, New York

MITCHELL R. HUMPHREYS, MD
Associate Professor, Department of Urology; Endourology Fellowship Director, Mayo Clinic, Phoenix, Arizona

ELIAS S. HYAMS, MD
Assistant Professor of Surgery, Division of Urology, Dartmouth-Hitchcock Medical Center, Lebanon, New Hampshire

GANESH KARTHA, MD
Department of Urology, Glickman Urological & Kidney Institute, The Cleveland Clinic, Cleveland, Ohio

JAMES E. LINGEMAN, MD
Professor, Department of Urology, Indiana University School of Medicine, Indianapolis, Indiana

MICHAEL E. LIPKIN, MD
Assistant Professor, Department of Urology, Duke University Medical Center, Durham, North Carolina

GIOVANNI SCALA MARCHINI, MD
Department of Urology, Glickman Urological & Kidney Institute, The Cleveland Clinic, Cleveland, Ohio

BRIAN R. MATLAGA, MD, MPH
Associate Professor of Urology, Brady Urological Institute, Johns Hopkins Hospital, Baltimore, Maryland

JOE MILLER, MD
Department of Urology, University of California San Francisco, San Francisco, California

MANOJ MONGA, MD
Department of Urology, Glickman Urological & Kidney Institute, The Cleveland Clinic, Cleveland, Ohio

STEPHEN Y. NAKADA, MD
Professor and Chairman of Urology, Department of Urology, University of Wisconsin School of Medicine and Public Health, Madison, Wisconsin

GYAN PAREEK, MD
Department of Urology, Warren Alpert Medical School of Brown University, Providence, Rhode Island

MARGARET S. PEARLE, MD, PhD
Professor of Urology and Internal Medicine, Department of Urology; Jane and Charles Pak Center for Mineral Metabolism, University of Texas Southwestern Medical Center, Dallas, Texas

KRISTINA L. PENNISTON, PhD, RD
Associate Scientist, Department of Urology, University of Wisconsin School of Medicine and Public Health, Madison, Wisconsin

GLENN M. PREMINGER, MD
Professor, Department of Urology; Chief, Division of Urology, Duke University Medical Center, Durham, North Carolina

OJAS SHAH, MD
Assistant Professor of Urology; Director, Endourology and Stone Disease; Chief of Urology, Bellevue Hospital; Residency Program Director, NYU Langone Medical Center, New York University School of Medicine, New York, New York

MARSHALL L. STOLLER, MD
Department of Urology, University of California San Francisco, San Francisco, California

YUNG K. TAN, MBBS, MRCS
Department of Urology, Columbia University Medical Center, New York, New York

Contents

Foreword **xi**

Samir S. Taneja

Preface **xiii**

Ojas Shah

New Insights Into the Pathogenesis of Renal Calculi **1**

Herman Singh Bagga, Thomas Chi, Joe Miller, and Marshall L. Stoller

The pathophysiology of the various forms of urinary stone disease remains a complex topic. Epidemiologic research and the study of urine and serum chemistries have created an abundance of data to help drive the formulation of pathophysiologic theories. This article addresses the associations of urinary stone disease with hypertension, cardiovascular disease, atherosclerosis, obesity, dyslipidemia, diabetes, and other disease states. Findings regarding the impact of dietary calcium and the formation of Randall's plaques are also explored and their implications discussed. Finally, further avenues of research are explored, including genetic analyses and the use of animal models of urinary stone disease.

Metabolic Evaluation of First-time and Recurrent Stone Formers **13**

David S. Goldfarb and Omotayo Arowojolu

Evaluation of stone formers should include careful attention to medications, past medical history, social history, family history, dietary evaluation, occupation, and laboratory evaluation. Laboratory evaluation requires at least serum chemistries and urinalysis. Twenty-four–hour urine collections are most appropriate for patients with recurrent stones or complex medical histories. However, these collections may be appropriate for some first-time stone formers, including those with comorbidities or large stones. Although twin studies demonstrate that heritability accounts for at least 50% of the kidney stone phenotype, the responsible genes are not clearly identified, and so genetic testing is rarely indicated.

Pharmacologic Treatment of Kidney Stone Disease **21**

Brian H. Eisner, David S. Goldfarb, and Gyan Pareek

This article reviews the data on pharmacologic treatment of kidney stone disease, with a focus on prophylaxis against stone recurrence. One of the most effective and important therapies for stone prevention, an increase in urine volume, is not discussed because this is a dietary and not a pharmacologic intervention. Also reviewed are medical expulsive therapy used to improve the spontaneous passage of ureteral stones and pharmacologic treatment of symptoms associated with ureteral stents. The goal is to review the literature with a focus on the highest level of evidence (ie, randomized controlled trials).

Diet and Alternative Therapies in the Management of Stone Disease **31**

Kristina L. Penniston and Stephen Y. Nakada

Although nonnutritional factors affect the risk for renal stone development, nutrition is widely viewed as contributory and is frequently included as part of the therapeutic regimen in secondary stone prevention. In this article, the therapeutic application of nutritional recommendations to address specific risk factors of urolithiasis is reviewed. The article focuses on calcium-containing and uric acid stones. The general approach to nutrition therapy is addressed first, and empiric and tailored approaches are discussed. How to assess a patient's nutrition risk for lithogenesis is reviewed, and the implementation or practice of nutrition therapy is discussed.

Imaging Techniques for Stone Disease and Methods for Reducing Radiation Exposure **47**

Michael E. Lipkin and Glenn M. Preminger

Imaging plays a critical role in the evaluation of patients with urolithiasis. It is essential for the diagnosis of stones and provides important information to aide in determining the appropriate treatment of renal or ureteral calculi. Imaging for urolithiasis has evolved over the past 30 years. Currently, noncontrast computed tomography remains the first-line imaging modality for the evaluation of patients with suspected urolithiasis. Proper imaging modality selection helps to minimize radiation exposure. Following the principles of *As Low As Reasonably Achievable* in the operating room can help reduce the amount of radiation patients are exposed to from fluoroscopy.

Shockwave Lithotripsy–New Concepts and Optimizing Treatment Parameters **59**

Naeem Bhojani and James E. Lingeman

The treatment of kidney stone disease has changed dramatically over the past 30 years. This change is due in large part to the arrival of extracorporeal shock wave lithotripsy (ESWL). ESWL along with the advances in ureteroscopic and percutaneous techniques has led to the virtual extinction of open surgical treatments for kidney stone disease. Much research has gone into understanding how ESWL can be made more efficient and safe. This article discusses the parameters that can be used to optimize ESWL outcomes as well as the new concepts that are affecting the efficacy and efficiency of ESWL.

Advances in Ureteroscopy **67**

Michael S. Borofsky and Ojas Shah

Recent innovations in imaging equipment and novel instrumentation have helped ureteroscopy evolve from a diagnostic to a therapeutic tool. In this review, the authors highlight several of the most recent advances in ureteroscopy that have helped allow unprecedented access, visualization, and treatment of upper urinary tract pathologic conditions.

Management of Stones in Abnormal Situations **79**

Yung K. Tan, Doh Yoon Cha, and Mantu Gupta

Stones in abnormal situations present a management conundrum to the urologist. Many of these situations are relatively rare and literature is scanty on the appropriate management. We review the current literature on the management of stones in the setting of pregnancy, calyceal diverticulum, urinary diversions, pelvic kidneys, transplant kidneys, autosomal dominant polycystic kidney disease, horseshoe kidneys, and other renal anomalies. The aims of treatment are complete stone-free status.

The modality of treatment should be individualized to the size and location of stone and type of abnormal situation confronted.

Advances in Percutaneous Nephrolithotomy **99**

Jodi A. Antonelli and Margaret S. Pearle

Percutaneous nephrolithotomy (PCNL) is the most morbid of the minimally invasive surgeical procedures for stone removal. Over the last 2 decades, refinements in technique and new technology have improved the efficacy and the efficiency of the procedure. Although PCNL has long been the procedure of choice for large and complex stones, it is increasingly being used for moderate stone burdens because of its high stone-free rates and because of the limitations of shock wave lithotripsy and ureteroscopy. The article reviews advances in the technique and technology applied to percutaneous access, tract dilation, stone visualization, stone fragmentation, stone clearance, and postoperative management.

The Emerging Role of Robotics and Laparoscopy in Stone Disease **115**

Mitchell R. Humphreys

The surgical management of urolithiasis has undergone a remarkable clinical evolution over the past three decades. The once common practice of open stone surgery has nearly been relegated to historical interest by modern technology. The introduction of minimally invasive techniques, laparoscopy and robot-assisted surgery, have emerged to complete the urologist's armamentarium. The benefits to patients when other endourologic procedures have failed include less pain, shorter hospitalization and convalescence, and improved cosmesis. This chapter explores the historical shift from open to minimally invasive management for stone disease and the unique risks and outcomes associated with these procedures in modern urology.

Cost-effectiveness Treatment Strategies for Stone Disease for the Practicing Urologist **129**

Elias S. Hyams and Brian R. Matlaga

Kidney stone disease is rising in prevalence in the United States and abroad, and the cost burden of this condition is substantial. Although cost-effectiveness considerations are typically made by policymakers, individual practitioners have become increasingly involved in these discussions, to affect the rising costs of care and to assert control of treatment options. This article reviews existing literature regarding the cost-effectiveness of medical and surgical treatments for stone disease and identifies areas in which additional investigation is needed.

Impact of Stone Disease: Chronic Kidney Disease and Quality of Life **135**

Ganesh Kartha, Juan C. Calle, Giovanni Scala Marchini, and Manoj Monga

This article reviews the impact of stone disease on chronic kidney disease and renal function; evaluating the natural progression of disease as well as the impact of surgical interventions. The impact of stone disease, medical therapy, and surgical therapy for stones on quality of life is discussed.

Index **149**

PROGRAM OBJECTIVE:

The goal of *Urologic Clinics of North America* is to keep practicing urologists and urology residents up to date with current clinical practice in urology by providing timely articles reviewing the state of the art in patient care.

TARGET AUDIENCE

Practicing urologists, urology residents and other health care professionals practicing in the discipline of urology.

ACCREDITATION

The Elsevier Office of Continuing Medical Education (EOCME) is accredited by the Accreditation Council for Continuing Medical Education (ACCME) to provide continuing medical education for physicians.

The EOCME designates this journal-based CME activity for a maximum of 12 *AMA PRA Category 1 Credit*(s)™. Physicians should claim only the credit commensurate with the extent of their participation in the activity.

All other health care professionals completing continuing education credit for this activity will be issued a certificate of participation.

DISCLOSURE OF CONFLICTS OF INTEREST

The EOCME assesses conflict of interest with its instructors, faculty, planners, and other individuals who are in a position to control the content of CME activities. All relevant conflicts of interest that are identified are thoroughly vetted by EOCME for fair balance, scientific objectivity, and patient care recommendations. EOCME is committed to providing its learners with CME activities that promote improvements or quality in healthcare and not a specific proprietary business or a commercial interest.

The planning committee, staff, authors and editors listed below have identified no financial relationships or relationships to products or devices they or their spouse/life partner have with commercial interest related to the content of this CME activity:
Jodi A. Antonelli, MD; Omotayo Arowojolu, BS; Herman Singh Bagga, MD; Naeem Bhojani, MD; Michael S. Borofsky, MD; Juan C. Calle, MD; Doh Yoon Cha, MD; Thomas Chi, MD; Jeannette Forcina; Mantu Gupta, MD; Elias S. Hyams, MD; Ganesh Kartha, MD; Indu Kumari; Jill McNair; Giovanni Scala Marchini, MD; Brian R. Matlaga, MD, MPH; Joe Miller, MD; Manoj Monga, MD; Stephen Y. Nakada, MD; Gyan Pareek, MD; Margaret S. Pearle, MD, PhD; Kristina L. Penniston, PhD, RD; Glenn M. Preminger, MD; Katelynn Steck; Marshall L. Stoller, MD and Yung K. Tan, MBBS, MRCS.

The planning committee, staff, authors and editors listed below have identified financial relationships or relationships to products or devices they or their spouse/life partner have with commercial interest related to the content of this CME activity:
Brian H. Eisner, MD has stock ownership in Ravine Group and is a consultant for Boston Scientific and Olympus.
David S. Goldfarb, MD is a consultant for Takeda and Keryx; is on the speaker's bureau, faculty or peer reviewer for Quintiles; and is an industry funded researcher/investigator for Amgen, Hospira and Reata.
Mitchell R. Humphreys, MD is a consultant for Luminis and Medafar.
James E. Lingeman, MD has stock ownership in Midwest Mobile Lithotripsy and Midstate Mobile Lithotripsy.
Michael E. Lipkin, MD is a consultant for Boston Scientific Corp and is on the speaker's bureau, faculty or peer reviewer for Lumenis Corp.
Ojas Shah, MD is a consultant for Boston Scientific Corp and is a consultant and on the speaker's bureau for Cook Medical; has received industry funded research/investigator for Watson Pharmaceuticals; and has stock ownership in New Jersey Kidney Stone Center and Metropolitan Lithotripsy.
Samir S. Taneja, MD is a consultant for Eigen, Gtx, and Steba Biotech, is an industry funded research/investigator for Gtx and Steba Biotech, and is on the Speakers' Bureau for Janssen.

UNAPPROVED/OFF-LABEL USE DISCLOSURE

The EOCME requires CME faculty to disclose to the participants:

1. When products or procedures being discussed are off-label, unlabelled, experimental, and/or investigational (not US Food and Drug Administration (FDA) approved; and
2. Any limitations on the information presented, such as data that are preliminary or that represent ongoing research, interim analyses, and/or unsupported opinions. Faculty may discuss information about pharmaceutical agents that is outside of DA-approved labelling. This information is intended solely for CME and is not intended to promote off-label use of these medications. If you have any questions, contact the medical affairs department of the manufacturer for the most recent prescribing information.

TO ENROLL

To enroll in the *Urologic Clinics of North America* Continuing Medical Education program, call customer service at 1-800-654-2452 or sign up online at http://www.theclinics.com/home/cme. The CME program is available to subscribers for an additional annual fee of $243 USD.

METHOD OF PARTICIPATION

In order to claim credit, participants must complete the following:

1. Complete enrolment as indicated above.
2. Read the activity.
3. Complete the CME Test and Evaluation. Participants must achieve a score of 70% on the test. All CME Tests and Evaluations must be completed online.

CME INQUIRIES/SPECIAL NEEDS

For all CME inquiries or special needs, please contact elsevierCME@elsevier.com.

UROLOGIC CLINICS OF NORTH AMERICA

UROLOGIC CLINICS OF NORTH AMERICA

FORTHCOMING ISSUES

May 2013
Diagnosis, Evaluation, and Treatment of Non-Muscle Invasive Bladder Cancer
Sam S. Chang, MD, *Guest Editor*

August 2013
Urologic Trauma and Reconstruction
Alan F. Morey, MD, and Steven J. Hudak, MD, *Guest Editors*

November 2013
Office Based Procedures
J. Stephen Jones, MD, *Guest Editor*

RECENT ISSUES

November 2012
Castrate-Resistant Prostate Cancer
Adam S. Kibel, MD, *Guest Editor*

August 2012
Controversies in Female Pelvic Reconstruction
Roger Dmochowski, MD, and Mickey Karram, MD, *Guest Editors*

May 2012
Evolving Treatment Paradigms for Renal Cancer
William C. Huang, MD, and Samir S. Taneja, MD, *Guest Editors*

NOW AVAILABLE FOR YOUR iPhone and iPad

Foreword

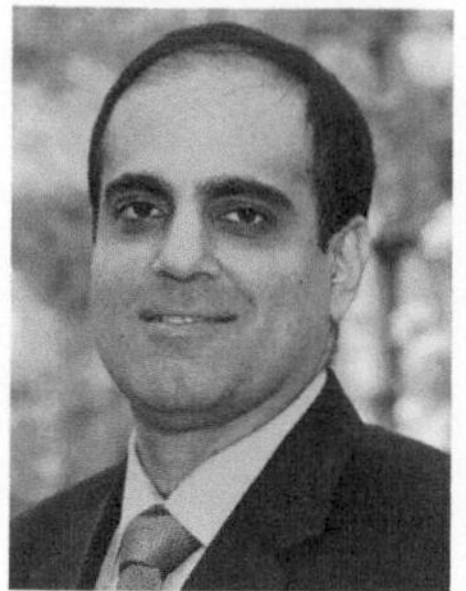

Samir S. Taneja, MD
Consulting Editor

Dating back to the days of traveling barbers treating bladder stones to the modern era of endourology, stone disease is, perhaps, the longest standing staple of urologic practice. With the advent of imaging, the number of urinary stones seen in practice grew to include asymptomatic stones for which treatment may or may not be indicated. Advances in imaging now offer insight into stone composition, in addition to accurate measurements of size and position.

In the contemporary era, the urologist's role is no longer to simply crush and remove, but instead, to treat the acute sequelae of stone passage, determine the necessity for treating the asymptomatic stone, and provide evaluation and management for the prevention of stone formation. In this regard, the management of stone disease represents one of the best examples of multidisciplinary care in Urology. As we move forward into the era of disease-based multidisciplinary approaches to health care, we can learn a great deal from the paradigms for care established by our colleagues who have chosen to specialize in the management of urinary stones.

In keeping with our goal of using *Urologic Clinics* as a means of demonstrating multidisciplinary approaches to urologic disease, this issue, guest edited by my colleague Ojas Shah, is constructed to review the comprehensive approach to the stone patient. Dr Shah has done a wonderful job of including current, relevant topics and inviting leading authorities within the discipline to contribute their perspective. The articles included range from surgical therapy to metabolic evaluation to dietary manipulation to cost-effectiveness in stone management. We are deeply indebted to each of the authors for their outstanding additions to this monograph.

In reviewing the content of this issue of *Urologic Clinics* I sincerely hope that you will gain insight into an aspect of stone disease management that you had previously not considered. Since most urologists treat stones surgically, it remains important for us as a urologic community to have a comprehensive understanding of the basis of stone formation, an evaluation of the metabolic derangements leading to stone disease, and the necessary preventive measures needed for the individual patient. In doing so, we will be well poised to provide complete care as the health care system evolves. Once again, I am deeply indebted to Dr Shah and all the contributing authors for a fabulous issue of *Urologic Clinics.*

Samir S. Taneja, MD
Division of Urologic Oncology
Smilow Comprehensive Prostate Cancer Center
Department of Urology
NYU Langone Medical Center
150 East 32nd Street, Suite 200
New York, NY 10016, USA

E-mail address:
samir.taneja@nyumc.org

Urol Clin N Am 40 (2013) xi
http://dx.doi.org/10.1016/j.ucl.2012.11.001

Preface

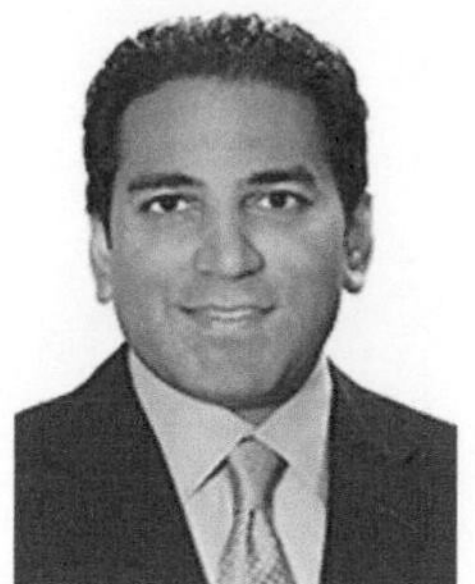

Ojas Shah, MD
Guest Editor

Upper urinary tract stones, which affect a large proportion of our population, are a significant source of morbidity and cost. With numerous risk factors, strategies to reduce stone recurrence and to minimize the need for surgical stone treatment are essential. Furthermore, a thorough understanding of the pathogenesis and pathophysiology of urolithiasis is critical in understanding the process for prevention. This issue of the *Urologic Clinics* provides new insights into kidney stone formation and the metabolic evaluation of first-time and recurrent stone formers to decrease stone recurrence.

In addition to medical therapy to decrease stone recurrence and aid in stone expulsion, the latest dietary and alternative therapy recommendations for stone prevention are discussed.

Over the last several years, new options in the diagnosis of stone disease have become available as well as strategies to optimize the older technologies. This issue updates the practitioner on the imaging techniques for urolithiasis, while providing the most up-to-date information on methods to reduce radiation exposure. Additionally, stone characterization with imaging is discussed, which has enhanced treatment outcomes by helping choose the most appropriate management based on stone size, location, density, and composition.

Despite efforts for stone prevention, stones continue to occur. Therefore, surgical treatments with the least morbidity and highest effectiveness are being investigated to optimize outcomes. Although shockwave lithotripsy technology has not advanced significantly in many years, new techniques involving acoustic coupling, shockwave rate, and shockwave energy sequence have led to improved outcomes. This issue also discusses new innovations in the minimally invasive surgical modalities of ureteroscopy and percutaneous renal surgery that has led to reduced morbidity and overall improved efficacy. The emerging role of laparoscopy and robotics in the setting of complex stone disease is also addressed. Additionally, management of stones in complex situations such as pregnancy, kidney transplantation, and anomalous kidney anatomy is discussed thoroughly.

In the new world of health care economics, in addition to the emphasis of investigating and improving the quality of life of stone formers, the treatment of stone disease is addressed from a cost-effectiveness perspective. This allows practitioners to develop treatment strategies that maximize success and stone-free rates with the minimal amount of procedures. One new and important concept also addressed in this edition is the impact of stone disease recurrence and treatment on the development of chronic kidney disease.

As the guest editor of this issue, I made it my goal to provide the reader with a valuable, comprehensive resource that familiarizes them with the current concepts and decision-making thought processes that have evolved in the multidisciplinary management of urolithiasis. I am extremely thankful for the hard work of the contributors to this issue. As recognized leaders in this field, their time and effort are appreciated and their insights are invaluable.

Ojas Shah, MD
Endourology and Stone Disease
Bellevue Hospital
NYU Langone Medical Center
New York University School of Medicine
150 East 32nd Street, 2nd Floor
New York, NY 10016, USA

E-mail address:
ojas.shah@nyumc.org

Urol Clin N Am 40 (2013) xiii
http://dx.doi.org/10.1016/j.ucl.2012.10.002

New Insights Into the Pathogenesis of Renal Calculi

Herman Singh Bagga, MD*, Thomas Chi, MD,
Joe Miller, MD, Marshall L. Stoller, MD

KEYWORDS

• Genitourinary system • Urinary calculi • Etiology • Review • Calcium

KEY POINTS

- Epidemiologic research and the study of urine and serum chemistries have created an abundance of data to help drive the formulation of pathophysiologic theories of stone formation.
- The abundance of associations between nephrolithiasis and metabolic disease states forces us to reconsider existing hypotheses of stone formation, including the etiology of Randall's plaques.
- Future steps in understanding the pathophysiology of urinary stone disease will likely include genetic studies and the use of animal models.

INTRODUCTION

Urolithiasis has been a documented medical affliction since at least ancient Egyptian civilization,[1] and continues to be responsible for an increasing number of practitioner visits worldwide.[2,3] Furthermore, the recurrence rates of symptomatic stones are high at more than 50% within 5 years of a first episode,[1] suggesting that identifiable high-risk cohorts may experience common pathways in the pathogenesis of stone formation that can be targeted for prevention efforts. This exciting field of research continues to grow. The goal of this article is to discuss new frontiers of understanding regarding the pathophysiology of urinary stone disease.

PHYSIOCHEMICAL ASPECTS OF URINARY STONE FORMATION

At the root of the pathophysiology of urolithiasis is the physiochemical formation of urinary stones. As the glomerular filtrate passes through the nephron, the urine becomes concentrated with stone-forming salts which, when supersaturated, can precipitate out of solution into crystals that can either be expulsed with voided urine or grow and aggregate under the relative influences of various stone-promoting or stone-inhibiting agents, resulting in stone formation.[5] Given an estimated transit time through the nephron of 5 to 7 minutes, traditional thought was that this did not allow sufficient time for free particles to aggregate enough to increase in size to occlude a tubular lumen and serve as a site of stone formation.[6] This theory suggested that some adhesion to tubular epithelial cells as fixed particles would be required to allow for crystal growth and subsequent stone formation. Although recalculation of nephron dimensions in the context of crystal conglomeration during acute increases in supersaturation have concluded that a free-particle theory of stone formation is a potential mechanism of disease,[7] research into the fixed particle mechanism has gained some favorable results. In particular, the theory has been evaluated that intraluminal deposits, mostly within the distal nephron, could serve as sites of stone formation.

Histopathologic evidence of plugs of mineral deposits has been noted in several stone-forming groups of patients, such as those with brushite stones, hyperparathyroidism, cystinuria, and distal renal tubular acidosis, and those with a history of intestinal surgery, including bypass surgery for obesity, small bowel resection, and ileostomy

Department of Urology, University of California San Francisco, 400 Parnassus Avenue, San Francisco, CA 94143-0738, USA
* Corresponding author.
E-mail address: hermanbagga@gmail.com

Urol Clin N Am 40 (2013) 1–12
http://dx.doi.org/10.1016/j.ucl.2012.09.006
0094-0143/13/$ – see front matter Published by Elsevier Inc.

creation. This theory is supported by observations of stone material growing from the ends of these plugs; however, whether these intraluminal deposits lead to stone formation remains unknown. Much research must be performed to elucidate this question, and most likely this is one of multiple pathways in the pathogenesis of urinary stone disease.[8,9]

RANDALL PLAQUES

Associations with Urinary Stone Disease

In contrast to the free and fixed particle theories of stone pathogenesis is the Randall plaque hypothesis. The theory evolved during a search for an initiating lesion for renal stones, which Alexander Randall thought originated in the renal papilla. Strong evidence was gained for this hypothesis during human autopsy studies in which calcium deposits were found in nearly 20% of renal papillae, with nearly one-third of these patients having a primary renal stone at the site. These deposits were coined "Randall plaques" and histologic analysis showed that the lesions were in the interstitial tissues of the papilla near segments of the nephron, rather than within the nephron lumen itself. Randall hypothesized the exposed plaque material served as a nidus for stone formation.[10,11] This hypothesis has regained popularity over the past decade, particularly in regard to the pathogenesis of idiopathic calcium oxalate stones, the most commonly encountered stone in clinical practice. Published observations by Miller and colleagues[12] during endoscopy confirmed that most stones in their study population of patients with idiopathic calcium oxalate stones, which were visually noted to be attached to and primarily originating from these Randall plaques (**Fig. 1**). Further evaluation from this group lent more credence to this observation. The group decided to also analyze free-floating stones encountered during ureteroscopy. More than half of these stones had mucus-covered, concavely cupped regions on one side of the stone that were found to contain apatite on micro-CT analysis of internal structure. This evidence supported the idea that these stones had also grown from a papillary plaque and then subsequently fallen off. Internal structure analysis of the remainder of the stones showed similar evidence of previous attachment to a Randall plaque at one end indicated by the presence of apatite. This finding also provided strong evidence that calcium oxalate stones arise from Randall plaques.[13]

Formation Theories

The origin of Randall plaques themselves remains an issue of debate. On histopathologic examination of the lesions, Evan and colleagues[14] suggested that these plaques arise from the basement membrane of the thin loops of Henle and subsequently protrude into the epithelium of the renal papillae after expanding through the interstitium. This theory has been based on examination of renal papillae from patients with idiopathic calcium oxalate stone formation. Using light microscopic analysis, the group first confirmed that Randall's plaques were limited only to the papillary interstitium and did not reside within the renal tubule, and then examined regions with limited versus heavy plaque burden to identify patterns of progression.[14] In separate studies, they have also noted small deposits within the basement membrane of the thin loops of Henle containing varying numbers of ring-like layers of proteins, suggesting the origin of stones to be within the basement membrane itself.[15,16]

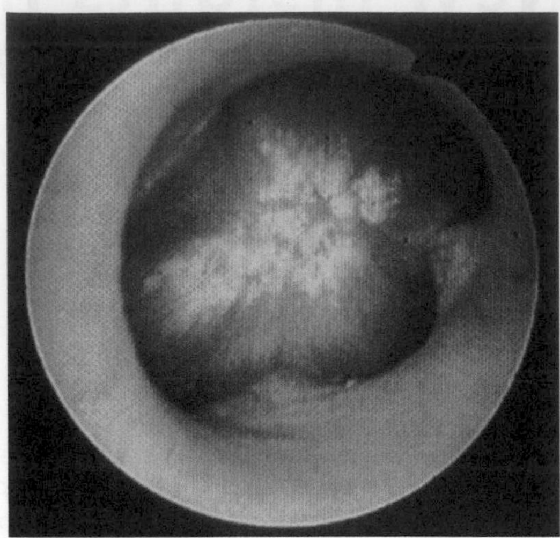

Fig. 1. A Randall plaque forming at a renal papilla, as visualized on endoscopy. No stone is currently attached.

Other analyses of Randall plaques from cadaveric samples with radiographic and immunohistochemical analysis, however, have noted the plaques to extend deep into the papilla, into the basement membrane of the collecting tubules and the vasa recta.[17] These observations have led to a vascular theory of Randall plaque formation and subsequent calcium oxalate stone development, which suggests that repair of injured papillary vasculature in an atherosclerotic-like fashion results in calcification near vessel walls that eventually erodes a calculus into the papilla through the renal papillary interstitium.

The vascular theory of Randall plaque formation is supported by 3 properties of renal physiology. The first is based on the idea that areas of turbulent flow are predisposed to inflammation and atherosclerosis. In the case of arterial plaques these locations include the bifurcation of the aorta, iliac arteries, and carotid arteries.[18] Laminar blood flow changes to turbulent flow at the tip of the renal papilla because of a 180° transition, likely predisposing the area to atherosclerotic-like reactions and subsequent plaque formation. Secondly, a 10-fold or higher increase in osmolality occurs between the renal cortex and the tip of the papilla.[19] In this hyperosmolar microenvironment, resident inflammatory cytokines and proteins can accumulate and promote plaque aggregation in response to vascular injury. Lastly, a decreasing gradient of oxygen-carrying capacity occurs from the renal cortex to the tip of the papilla.[20] In severe cases, as with diabetes mellitus, this can translate to events such as papillary necrosis and sloughed papillae that may obstruct the ureter and create a microenvironment of inflammation. These 3 factors can promote an atherosclerotic-like response to inflammation with perivascular calcification, which may lead to Randall plaque formation.

Given a known association of esterified cholesterol with atherosclerotic processes, this vascular theory was investigated with cholesterol extraction studies on calcium oxalate stones. Analysis noted high esterified-to-free cholesterol ratios in stones with high calcium oxalate composition, providing some support for this hypothesis.[21] Indirect evidence of the interaction between the vascular system and urinary stone formation has also been noted after the interesting finding that urinary stones tend to be largely unilateral and on the dependent sleeping side of patients.[22] These observations prompted renal perfusion studies of patients in various sleep positions, with results noting that renal perfusion is also position-dependent. Increased renal blood flow on the dependent sleeping side of patients may lead to increased turbulence and accumulation of inflammatory elements contributing to a vascular event leading to urinary stone formation.[23] This association may implicate increased renal blood flow as a contributory cause of urinary stone disease. This mechanism may work in concert with hyperfiltration, leading to increased solute deposition and subsequent accumulation of stone-forming elements. These observations open the doorway to explore the associations between vascular disease and urolithiasis.

VASCULAR DISEASE ASSOCIATIONS WITH UROLITHIASIS

To explore new frontiers in the pathogenesis of urinary stone disease, it is helpful to explore associations between urolithiasis and other phenomena, such as vascular disease. The link between urolithiasis and vascular disease is well documented in the literature. Nephrolithiasis has been associated with a 31% increased risk of myocardial infarction (MI), as documented by Rule and colleagues[24] in a study of more than 4500 stone formers compared with nearly 11,000 control patients with 9 years of follow-up. The risk was noted to be independent of kidney disease or other common risk factors for MI. Data from a large cohort of nearly 10,000 women participating in the Study of Osteoporotic Fractures has similarly revealed that patients with a history of nephrolithiasis have an increased relative risk (RR) of MI (RR, 1.78) and angina (RR, 1.63).[25]

Although the precise mechanisms underlying these associations remain to be elucidated, one speculation is that the disease processes may have shared risk factors that have not been fully identified. One potential risk factor could be atherosclerosis, as supported by the vascular theory of Randall plaque formation. The association between nephrolithiasis and subclinical atherosclerosis was recently investigated within the Coronary Adult Risk Development in Young Adults (CARDIA) cohort, which identified a significant association between kidney stones and carotid artery atherosclerosis (odds ratio [OR], 1.6), even after adjusting for known major atherosclerotic risk factors. This study provided further support for possible common systemic pathophysiology that may be shared between vascular and urinary stone disease.[26]

Perhaps most well studied is the association between urinary stone disease and hypertension, which was recognized as early as the 1760s when Morgagni described a patient with clinical and anatomic findings suggestive of both diseases.[27] More recent studies have confirmed these observations. In their prospective analysis of 503 men, Cappuccio and colleagues[27] noted an RR of 1.96 for the development of kidney stones in hypertensive men compared with normotensive men at 8 years. Similarly, in another prospective analysis, Borghi and colleagues[28] noted an OR of 5.5 linking a baseline history of hypertension to the formation of a kidney stone at 5 years of follow-up. This risk seemed particularly pronounced for individuals who were overweight. The link between hypertension and urinary stone disease seems to be potentially bidirectional, as supported by studies that have demonstrated stone formation to predate the onset of hypertension. In their prospective study of a cohort of more than 50,000 men, Madore and colleagues[29] noted an association between nephrolithiasis and risk of hypertension (OR, 1.31), and reported that in men who had both disorders, 79.5% experienced the occurrence of nephrolithiasis before or concomitant to their diagnosis of hypertension. A similar association was seen in women, with an RR of 1.36 for developing a new diagnosis of hypertension in those with a history of nephrolithiasis, as demonstrated from data secured from the Nurses' Heath study, a cohort with nearly 90,000 women.[30]

Although an association seems to exist between hypertension and urinary stone disease, the pathophysiology responsible for this link remains unclear. Multiple theories have been proposed, some highlighting the contribution of urinary composition to the mechanism of disease. Strazzullo and colleagues[31] in a case-controlled study of 110 patients, evaluated calcium metabolism in cohorts with and without essential hypertension, noting higher urinary calcium excretion rates in hypertensive individuals despite similar total and ionized serum calcium levels. The response to intravenous calcium infusion was also investigated, showing that hypertensive patients excreted more calcium at all serum calcium concentrations, suggesting that a form of urinary leak of calcium could be occurring within hypertensive patients. Cappuccio and colleagues[32] similarly recorded abnormalities of calcium metabolism in hypertensive patients, specifically highlighting increased parathyroid gland activity, urinary cyclic AMP, and intestinal calcium absorption. Increased levels of urinary uric acid[33] and decreased levels of urinary citrate[34] have also been seen in studies of hypertensive individuals. These risk factors for the development of urinary stones are well established.[35,36] Differences in urinary composition of magnesium and oxalate may also contribute to the link between hypertension and urinary stone disease.[28] Diet has also been implicated as a potential link between hypertension and a predisposition for urolithiasis. In particular, the known effects of increased dietary sodium, known to promote urolithiasis via hypercalciuria[37] and also promote hypertension,[38] has led to its consideration as a potential parsimonious factor.

Animal models have also demonstrated this association between hypertension and urinary stone disease. Although otherwise rare in animals, Wexler and McMurtry[39] showed that strains of spontaneously hypertensive rats that were born normotensive and developed hypertension with maturation were prone to the development of urinary stone disease. The substrain most prone to urolithiasis also became obese with maturity and stereotypically formed microscopic stones within the kidney. These stones began in a subepithelial location before detaching and serving as a nidus for further stone growth, a mechanism reminiscent of current Randall plaque theories of stone formation. This finding also implicates other metabolic associations with urinary stone disease, such as obesity.

OBESITY, DIABETES, AND URINARY STONE DISEASE

Several studies have found significant associations between weight and body mass index (BMI) and urinary stones. Taylor and colleagues,[40] in an analysis of 3 large prospective cohorts of nearly 250,000 individuals, showed that the RR of incident kidney stone formation for people weighing more than 100 kg, compared with those weighing less than 68.2 kg, was 1.44 in men, 1.89 in older women, and 1.92 in younger women. Using a BMI cutoff of 30, the RRs were 1.33, 1.90, and 2.09, respectively. Similarly, in a study of more than 800 renal stone formers, Del Valle and colleagues[41] showed that most patients (nearly 60%) were either overweight or obese. In 2006, Taylor and Curhan[42] investigated the relationship of BMI as a continuous variable to stone formation, and noted that even in nonobese patients (BMI <30), an increasing BMI lent itself to a higher risk of urolithiasis. The effect was most significant in women, wherein those with a BMI of 23 to 24.9 had a 25% increased incidence of stones compared with those with a BMI of 21 to 22.9. Those with a BMI of 27.5 to 29.9 had a 65% to 75% increased incidence. Similar results were seen in men, wherein those with a BMI of 25 to 29.9 had a 15% to 25% increase in stone incidence compared with those with a BMI of 21 to 22.9. These findings support the idea that increasing weight and BMI are directly correlated to susceptibility to urinary stone formation.

Multiple groups have investigated urine chemistries to better characterize the links between BMI and urinary stone disease. Ekeruo and colleagues,[43] for example, noted that obese (BMI >30) urinary stone formers most commonly had evidence of hypocitraturia (54%) and hyperuricosuria (43%) compared with nonobese stone formers. Taylor and Curhan[42] and Powell and colleagues[44] similarly investigated urine chemistries, showing increased urinary excretion of oxalate, uric acid, phosphate, sodium, sulfate, and cysteine[44] in obese versus nonobese patients. Urinary composition in the obese population seems to contain higher levels of substances known to precipitate urinary stones compared with the nonobese population.

The close association between obesity and diabetes, another known risk factor for urolithiasis, may compound the influence of obesity on the development of urinary stones. Obesity has been shown to carry with it a well-established increased risk for diabetes mellitus.[45,46] In several large-scale studies, patients with diabetes have been closely linked to increased risk of formation of all types of urinary calculi[47,48] and increased risk of uric acid stone formation in particular.[49] Several pathophysiologic mechanisms have been suggested to explain these observations. One explanation offered by Canda and Isgoren[50] stems from their observation of decreased function of interstitial cells and neural tissue within the urothelial tissue of diabetic rabbits. They suggested that these perturbations of function could affect ureteral peristalsis and promote urinary stone formation by virtue of urinary stasis. Other authors, however, suggest that the insulin resistance seen in diabetics is the underlying mechanism through which stones form. Insulin resistance has been noted to impair renal ammoniagenesis, resulting in acidic urine. It also promotes reabsorption of uric acid in the proximal tubule, resulting in hyperuricemia. Both of these factors could contribute to an increased propensity for uric acid urolithiasis.[51] Hyperglycemia has also been associated with increased urinary calcium[52] and oxalate[53] excretion. Taken together, these metabolic changes may explain the consistent association seen between diabetes and urinary stone disease.

DYSLIPIDEMIA AND URINARY STONE DISEASE

The links between dyslipidemia and urinary stone disease have also been investigated. Kadlec and colleagues,[54] in their retrospective review of nearly 600 endourologic stone procedures for which stone composition data were available, noted that more than 30% of their cohort was characterized as dyslipidemic (defined by the use of a cholesterol-lowering medication). Of these patients with dyslipidemia, nearly 70% had calcium oxalate stones and 15% had uric acid stones. A recent study by Inci and colleagues[55] similarly found that total cholesterol levels were significantly higher in stone formers compared with patients who do not form stones, with the association noted to be particularly prominent for calcium oxalate and uric acid stone formers.

To evaluate the potential pathophysiologic mechanisms linking dyslipidemia with urinary stone disease, related research on atorvastatin may be useful to consider. Atorvastatin is a commonly prescribed drug used to decrease serum cholesterol levels. Tsujihata and colleagues[56,57] reported that the administration of atorvastatin to stone-forming rats significantly lowered crystalline deposits on quantitative light microscopy analysis of excised kidney specimens. They hypothesized that anti-inflammatory and antioxidative effects of the drug were responsible, through preventing renal tubular cell injury from oxalate and subsequently inhibiting renal crystal retention. In their experimental model, they found that urinary levels of biomarkers for renal tubular cell injury (*N*-acetyl glucosamidase) and oxidative stress (8-OHdG) were decreased significantly by atorvastatin treatment. Furthermore, atorvastatin treatment decreased the apoptosis of renal tubular cells. These results suggest that common pathophysiology shared between dyslipidemia and urinary stone formation may be related to inflammation and subsequent cellular injury of renal tubular cells.

THE METABOLIC SYNDROME AND UNIFICATION OF THE METABOLIC LINKS TO URINARY STONE DISEASE

Metabolic syndrome is the term given to a combination of risk factors that may include impaired fasting glucose, elevated blood pressure, central obesity, and dyslipidemia in the form of high serum triglycerides or low high-density lipoprotein cholesterol levels. The presence of at least 3 of these traits establishes a diagnosis.[58] This syndrome has been strongly associated with various disease states, most notably diabetes and cardiovascular disease, with a documented relative risk of 3 for diabetes, and 1.78 for cardiovascular disease and death.[59,60]

More recently, metabolic syndrome has become the subject of increased urologic research because of continued observations that it is associated with an increased risk of urinary stone disease. West and colleagues[61] examined the association between the number of metabolic syndrome traits and risk of nephrolithiasis using a national sample of patients in the United States. Prevalence of kidney stones increased with the number of traits, from 3% with 0 traits to 9.8% with 5 traits. The presence of 2 or more traits significantly increased the odds of stone disease, and the presence of 4 or more traits was associated with an approximate 2-fold increase. In a study of Italian adults, Rendina and colleagues[62] similarly found an approximate 2-fold increase in the risk of stone disease for patients with metabolic syndrome. In an analysis of the individual components of the syndrome, they found that the only syndrome trait independently associated with increased stone risk on its own was hypertension. The risk of nephrolithiasis with hypertension was reported with an OR of 2.1 for men and 4.9 for women. The presence of hypertension with any other trait of metabolic syndrome further increased the risk of urolithiasis, with an OR of 2.2 compared with those individuals with hypertension alone. Jeong and colleagues[63] confirmed a similar pattern in an American population, finding metabolic syndrome and the trait of hypertension as independent risk factors for the presence of urinary stones. The other components of metabolic syndrome did not independently carry a risk for kidney stone disease. Patients with metabolic syndrome had an OR of 1.25 for stone disease, and those with hypertension had an OR of 1.47. These studies suggest that synergistic effects of the components of the syndrome lead to an increased risk of urolithiasis. Therefore, the pathophysiology explaining increased urinary stone risk related to metabolic syndrome likely goes beyond simple cumulative effects on urine chemistry by the individual components of the syndrome. Underlying shared systemic influences are likely at play. The vascular theory of stone development is one hypothesis that attempts to link the components of the metabolic syndrome with urinary stone disease by considering a possible common systemic malfunction of inflammation and tissue damage as an underlying mechanism. However, further research is needed to investigate this hypothesis further, and to consider other possible unifying mechanisms of disease. This research will likely need to go beyond epidemiologic and urine composition studies to tease out the mechanisms behind the individual disease states themselves.

INTESTINAL CALCIUM ABSORPTION AND URINARY STONE DISEASE

The physiochemical understanding of stone formation has identified hypercalciuria as a clear risk factor for calcium-based stone formation, with increasing saturation of calcium within urine pushing crystallization and resultant stone formation. Absorption of calcium within the intestine has been associated with hypercalciuria,[64,65] highlighting the importance of understanding the pathophysiologic mechanisms behind this aspect of calcium metabolism. A recent study by Sorensen and colleagues[66] evaluated a cohort of nearly 10,000 women followed for 20 years who were administered radioactive oral calcium assays. The impact of dietary and supplemental calcium on intestinal fractional calcium absorption and the development of urinary stone disease was determined within the cohort. Fractional calcium absorption was found to be associated with increased risk of stone formation; however, it decreased with increased dietary calcium intake. As a result, increased intake of calcium decreased the likelihood of nephrolithiasis. The effect was noted to be a decrease of at least 45% for all levels of dietary calcium intake compared with patients in the lowest quintile of intake. This observation was thought to be from active absorption of intestinal calcium at low calcium intakes compared with passive paracellular diffusion of calcium at higher intake levels, which tends to be more linear.[67] With decreased intestinal calcium to bind to oxalate in the gut of these individuals, the oxalate is absorbed and ultimately excreted in greater concentration into the already hypercalciuric urine, increasing the likelihood for calcium oxalate stone formation.[66]

This understanding of the pathogenesis of urinary stones is not only important for this disease process but also has important implications in other disease processes. For example, several epidemiologic studies have noted an increased risk of osteoporotic fractures in patients with urinary stone disease.[68–70] This association is thought to be related to multiple risk factors, including metabolic acidosis, mutual genetic factors, and abnormal bone remodeling in hypercalciuric stone formers thought to be from elevated vitamin D levels and aberrant local cytokine and growth factor signals seen in both of these patient populations.[68] Sorensen and colleagues[66] in their study noted that women with a history of nephrolithiasis were less likely to supplement calcium in their diet, and those who did, did so at low doses. Given that low dietary calcium is associated with osteoporotic fracture risk,[71] this suggests that another simple and modifiable reason for the association between urolithiasis and osteoporotic fractures is low calcium intake by stone formers. Although the influence of calcium intake on urinary stone formation is still a subject of debate, based on these data, the authors do not recommend the restriction of dietary calcium supplementation, because no clear increased risk for urinary stones has been shown. However, calcium supplementation is important for reducing the risk of osteoporotic fracture and for maintaining bone health.[72,73]

HEAVY METALS AND URINARY STONE DISEASE

Traditionally, calcium hydroxyapatite is regarded as the predominant nidus for calcium-based urinary stone formation. A recent study has found that other heavy metal compounds may act comparably. Strontium is a heavy metal that is processed by the human body in much the same way as calcium, as demonstrated in intestinal absorption and renal filtration studies.[74,75] This similarly divalent cation has been observed to substitute for calcium during the process of biomineralization in bone studies, incorporating into hydroxyapatite in bones through replacing a proportion of the calcium ions.[76] These observations, and the finding that hypercalciuric stone formers were noted to have increased strontium absorption compared with normocalciuric patients,[77] have recently led to investigations regarding strontium incorporation into uroliths. Using synchrotron radiation imaging techniques on human stone samples, a recent study showed that 80% of strontium in these stones appeared as strontium apatite and 20% as strontium carbonate.[78] Although strontium research in urolithiasis is still in its infancy, this study suggests that strontium hydroxyapatite may serve as a nidus for calcium-based stone formation and could potentially serve as a valuable marker to study calcium-based stone pathogenesis.

Still elusive is a clear understanding of the initiating factors for the calcification process of urinary stone disease. For example, although Randall plaques are accepted as a nucleus for calcium oxalate stone formation,[10–14] the process through which crystals enucleate to form the plaque remains unclear. To search for potentially responsible elements, a group in France led by Carpentier and Bazin[79] performed x-ray diffraction and fluorescence studies on human Randall plaques and kidney stones to determine their chemical compositions and the nature and amount of trace elements in each. They demonstrated that zinc levels were dramatically increased in the carbapatite of Randall plaques compared with the carbapatite of kidney stones. This finding suggested a role for zinc in the formation of Randall plaques in the medullar interstitium.

The Role of Calcifying Nanoparticles

Calcifying nanoparticles (CNPs), also known as *nanobacteria*, were discovered more than 25 years ago as cell culture contaminants.[80] They were originally described as novel microorganisms, and were isolated from human and bovine blood and blood products. They were characterized as fastidious and cytotoxic, and carbonate apatite–forming.[81] The nature of these particles has since been debated, with contrasting theories—some describing them as a self-replicating form of life, and others describing them as a nonliving physicochemical phenomenon in the form of mineralo-protein complexes. Those who favor their existence as nanobacteria often cite characteristics such as morphologic similarities to bacteria; presence of DNA, RNA, and bacterial proteins; and their susceptibility to antimetabolic antimicrobials. In contrast, arguments favoring their existence as mineralo-protein complexes include their extremely small size, the absence of an accurately sequenced genome, morphologic similarities to other mineralo-protein complexes, resistance to DNase and RNase activity, and proposed chemical models of formation.[82]

Regardless of their origin, careful study has implicated these particles in the pathogenesis of multiple disease states, including polycystic kidney disease, cholelithiasis, prostatitis, HIV infection, atherosclerotic disease, and cardiovascular calcification.[82] However, perhaps the most studied association is between these particles and urinary stone disease. Several investigators have isolated evidence of CNPs in 62% to 100% of urinary stone samples in various studies.[81,83,84] Similarly, serum studies of patients with nephrolithiasis have also noted evidence of CNPs, with Chen and colleagues[85] evaluating a 27-patient cohort and showing CNPs in the serum of 92% of patients with nephrolithiasis, compared with 0% of controls. The mechanism through which CNPs influence urinary stone disease has been suggested to be related to an etiologic role they may play in Randall plaques. This theory was supported by Ciftçioglu and colleagues,[81] who detected CNPs in more than 70% of kidney papillae samples with Randall plaques, while conversely noting that more than 80% of papillae samples without Randall plaques were free of CNPs.

Although the precise mechanisms through which CNPs may be related to urinary stone disease remain elusive, evaluation of their involvement with atherosclerotic disease and cardiovascular calcification may provide some clues. The links between CNPs and these forms of cardiovascular disease have been evaluated in multiple studies. Puskás and colleagues[86] serologically identified CNPs in most atherosclerotic plaques they examined, whereas their presence was lacking in control areas of the same vessels. Furthermore, CNPs were extracted and cultivated from most calcified sclerotic aortic and carotid samples, suggesting their involvement in atherosclerotic pathogenesis and subsequent blood vessel calcification. Similarly, Miller and colleagues[87] and Bratos-Pérez and colleagues[88] noted the presence of CNPs in calcified cardiac vessels and arterial plaques, and stenotic aortic valves, respectively. In an effort to investigate the nature of CNP arterial toxicity, Schwartz and colleagues[89] exposed a rabbit model with unilaterally damaged carotid arteries to mineralized CNPs from kidney stones. Damaged arteries exposed to the CNPs became occluded and calcified, whereas the arteries with a healthy endothelium were resistant to exposure to the CNPs in this respect. These interesting findings note a connection between endothelial damage of blood vessels and calcification, with CNPs as a pathogenic factor. Although further studies are required to definitively establish association and theories of pathogenesis, this is one potential mechanism through which CNPs could be involved in the formation of urinary stones.

GENETIC LINKS TO URINARY STONE DISEASE

Genetic links to urolithiasis have been long established in certain heritable disorders, such as primary hyperoxaluria and the AGXT gene[90]; cystinuria and the SLC3A1 and SLC7A9 genes[91]; and xanthinuria and the XDH gene.[92] Familial and twin studies have suggested that calcium-based urolithiasis may also be genetically linked, with the latter studies implicating a 50% heritability for calcium nephrolithiasis.[93] This suspected heritability has prompted genome-wide association studies to determine candidate genes that may underlie stone formation. These studies have implicated genes encoding the calcium-sensing receptor (CASR), osteopontin (OPN), vitamin D receptor (VDR), and the claudin family of genes (particularly CLDN14) in calcium urolithiasis.[93,94] CASR protein inhibits calcium absorption in the ascending limb in response to increased interstitial calcium. Mutations in this gene have been found to be associated with idiopathic calcium stone formation and primary hyperparathyroidism.[93,94] Polymorphisms of the OPN gene, which encodes a urinary crystallization inhibitor, have been implicated in calcium urolithaisis.[93] The VDR gene has also been linked to nephrolithiasis. Polymorphisms resulting in less active versions of the gene have been hypothesized to result in increased citrate reabsorption and therefore less inhibition of stone formation.[94,95] The CLDN14 gene was identified in a population of subjects from Iceland and The Netherlands. Polymorphisms in this gene were associated with patients showing higher urinary calcium exretion.[95]

These genome-wide association studies rely on large population-based cohorts with carefully sequenced genomic data to identify subtle variations in genetic expressions. They imply that calcium-based urinary stone disease may not simply be affected by a few major genes, but rather that many genetic polymorphisms may have a sum effect resulting in increased individual susceptibility to stone formation.[93] The identification of a limited set of common genetic defects that contribute to a large proportion of stone disease remains elusive, most likely because of the contributions of diet, obesity, and other environmental factors in the pathogenesis of urinary stone disease. The search for genetic links to urolithiasis is currently in its infancy but certainly holds great promise for future research into origins of urinary stone formation.

ANIMAL MODELS OF URINARY STONE DISEASE

Animal models have long been used to dissect complex disease processes into simpler components to allow for study and testing of scientific hypotheses. The known presence of various types of urinary stones and the complex, likely multifactorial causes of pathogenesis within stone types makes the use of appropriate models particularly important in urolithiasis research. As an era of whole genome sequencing is ushered in and more candidate genetic changes leading to the development of stone disease are identified, more animal models will surely need to be developed to better study the pathogenic mechanisms of stone disease in an in vivo fashion. A variety of animal models have historically been used in the investigation of urinary stone disease, including mice, rabbits, rats, and pigs. However, most studies in the literature to date have preferentially used rat models, likely because of the similarities between experimentally induced nephrolithiasis in rats with human kidney stones and the ease of inducing urolithiasis under experimental conditions. Rats have a nearly identical oxalate metabolism, can be induced to have calcium oxalate nephrolithiasis with hyperoxaluria, and produce kidney stones located on renal papillary surfaces with a similar organic and crystal matrix to humans. All of these characteristics make the rat a reasonable animal model for urolithiasis.[96–99] Disadvantages of a rat model, however, include the high costs of breeding, care, and performance of gene knockout experiments. Many of these models also rely on the feeding of ethylene glycol to induce urinary stones, which may not be representative of a physiologic mechanism through which stones normally form. Some have also noted the potential existence of uncharacterized promoters or inhibitors of stone formation in rat metabolic pathways as downsides.[97]

A novel model of stone disease using the common fruit fly, *Drosophila melanogaster,* was recently developed. The feasibility of this model was seeded in the observation that the *Drosophila* Malpighian tubule, as the site of solute transport and excretion of calcium, uric acid, and phosphorus, is the functional equivalent of the human kidney convoluted tubule.[100] The use of a *Drosophila* model was first published by Chen and colleagues.[97] This team dissected and analyzed *Drosophila* Malpighian tubules with electron microscopy and x-ray spectroscopy after feeding the flies prolithogenic agents. The investigators subsequently confirmed the presence of deposited calcium oxalate crystals within the tubules. Furthermore, they were able to demonstrate appropriate changes in crystal deposition with antilithogenic agents, such as potassium citrate. Additional studies to support the translational utility of this model are currently underway by other research groups.

SUMMARY

The pathophysiology of the various forms of urinary stone disease is a complex topic. Epidemiologic research to identify high-risk cohorts and the study of urine and serum chemistries have been important in raising hypothesis-generating questions. However, many of the answers are still outstanding. Multiple, varied mechanisms have been proposed to explain the observations. Although this is valuable, the development and study of unifying theories to couple these proposed mechanisms remains the next great frontier of discovery. Genetic studies and the use of animal models will likely be important as the next steps are taken in understanding this intriguing disease and its diverse origins.

REFERENCES

1. Eknoyan G. History of urolithiasis. Clin Rev Bone Miner Metabol 2004;2:177–85.
2. Ramello A, Vitale C, Marangella M. Epidemiology of nephrolithiasis. J Nephrol 2000;13(Suppl 3):S45–50.
3. Stamatelou KK, Francis ME, Jones CA, et al. Time trends in reported prevalence of kidney stones in the United States: 1976-1994. Kidney Int 2003;63:1817–23.
4. Uribarri J, Oh MS, Carroll HJ. The first kidney stone. Ann Intern Med 1989;111:1006–9.
5. Stoller ML, Meng MV. Urinary stone disease. Totowa (NJ): Humana Press; 2007.
6. Finlayson B, Reid F. The expectation of free and fixed particles in urinary stone disease. Invest Urol 1978;15:442–8.
7. Kok DJ, Khan SR. Calcium oxalate nephrolithiasis, a free or fixed particle disease. Kidney Int 1994;46:847–54.
8. Evan AP, Unwin RJ, Williams JC Jr. Renal stone disease: a commentary on the nature and significance of Randall's plaque. Nephron Physiol 2011;119:p49–53.
9. Coe FL, Evan AP, Lingeman JE, et al. Plaque and deposits in nine human stone diseases. Urol Res 2010;38:239–47.
10. Randall A. The origin and growth of renal calculi. Ann Surg 1937;105:1009–27.
11. Randall A. Papillary pathology as a precursor of primary renal calculus. J Urol 1940;44:580.
12. Miller NL, Gillen DL, Williams JC, et al. A formal test of the hypothesis that idiopathic calcium oxalate stones grow on Randall's plaque. BJU Int 2009;103:966–71.
13. Miller NL, Williams JC Jr, Evan AP, et al. In idiopathic calcium oxalate stone-formers, unattached stones show evidence of having originated as attached stones on Randall's plaque. BJU Int 2010;105:242–5.
14. Evan AP, Lingeman JE, Coe FL, et al. Randall's plaque of patients with nephrolithiasis begins in basement membranes of thin loops of Henle. J Clin Invest 2003;111:607–16.
15. Evan AP, Coe FL, Rittling SR, et al. Apatite plaque particles in inner medulla of kidneys of calcium oxalate stone formers: osteopontin localization. Kidney Int 2005;68:145–54.
16. Evan AP, Bledsoe S, Worcester EM, et al. Renal inter-α-trypsin inhibitor heavy chain 3 increases in calcium oxalate stone-forming patients. Kidney Int 2007;72(12):1503–11.
17. Stoller ML, Low RK, Shami GS, et al. High resolution radiography of cadaveric kidneys: unraveling the mystery of Randall's plaque formation. J Urol 1996;156:1263–6.
18. Olgun A, Akman S, Erbil MK. The role of RBC destruction in vascular regions with high turbulence on atherosclerosis. Med Hypotheses 2004;63:283–4.
19. Kwon MS, Lim SW, Kwon HM. Hypertonic stress in the kidney: a necessary evil. Physiology (Bethesda) 2009;24:186–91.
20. O'Connor PM. Renal oxygen delivery: matching delivery to metabolic demand. Clin Exp Pharmacol Physiol 2006;33:961–7.
21. Stoller ML, Meng MV, Abrahams HM, et al. The primary stone event: a new hypothesis involving a vascular etiology. J Urol 2004;171:1920–4.
22. Shekarriz B, Lu HF, Stoller ML. Correlation of unilateral urolithiasis with sleep posture. J Urol 2001;165:1085–7.
23. Rubenstein JN, Stackhouse GB, Stoller ML. Effect of body position on renal parenchyma perfusion as measured by nuclear scintigraphy. Urology 2007;70:227–9.
24. Rule AD, Roger VL, Melton LJ, et al. Kidney stones associate with increased risk for myocardial infarction. J Am Soc Nephrol 2010;21:1641–4.

25. Eisner BH, Cooperberg MR, Kahn AJ, et al. Nephrolithiasis and the risk of heart disease in older women. J Urol 2009;181:517–8.
26. Reiner AP, Kahn A, Eisner BH, et al. Kidney stones and subclinical atherosclerosis in young adults: the CARDIA study. J Urol 2011;185:920–5.
27. Cappuccio FP, Siani A, Barba G, et al. A prospective study of hypertension and the incidence of kidney stones in men. J Hypertens 1999;17:1017–22.
28. Borghi L, Meschi T, Guerra A, et al. Essential arterial hypertension and stone disease. Kidney Int 1999;55:2397–406.
29. Madore F, Stampfer MJ, Rimm EB, et al. Nephrolithiasis and risk of hypertension. Am J Hypertens 1998;11:46–53.
30. Madore F, Stampfer MJ, Willett WC, et al. Nephrolithiasis and risk of hypertension in women. Am J Kidney Dis 1998;32:802–7.
31. Strazzullo P, Nunziata V, Cirillo M. Abnormalities of calcium metabolism in essential hypertension. Clin Sci (Lond) 1983;65(2):137–41.
32. Cappuccio FP, Kalaitzidis R, Duneclift S, et al. Unravelling the links between calcium excretion, salt intake, hypertension, kidney stones and bone metabolism. J Nephrol 2000;13:169–77.
33. Losito A, Nunzi EG, Covarelli C, et al. Increased acid excretion in kidney stone formers with essential hypertension. Nephrol Dial Transplant 2008;24: 137–41.
34. Taylor EN, Mount DB, Forman JP, et al. Association of prevalent hypertension with 24-hour urinary excretion of calcium, citrate, and other factors. Am J Kidney Dis 2006;47:780–9.
35. Coe FL, Parks JH, Asplin JR. The pathogenesis and treatment of kidney stones. N Engl J Med 1992;327(16):1141–52.
36. Moe OW. Kidney stones: pathophysiology and medical management. Lancet 2006;367(9507): 333–44.
37. Muldowney FP, Freaney R, Moloney MF. Importance of dietary sodium in the hypercalciuria syndrome. Kidney Int 1982;22:292–6.
38. Luft FC. Sodium intake and essential hypertension. Hypertension 1982;4(5 Pt 2):III14–9.
39. Wexler BC, McMurtry JP. Kidney and bladder calculi in spontaneously hypertensive rats. Br J Exp Pathol 1981;62:369.
40. Taylor EN, Stampfer MJ, Curhan GC. Obesity, weight gain, and the risk of kidney stones. JAMA 2005;293:455–62.
41. Del Valle EE, Negri AL, Spivacow FR, et al. Metabolic diagnosis in stone formers in relation to body mass index. Urol Res 2012;40:47–52.
42. Taylor EN, Curhan GC. Body size and 24-hour urine composition. Am J Kidney Dis 2006;48:905–15.
43. Ekeruo WO, Tan YH, Young MD, et al. Metabolic risk factors and the impact of medical therapy on the management of nephrolithiasis in obese patients. J Urol 2004;172:159–63.
44. Powell CR, Stoller ML, Schwartz BF, et al. Impact of body weight on urinary electrolytes in urinary stone formers. Urology 2000;55:825–30.
45. Thamer C, Machann J, Stefan N, et al. High visceral fat mass and high liver fat are associated with resistance to lifestyle intervention. Obesity (Silver Spring) 2007;15:531–8.
46. Blüher S, Markert J, Herget S, et al. Who should we target for diabetes prevention and diabetes risk reduction? Curr Diab Rep 2012;12:147–56.
47. Taylor EN, Stampfer MJ, Curhan GC. Diabetes mellitus and the risk of nephrolithiasis. Kidney Int 2005; 68:1230–5.
48. Chung SD, Chen YK, Lin HC. Increased risk of diabetes in patients with urinary calculi: a 5-year followup study. J Urol 2011;186:1888–93.
49. Daudon M, Traxer O, Conort P, et al. Type 2 diabetes increases the risk for uric acid stones. J Am Soc Nephrol 2006;17:2026–33.
50. Canda AE, Isgoren AE. Re: Increased risk of diabetes in patients with urinary calculi: a 5-year followup study: S.-D. Chung, Y.-K. Chen and H.-C. Lin J Urol 2011; 186: 1888-1893. J Urol 2012;187: 2279–80.
51. Abate N, Chandalia M, Cabo-Chan AV. The metabolic syndrome and uric acid nephrolithiasis: novel features of renal manifestation of insulin resistance. Kidney Int 2004;65(2):386–92.
52. Lemann J, Piering WF, Lennon EJ. Possible role of carbohydrate-induced calciuria in calcium oxalate kidney-stone formation. N Engl J Med 1969;280: 232–7.
53. Eisner BH, Porten SP, Bechis SK, et al. Diabetic kidney stone formers excrete more oxalate and have lower urine pH than nondiabetic stone formers. J Urol 2010;183:2244–8.
54. Kadlec AO, Greco K, Fridirici ZC, et al. Metabolic syndrome and urinary stone composition: what factors matter most? Urology 2012;80(4):805–10.
55. Inci M, Demirtas A, Sarli B, et al. Association between body mass index, lipid profiles, and types of urinary stones. Ren Fail 2012;34(9):1140–3.
56. Tsujihata M, Momohara C, Yoshioka I, et al. Atorvastatin inhibits renal crystal retention in a rat stone forming model. J Urol 2008;180:2212–7.
57. Tsujihata M, Yoshioka I, Tsujimura A, et al. Why does atorvastatin inhibit renal crystal retention? Urol Res 2011;39:379–83.
58. Grundy SM, Cleeman JI, Daniels SR, et al. Diagnosis and management of the metabolic syndrome: an American Heart Association/National Heart, Lung, and Blood Institute Scientific Statement. Circulation 2005;112:2735–52.
59. Ford ES. Risks for all-cause mortality, cardiovascular disease, and diabetes associated with the

metabolic syndrome: a summary of the evidence. Diabetes Care 2005;28:1769–78.

60. Gami AS, Witt BJ, Howard DE, et al. Metabolic syndrome and risk of incident cardiovascular events and death. J Am Coll Cardiol 2007;49: 403–14.
61. West B, Luke A, Durazo-Arvizu RA, et al. Metabolic syndrome and self-reported history of kidney stones: the National Health and Nutrition Examination Survey (NHANES III) 1988-1994. Am J Kidney Dis 2008;51:741–7.
62. Rendina D, Mossetti G, De Filippo G, et al. Association between metabolic syndrome and nephrolithiasis in an inpatient population in southern Italy: role of gender, hypertension and abdominal obesity. Nephrol Dial Transplant 2009;24:900–6.
63. Jeong IG, Kang T, Bang JK, et al. Association between metabolic syndrome and the presence of kidney stones in a screened population. Am J Kidney Dis 2011;58:383–8.
64. Pak CY, East DA, Sanzenbacher LJ, et al. Gastrointestinal calcium absorption in nephrolithiasis. J Clin Endocrinol Metab 1972;35:261–70.
65. Worcester EM, Coe FL. New insights into the pathogenesis of idiopathic hypercalciuria. Semin Nephrol 2008;28:120–32.
66. Sorensen MD, Eisner BH, Stone KL, et al. Impact of calcium intake and intestinal calcium absorption on kidney stones in older women: the study of osteoporotic fractures. J Urol 2012;187:1287–92.
67. Ireland P, Fordtran JS. Effect of dietary calcium and age on jejunal calcium absorption in humans studied by intestinal perfusion. J Clin Invest 1973; 52:2672–81.
68. Maalouf NM, Kumar R, Pasch A, et al. Nephrolithiasis-associated bone disease: pathogenesis and treatment options. Kidney Int 2011;79(4): 393–403.
69. Lauderdale DS, Thisted RA, Wen M, et al. Bone mineral density and fracture among prevalent kidney stone cases in the Third National Health and Nutrition Examination Survey. J Bone Miner Res 2001;16:1893–8.
70. Melton LJ, Crowson CS, Khosla S, et al. Fracture risk among patients with urolithiasis: a population-based cohort study. Kidney Int 1998;53:459–64.
71. Garriguet D. Bone health: osteoporosis, calcium and vitamin D. Health Rep 2011;22:7–14.
72. Dawson-Hughes B, Harris SS, Krall EA. Effect of calcium and vitamin D supplementation on bone density in men and women 65 years of age or older. N Engl J Med 1997;337(10):670–6.
73. Tang BM, Eslick GD, Nowson C, et al. Use of calcium or calcium in combination with vitamin D supplementation to prevent fractures and bone loss in people aged 50 years and older: a meta-analysis. Lancet 2007;370:657–66.
74. Samachson J, Scheck J, Spencer H. Radiocalcium absorption at different times of day. Am J Clin Nutr 1966;18:449–51.
75. Vezzoli G, Baragetti I, Zerbi S, et al. Strontium absorption and excretion in normocalciuric subjects: relation to calcium metabolism. Clin Chem 1998; 44(3):586–90.
76. Li C, Paris O, Siegel S, et al. Strontium is incorporated into mineral crystals only in newly formed bone during strontium ranelate treatment. J Bone Miner Res 2010;25:968–75.
77. Vezzoli G, Rubinacci A, Bianchin C. Intestinal calcium absorption is associated with bone mass in stone-forming women with idiopathic hypercalciuria. Am J Kidney Dis 2003;42(6):1177–83.
78. Blaschko SD, Miller J, Chi T, et al. Micro-composition of human urinary calculi using advanced imaging techniques. J Urol 2012. [Epub ahead of print].
79. Carpentier X, Bazin D, Combes C, et al. High Zn content of Randall's plaque: a μ-X-ray fluorescence investigation. J Trace Elem Med Biol 2011;25:160–5.
80. Kajander EO, Kuronen I, Akerman KK, et al. Nanobacteria from blood: the smallest culturable autonomously replicating agent on Earth. Proceedings of SPIE 1997;3111:420–8.
81. Ciftçioglu N, Björklund M, Kuorikoski K, et al. Nanobacteria: an infectious cause for kidney stone formation. Kidney Int 1999;56:1893–8.
82. Kutikhin A, Brusina, Yuzhalin A. The role of calcifying nanoparticles in biology and medicine. Int J Nanomedicine 2012;7:339–50.
83. Kajander EO, Ciftçioglu N. Nanobacteria: an alternative mechanism for pathogenic intra- and extracellular calcification and stone formation. Proc Natl Acad Sci U S A 1998;95:8274–9.
84. Khullar M, Sharma SK, Singh SK, et al. Morphological and immunological characteristics of nanobacteria from human renal stones of a north Indian population. Urol Res 2004;32:190–5.
85. Chen L, Huang XB, Xu QQ, et al. Cultivation and morphology of nanobacteria in sera of patients with kidney calculi. Beijing Da Xue Xue Bao 2010; 42(4):443–6 [in Chinese].
86. Puskás LG, Tiszlavicz L, Rázga Z, et al. Detection of nanobacteria-like particles in human atherosclerotic plaques. Acta Biol Hung 2005;56:233–45.
87. Miller VM, Rodgers G, Charlesworth JA, et al. Evidence of nanobacterial-like structures in calcified human arteries and cardiac valves. Am J Physiol Heart Circ Physiol 2004;287:H1115–24.
88. Bratos-Pérez MA, Sánchez PL, García de Cruz S, et al. Association between self-replicating calcifying nanoparticles and aortic stenosis: a possible link to valve calcification. Eur Heart J 2008;29: 371–6.
89. Schwartz MA, Lieske JC, Kumar V, et al. Human-derived nanoparticles and vascular response to

injury in rabbit carotid arteries: proof of principle. Int J Nanomedicine 2008;3:243–8.

90. Cellini B, Oppici E, Paiardini A, et al. Molecular insights into primary hyperoxaluria type 1 pathogenesis. Front Biosci 2012;17:621–34.
91. Eggermann T, Venghaus A, Zerres K. Cystinuria: an inborn cause of urolithiasis. Orphanet J Rare Dis 2012;7:19.
92. Arikyants N, Sarkissian A, Hesse A, et al. Xanthinuria type I: a rare cause of urolithiasis. Pediatr Nephrol 2007;22:310–4.
93. Vezzoli G, Terranegra A, Arcidiacono T, et al. Genetics and calcium nephrolithiasis. Kidney Int 2010;80:587–93.
94. Sayer JA. Renal stone disease. Nephron Physiol 2011;118:p35–44.
95. Thorleifsson G, Holm H, Edvardsson V, et al. Sequence variants in the CLDN14 gene associate with kidney stones and bone mineral density. Nat Genet 2009;41:926–30.
96. Evan AP, Bledsoe SB, Smith SB, et al. Calcium oxalate crystal localization and osteopontin immunostaining in genetic hypercalciuric stone-forming rats. Kidney Int 2004;65:154–61.
97. Chen YH, Liu HP, Chen HY, et al. Ethylene glycol induces calcium oxalate crystal deposition in Malpighian tubules: a Drosophila model for nephrolithiasis/urolithiasis. Kidney Int 2011;80:369–77.
98. Khan SR. Animal models of kidney stone formation: an analysis. World J Urol 1997;15:236–43.
99. Khan SR. Nephrocalcinosis in animal models with and without stones. Urol Res 2010;38:429–38.
100. Dow JA, Romero MF. Drosophila provides rapid modeling of renal development, function, and disease. Am J Physiol Renal Physiol 2010;299: F1237–44.

Metabolic Evaluation of First-time and Recurrent Stone Formers

David S. Goldfarb, MD[a,b,*], Omotayo Arowojolu, BS[a]

KEYWORDS

• Diagnosis • Calcium oxalate • Humans • Kidney calculi/urine • Nephrolithiasis • Uric acid • Urolithiasis

KEY POINTS

- Evaluation of stone formers should include careful attention to medications, past medical history, social history, family history, dietary evaluation, occupation, and laboratory evaluation.
- Kidney stones are associated with obesity, hypertension, and metabolic syndrome, and may be a harbinger of diabetes.
- Twenty-four–hour urine collections are most often appropriate for patients with recurrent stones or complex medical histories. They may be appropriate for some first-time stone formers, including those with comorbidities or large stones.
- Uric acid stones are usually associated with low urine pH, whereas calcium phosphate stones are most often associated with high urine pH. Very high urine pH suggests infection with urease-producing organisms.
- Young age and infrequent features, such as decreased glomerular filtration rate, proteinuria, or extremely high urine oxalate excretion, should lead to consideration of some rare genetic causes of stone disease, such as Dent disease and primary hyperoxaluria.

INTRODUCTION

Approximately 1 in 11 people in the United States will be affected by kidney stones at least once in their lifetime. The prevalence rate seems to continue to increase, as demonstrated by the National Health and Nutrition Examination Survey III cohort (1988–1994 and 2007–2010).[1] This increase in prevalence of kidney stones has also been seen globally. It may be attributable to changing dietary practices, increasing prevalence of diabetes and obesity, migration from cooler rural settings to warmer urban settings, and even global warming. These increasing prevalence rates are also associated with an increase in the cost of kidney stone management to an estimated $2.1 billion in 2000.[2,3]

The high cost of kidney stones and the associated social expenditures, such as missed work, play a role in medical decision making for both patients and physicians.[4] To decrease the cost and prevalence of kidney stones, it is important to provide patients with recommendations for

Disclosure: Dr Goldfarb is a consultant to Keryx and Takeda. He received honoraria for talks from Quintiles. He performed research for Reata and Amgen.
Dr Goldfarb is the principal investigator of the cystinuria project of the Rare Kidney Stone Consortium funded by the National Institute of Diabetes, Digestive Diseases and Kidney Diseases and the Office of Rare Diseases Research via grant U54-DK08390.
[a] New York University School of Medicine, 550 First Avenue, New York, NY 10016, USA; [b] Nephrology Section, New York Harbor VA Healthcare System, 100 East 77th Street, New York, NY, USA
* Corresponding author. Nephrology Section, New York DVAMC, 423 East 23 Street/111G, New York, NY 10010.
E-mail address: David.Goldfarb@va.gov

Urol Clin N Am 40 (2013) 13–20
http://dx.doi.org/10.1016/j.ucl.2012.09.007
0094-0143/13/$ – see front matter Published by Elsevier Inc.

prevention and control of kidney stone formation. Whether patients should receive a limited or a comprehensive metabolic evaluation regarding their kidney stone risk factors is a question frequently debated. With a relative lack of evidence-based guidelines for metabolic evaluation, it seems preferable to the authors to customize each patient's evaluation both to the individual patient's risk factors as well as other comorbidities. For instance, recent studies indicate that the prevalence of kidney stones is significantly associated with diabetes.[5] Recognizing the links between metabolic syndrome and stones allows the physician to highlight a stone as a harbinger of insulin resistance. To address these comorbidities, current recommendations include a change in diet, exercise, weight loss, and a shift toward more dietary calcium, fluids, and less sodium.[6,7] This article discusses the newest recommendations in the field for the metabolic evaluation of both first-time and recurrent kidney stone formers.

EVALUATION

The following discussion of evaluation applies both to first-time and recurrent stone formers. Much of these recommendations represent the practice of the authors and other lithologists and are not necessarily the result of high-grade evidence. Guidelines have been promulgated by the European Association of Urology[8] and by a consensus panel of the National Institutes of Health[9] and are not necessarily out of date.[10] Guidelines are likely to be formulated by the American Urological Association in collaboration with the American Society of Nephrology in the coming year.

HISTORY

The past medical history, family history, and social history are all essential to determine risk factors for each patient after a first stone is passed. These histories are predictors of future recurrent stones and can help to draw conclusions that will aid in behavior modification and metabolic evaluation.

Past Medical History

Stones can be associated with a variety of medical conditions. Gastrointestinal (GI) abnormalities, like chronic inflammatory bowel disease or chronic diarrhea, can cause low urine volume and acid urine pH, which are risk factors for uric acid stones, and hypocitraturia or hyperoxaluria, which are risk factors for calcium oxalate stone formation.[11] Ileal resection caused by GI tract abnormalities is a common cause of kidney stones and can be associated with chronic kidney disease; therefore, a comprehensive evaluation is necessary after the first stone. Other pertinent surgical history includes bariatric surgery. Patients with Roux-en-Y bypass are at risk for hyperoxaluria, metabolic bone disease, and nephrolithiasis.[12] A history of gallstone disease and high serum triglycerides is also associated with kidney stones, although the pathophysiology is uncertain.[5] Sarcoidosis leads to hypercalciuria and hypercalcemia.

Hypertension and diabetes are often associated with metabolic syndrome, whose features include abdominal obesity and insulin resistance. Metabolic syndrome is associated with an increased risk of uric acid stone formation caused by the associated unduly acid urine caused by insulin resistance.[12,13] These disorders might also be associated with more calcium oxalate stones because a greater body mass index is associated with greater urinary oxalate excretion.

Chronic kidney disease is probably associated with a reduction in stone risk because of the urinary concentration defects and the reduction in urine calcium excretion as the result of secondary hyperparathyroidism. However, some kidney diseases are associated with stone disease, such as polycystic kidney disease and medullary sponge kidney. Sjögren syndrome and other tubulointerstitial nephritides are associated with stones as the result of renal tubular acidosis (RTA).

A full list of current and past medications and supplements will be useful in the differential diagnosis of stone formation and will provide information about comorbidities. Certain medications can increase kidney stone recurrence risk. These medications include some protease inhibitors for human immunodeficiency virus (HIV), such as atazanavir; carbonic anhydrase inhibitors (acetazolamide, topiramate); triamterene; and felbamate an antiepileptic medication.[14] Supplements that may increase patients' risk include vitamin C and calcium supplements.[15–17] On the other hand, vitamin B6 and dietary calcium do not increase the risk for kidney stones and may help reduce the risk. Vitamin D does not seem to affect 24-hour urine calcium excretion and has not been shown to increase the risk of stones.[18]

Family History

A family history of kidney stones may suggest further evaluations. Twin studies demonstrate higher concordance for stones among monozygotic twin pairs compared with dizygotic twins, leading to an estimate that 56% of the stone phenotype is attributable to genetic factors.[19] However, the genetic basis for this strong genetic influence remains uncertain, and genetic testing is almost never part of a clinical evaluation. The exception is genotyping for primary hyperoxaluria and Dent disease in appropriate circumstances (see later discussion). Because these disorders have autosomal recessive inheritance, family history will be negative. Infrequently, autosomal-dominant polycystic kidney disease can be associated with stones and be diagnosed via any renal imaging study. RTA may also be familial and may be associated and present with stones.

Social History

Social history, particularly occupational history, is another important component of the evaluation. Patients with professions that do not allow frequent hydration or use of toilet facilities have a decreased urine output and are susceptible to stone formation. Some examples of these occupations include professional drivers (cargo transporters, taxicab drivers, chauffeurs) and primary school teachers. People who live in climates with elevated temperatures, where patients are prone to water depletion, may also have difficulty maintaining a dilute urine. Examples include people with patients in construction, athletics, or other outdoor professions. Knowing a patient's occupation can provide insight into recommendations that will keep the patient hydrated and urine dilute with a high volume.

Diet History

Understanding a patient's diet will allow one to understand possible risk factors for stone formation and then to prescribe dietary modifications to prevent recurrent stone formation. A diet high in salt contributes to excessive calcium excretion. Young people particularly have less control of their diets and often ingest more processed and packaged foods high in sodium content. Often people are unaware of their high sodium intake until it is revealed by 24-hour urine collections. Animal protein (not just beef as many lay people think) can cause hypercalciuria, hyperoxaluria, and hyperuricosuria—all factors increasing the risk of calcium kidney stone formation and often contributing to stones in athletes and body builders. Protein also increases net acid excretion and contributes to the low urine pH of uric acid stone formers. The Atkins diet and other high-protein diets are not recommended as weight loss regimens for patients with kidney disease (unless, perhaps, potassium citrate is prescribed).[20]

More grapefruit juice consumption is associated with a higher risk for stones in both men and women for unclear reasons, and beverages high in fructose are also associated with stones.[21–23] Dietary oxalate content can be assessed by asking about the ingestion of nuts, dark greens (particularly spinach), concentrated and dried fruits, and chocolate. Low dietary calcium intake is consistently associated with more stones, perhaps because it allows more dietary oxalate to be absorbed by the intestine.[24,25] Although vegetarians may have higher urinary oxalate excretion, they have fewer stones because they have higher urine volume and urinary citrate excretion.[26]

The Dietary Approaches to Stop Hypertension (DASH) diet is high in fruits and vegetables, moderate in low-fat dairy, and low in animal protein.[27] The diet also contains sources of oxalate, such as nuts, legumes, and whole grains; but its variants include reduced intake of sodium, sweetened beverages, and red and processed meats.[28] A high DASH score is associated with a reduced risk of kidney stones.[28]

PHYSICAL EXAMINATION

Although kidney stones have no specific manifestations on physical examination, a full physical examination is important in patients with renal colic for ruling out other conditions. Because of the correlation between hypertension and stone formation, blood pressure (BP) should be measured during the physical examination.[29] High blood pressure is a significant predictor of kidney stone morbidity.[5] If treatment with thiazide-like drugs is contemplated, monitoring BP will be important.

LABORATORY EVALUATION

The most crucial component of a patient's evaluation is the laboratory evaluation of blood and urine. **Box 1** includes the relevant tests.

Blood Tests

A basic metabolic panel should be obtained for all stone formers. In addition to this routine chemistry test, measurement of serum phosphorus and uric acid may also be useful. Kidney function is assessed at baseline and over the years of the patient's history of stones. Correlations between decreases in estimated glomerular filtration rate and kidney stones have been demonstrated, although the nature of this relationship is not well established.[30] The decreased glomerular filtration rate associated with stones could be caused by the stone disease itself, for instance, caused by nephrocalcinosis; to recurrent episodes of ureteral obstruction; or to repeated urologic interventions.

Box 1
Laboratory evaluation of nephrolithiasis

Stone composition by x-ray crystallography or infrared spectroscopy

Serum chemistry

Calcium

Glucose

Sodium

Potassium

Chloride

Bicarbonate

Blood urea nitrogen

Creatinine

Phosphorus

Uric acid

Intact parathyroid hormone (if high normal to high serum calcium)

25-hydroxy-vitamin D (if low urine calcium or serum calcium)

Urinalysis

pH

Specific gravity

Protein

Microscopic

24-hour urine

For patients with recurrent stones

Some first-time stone formers

As glomerular filtration declines, risk may also decrease. Electrolytes are evaluated because hypokalemia and hypobicarbonatemia are features of RTA. Therapy with thiazides and potassium citrate will also require periodic monitoring of electrolytes.

If serum calcium levels are borderline or elevated (greater than 10.0 mg/dL, especially if hypercalciuria is present), measurement of the intact parathyroid hormone (PTHi) level is recommended to rule out primary hyperparathyroidism as a contributing cause for stone formation. Hypophosphatemia may also be present. Primary hyperparathyroidism may be present if both serum calcium and PTHi are at the high ends of their normal ranges, in which case ionized calcium may help confirm the diagnosis.[31] However, secondary hyperparathyroidism should be suspected if PTHi is high and serum calcium is at the low end of the normal range. This situation should be suspected if urine calcium is low or bone mineral density (BMD) decreased, in which case the measurement of 25-hydroxy-vitamin D may be indicated.

A uric acid measurement may be useful in managing associated gout; when prescribing xanthine dehydrogenase inhibitors, allopurinol or febuxostat; and in monitoring therapy with thiazides.[32,33]

Hypophosphatemia may suggest not only hyperparathyroidism but also phosphaturia related to mutations in proximal tubular phosphate reabsorption.[34] A measure of glucose and hemoglobin A1c can sometimes detect previously unrecognized diabetes, another risk factor for stone formation, which has health implications far beyond those of nephrolithiasis.[35]

Urine Tests

Urinary tests for all stone formers should begin with urinalysis. The specific gravity, urine pH, and presence of protein, blood cells, or bacteria will aid in the differential diagnosis of the causes of kidney disease and renal colic. A urine sediment may reveal crystals and may lead to the recognition of drug-induced crystalluria.[14] Uric acid crystals are seen in acidic urine, usually 5.5 or less, and calcium phosphate crystals in more alkaline urine, usually 6.5 to 7.0; identification can be aided if crystals are dissolved or precipitated by manipulating the urine pH *ex vivo*. Besides infection with urease-producing organisms, higher urine pH may be associated with distal RTA. Hexagonal crystals are pathognomonic for cystinuria. Struvite crystals are associated with organisms, such as *Proteus*, which produce urease and lead to high urine pH (7–9) and are a rectangular coffin-lid shape. Calcium oxalate dihydrate crystals are a tetrahedral envelope shape, whereas the monohydrate is often described as dumbbells. Urine culture should also be obtained to test for bacteria, pyuria, and infection.

Twenty-four–Hour Urine Collections

The difference in the evaluation of first-time versus recurrent stone formers has long centered on the appropriate application of 24-hour urine collections. Some reviews and consensus statements have suggested that the tests are appropriate and cost-effective only for recurrent stone formers.[9,36] The authors do not disagree with this recommendation. It is true that the frequency of recurrence and metabolic activity of stone formation cannot be judged in first-time stone formers who present with a solitary stone. It is also clear from the authors' clinical experience that most first-time stone formers, particularly younger people, are reluctant to adhere to recommendations regarding dietary manipulation or prescription of drugs. In such cases, generic recommendations to increase fluid intake to 3 L/d may suffice if other comorbidities discussed earlier are absent.

However, there are other people with stones who might warrant the more thorough evaluation that includes 24-hour urine collections. Perhaps people presenting with larger stones, stones requiring a trip to the operating room, or older people with other comorbidities, such as heart disease or warfarin use, should have a more detailed evaluation. Such patients are among the ones most motivated to prevent stones and can best do so when presented with the results of their own risk assessments and corresponding prescriptions, not simply the generic advice proffered to most stone formers. The European Association of Urology prescribes 24-hour collections in complicated patients: those with multiple stones or other risk factors for recurrence.[8]

In any case, it is important to emphasize that today there remains a surprising dearth of data demonstrating that prescribing preventative regimens based on urine collections is superior to offering generic advice not specific to the individual. Despite that lack of evidence, it seems evident to the authors that 24-hour urine collections are a useful tool for understanding each patient's specific urine composition to access the risk factors for recurrence and make recommendations for prevention. Spot urine collections are not as accurate because of the daily variability of urine composition caused by dietary and other circadian variations throughout the day but may be useful when 24-hour collections are not possible.[37]

Urine collections are usually performed on the patients' self-selected diets. The analytes measured should include calcium; oxalate; phosphate; urate; urine volume; pH; and measures revealing dietary intake of sodium, potassium and protein. Based on the results, a laboratory specializing in the assessment of stone risk can calculate supersaturation of crystal-forming phases, so that changes in multiple urinary variables can be translated into a single number correlating with the stone risk. Stone composition usually correlates with urinary supersaturation.[38] For patients with hypercalciuria, protocols used in the past to classify the cause of the abnormality and then treat based on the results have not been shown to lead to a superior method of stone prevention, are costly and unwieldy, and are, therefore, not recommended.

At least two 24-hour urine collections should be completed before treatment is prescribed because of the additional diagnoses that multiple collections reveal.[39] Additional 24-hour urine collections should be performed 4 to 6 weeks after any prescribed intervention to judge efficacy and provide patients with feedback regarding achieved success in making modifications. Laboratories that specialize in evaluating patients with stones may perform a qualitative screen for cystine for all patients new to the laboratory.

In **Box 2**, the authors briefly explicate the results of these collections. For further discussion, the reader is referred to articles in this volume regarding corresponding dietary and pharmacologic therapy.

IMAGING

Every patient presenting with kidney stones should have, if not done previously in an emergency department, an imaging study to determine the stone burden present.[45] This counting will be useful in following stone disease and judging whether prevention regimens have been successful, in ensuring that other stones do not warrant urologic intervention, in demonstrating that hydronephrosis has resolved, and to rule out polycystic kidney disease or other anatomic variants. Most often, computed tomography is done during emergency department visits. Although ultrasound is less sensitive and specific for stones than computed tomography, it is less expensive and does not result in exposure to radiation; therefore, it often suffices for periodic follow-up. Plain radiography is very inexpensive and entails very-low-dose radiation and may be appropriate when a known calcium stone, large enough to appear on the film, is being followed. The authors usually repeat ultrasound or plain radiography at yearly intervals for a few years after an episode of symptomatic obstruction and continue indefinitely only if metabolic activity persists.

Medullary sponge kidney is not an uncommon cause of stones and nephrocalcinosis. However, as radiocontrast administration is now relatively infrequent in stone formers, the diagnosis is likely to be made much less often.[46] It can be suspected when family members are affected and nephrocalcinosis is demonstrated. Because the disorder has no specific therapy other than addressing urine chemistry, contrast administration to find it is not recommended.

STONE COMPOSITION

Composition of stones should always be determined by x-ray crystallography or infrared spectroscopy. Both tests are relatively inexpensive and can lead to important diagnoses, especially in detecting unusual causes of stones, such as

Box 2
Twenty-four–hour urine variables

Variables directly affecting supersaturation of stone-forming salts

Calcium: A clear demarcation of hypercalciuria cannot be clearly drawn. Risk of stones increases with increasing urine calcium excretion, even at values less than traditionally considered hypercalciuria.[40] Variations in urine calcium often correlate with urine sodium excretion and may correlate less with dietary calcium.

Oxalate: As with calcium, risk for stones increases with increasing oxalate excretion even at levels considered normal.[41] Dietary oxalate is only one determinant of urine oxalate excretion, with influences of body size, calcium intake, and colonization with *Oxalobacter formigenes*.

Volume: Low urine volume (<2 L) is often related to occupation, activities, and perceived thirst.

pH: Persistently low urine pH (<5.8) is commonly associated with uric acid stones and hypocitraturia.[42] Higher urine pH (>6.2) is commonly associated with calcium phosphate stones and RTA.[43] Values greater than 8.0 may suggest infection with urease-producing organisms.

Uric acid: Hyperuricosuria may be a risk factor for calcium stones, although contributes less strongly than pH to uric acid stones, and is usually the result of increased ingestion of animal protein.

Citrate: Hypocitraturia results from increased acid load, such as that resulting from increased animal protein intake or metabolic acidosis, but may also be hereditary.[44]

Dietary variables affecting relevant urine chemistries

Sodium: Increased salt intake is endemic in the Western world and often is far beyond what patients imagine they are eating. It is an important variable contributing to increased calcium excretion.

Urea, sulfate: These variables reflect animal protein intake. Urea can be used to calculate protein catabolic rate to estimate protein intake. Sulfate is a correlate of dietary acid ingestion and usually approximates urine ammonium, unless nondietary causes of metabolic acidosis, such as diarrhea, are present.

Phosphorus: Excretion of phosphorus is related to dietary animal protein as well as diary intake. Whether reduction of phosphorus intake is specifically useful for stone prevention is not known.

cystinuria or crystallization of drugs. Prescription of citrate for stone prevention can occasionally lead to increases in urine pH and might change calcium oxalate or cystine stone formers into calcium phosphate stone formers. This phenomenon is relatively infrequent because citrate prevents calcium phosphate precipitation and lowers urine calcium, but vigilance for this transformation should be maintained.[43]

EVALUATION OF BMD

For patients with hypercalciuria and calcium stones, measurement of BMD may be useful. The strong link between hypercalciuria, low BMD, and increased fracture rate leads to the consideration of performing dual-energy x-ray absorptiometry in such patients.[47,48] Highlighting this relationship may be of particular significance in postmenopausal women with stones who have not had BMD assessed previously. However, this relationship is also present in men. Calculation of bone fracture risk using the FRAX® tool (www.shef.ac.uk/FRAX) may also be useful. The FRAX score incorporates both the patient's risk factors and BMD to determine the 10-year probability of a fracture. Common risk factors that affect fracture risk are age, gender, history of fracture, alcohol use, smoking, and low body mass index. The authors find that describing these links often offers patients additional motivations to increase dairy intake or take thiazides. The latter drugs reduce urine calcium excretion and are associated with the prevention of recurrent stones as well as increased BMD and reduced fracture rates.[49] Bisphosphonates may also reduce urine calcium excretion and prevent stones, although the evidence of this effect is less clear.[50] However, the possibility of prescribing these drugs when osteoporosis is found constitutes an indication for measuring BMD in stone formers.

DETECTION OF UNUSUAL CAUSES OF STONE DISEASE

As the pathophysiology and genetics of kidney stone disease are uncovered, it has become clear that some cases of genetic nephrolithiasis are escaping detection because of a lack of familiarity of clinicians with their presentations. The Rare Kidney Stone Consortium (see www.rarekidneystones.org) has been highlighting this deficiency to improve diagnosis of cystinuria, primary hyperoxaluria, Dent disease, claudin mutations, and adenine phosphoribosyltransferase deficiency (a cause of dihydroxyadenine stones).[51] Stone composition is always important, but young age, decreased glomerular filtration rate, proteinuria, and extremes of oxaluria are among the variables that should lead to more complete evaluation.

SUMMARY

Kidney stones are preventable. To maximize the efficacy of preventative regimens, the appropriate data need to be gathered. A thorough history should be directed toward assessing the past medical history, social history, occupation, activities, family history, and diet. Stone composition is always appropriate. Laboratory evaluation requires serum chemistries and urinalysis. Twenty-four–hour urine collections are most appropriate for recurrent stone formers; but some patients who are motivated to prevent recurrence and have large or complicated stones that required urologic intervention might also be appropriate candidates for complete metabolic assessment. The links between metabolic syndrome, hypertension, and obesity and stones suggest that stones may be a harbinger of important morbidity, particularly an increased risk of diabetes.

REFERENCES

1. Scales CD Jr, Smith AC, Hanley JM, et al. Prevalence of kidney stones in the United States. Eur Urol 2012;62:160–5.
2. Lotan Y, Cadeddu JA, Roerhborn CG, et al. Cost-effectiveness of medical management strategies for nephrolithiasis. J Urol 2004;172:2275–81.
3. Romero V, Akpinar H, Assimos DG. Kidney stones: a global picture of prevalence, incidence, and associated risk factors. Rev Urol 2010;12:e86–96.
4. Lotan Y. Economics and cost of care of stone disease. Adv Chronic Kidney Dis 2009;16:5–10.
5. Akoudad S, Szklo M, McAdams MA, et al. Correlates of kidney stone disease differ by race in a multi-ethnic middle-aged population: the ARIC study. Prev Med 2010;51:416–20.
6. Nouvenne A, Meschi T, Prati B, et al. Effects of a low-salt diet on idiopathic hypercalciuria in calcium-oxalate stone formers: a 3-mo randomized controlled trial. Am J Clin Nutr 2010;91:565–70.
7. Sorensen MD, Kahn AJ, Reiner AP, et al. Impact of nutritional factors on incident kidney stone formation: a report from the WHI OS. J Urol 2012;187:1645–9.
8. Tiselius HG, Ackermann D, Alken P, et al. Guidelines on urolithiasis. Eur Urol 2001;40:362–71.
9. National Institutes of Health consensus development conference on prevention and treatment of kidney stones. Bethesda, Maryland, March 28–30, 1988. J Urol 1989;141:705–808.
10. Goldfarb DS. Reconsideration of the 1988 NIH consensus statement on prevention and treatment of kidney stones: are the recommendations out of date? Rev Urol 2002;4:53–60.
11. Finkielstein VA, Goldfarb DS. Strategies for preventing calcium oxalate stones. CMAJ 2006;174:1407–9.
12. Sakhaee K, Maalouf NM, Sinnott B. Kidney stones 2012: pathogenesis, diagnosis, and management. J Clin Endocrinol Metab 2012;97:1847–60.
13. Maalouf NM. Metabolic syndrome and the genesis of uric acid stones. J Ren Nutr 2011;21:128–31.
14. Daudon M, Jungers P. Drug-induced renal calculi: epidemiology, prevention and management. Drugs 2004;64:245–75.
15. Worcester EM, Coe FL. Clinical practice. Calcium kidney stones. N Engl J Med 2010;363:954–63.
16. Curhan GC, Willett WC, Rimm EB, et al. A prospective study of the intake of vitamins C and B6, and the risk of kidney stones in men. J Urol 1996;155:1847–51.
17. Curhan GC, Willett WC, Speizer FE, et al. Intake of vitamins B6 and C and the risk of kidney stones in women. J Am Soc Nephrol 1999;10:840–5.
18. Leaf DE, Korets R, Taylor EN, et al. Effect of vitamin D repletion on urinary calcium excretion among kidney stone formers. Clin J Am Soc Nephrol 2012;7:829–34.
19. Goldfarb DS, Fischer ME, Keich Y, et al. A twin study of genetic and dietary influences on nephrolithiasis: a report from the Vietnam Era Twin (VET) Registry. Kidney Int 2005;67:1053–61.
20. Friedman AN. High-protein diets: potential effects on the kidney in renal health and disease. Am J Kidney Dis 2004;44:950–62.
21. Curhan GC, Willett WC, Rimm EB, et al. Prospective study of beverage use and the risk of kidney stones. Am J Epidemiol 1996;143:240–7.
22. Curhan GC, Willett WC, Speizer FE, et al. Beverage use and risk for kidney stones in women. Ann Intern Med 1998;128:534–40.
23. Taylor EN, Curhan GC. Fructose consumption and the risk of kidney stones. Kidney Int 2008;73:207–12.
24. Curhan GC, Willett WC, Rimm EB, et al. A prospective study of dietary calcium and other nutrients and the risk of symptomatic kidney stones. N Engl J Med 1993;328:833–8.
25. Massey LK, Roman-Smith H, Sutton RA. Effect of dietary oxalate and calcium on urinary oxalate and risk of formation of calcium oxalate kidney stones. J Am Diet Assoc 1993;93:901–6.
26. Meschi T, Maggiore U, Fiaccadori E, et al. The effect of fruits and vegetables on urinary stone risk factors. Kidney Int 2004;66:2402–10.

27. Taylor EN, Stampfer MJ, Mount DB, et al. DASH-style diet and 24-hour urine composition. Clin J Am Soc Nephrol 2010;5:2315–22.
28. Taylor EN, Fung TT, Curhan GC. DASH-style diet associates with reduced risk for kidney stones. J Am Soc Nephrol 2009;20:2253–9.
29. Strazzullo P, Mancini M, Cappuccio FP. Kidney stones and hypertension: population based study of an independent clinical association. BMJ 1990; 300:1234.
30. Rule AD, Bergstralh EJ, Melton LJ III, et al. Kidney stones and the risk for chronic kidney disease. Clin J Am Soc Nephrol 2009;4(4):804–11.
31. Parks JH, Coe FL, Evan AP, et al. Clinical and laboratory characteristics of calcium stone-formers with and without primary hyperparathyroidism. BJU Int 2009;103:670–8.
32. Mugiya S, Nagata M, Un-No T, et al. Endoscopic management of impacted ureteral stones using a small caliber ureteroscope and a laser lithotriptor. J Urol 2000;164:329–31.
33. Basting RF, Corvin S, Antwerpen C, et al. Use of water jet resection in renal surgery: early clinical experiences. Eur Urol 2000;38:104–7.
34. Prie D, Huart V, Bakouh N, et al. Nephrolithiasis and osteoporosis associated with hypophosphatemia caused by mutations in the type 2a sodium-phosphate cotransporter. N Engl J Med 2002;347: 983–91.
35. Obligado SH, Goldfarb DS. The association of nephrolithiasis with hypertension and obesity: a review. Am J Hypertens 2008;21:257–64.
36. Uribarri J, Oh MS, Carroll HJ. The first kidney stone. Ann Intern Med 1989;111:1006–9.
37. Asplin JR. Evaluation of the kidney stone patient. Semin Nephrol 2008;28:99–110.
38. Lingeman J, Kahnoski R, Mardis H, et al. Divergence between stone composition and urine supersaturation: clinical and laboratory implications. J Urol 1999;161:1077–81.
39. Parks JH, Goldfisher E, Asplin JR, et al. A single 24-hour urine collection is inadequate for the medical evaluation of nephrolithiasis. J Urol 2002; 167:1607–12.
40. Taylor EN, Curhan GC. Demographic, dietary, and urinary factors and 24-h urinary calcium excretion. Clin J Am Soc Nephrol 2009;4:1980–7.
41. Taylor EN, Curhan GC. Determinants of 24-hour urinary oxalate excretion. Clin J Am Soc Nephrol 2008;3:1453–60.
42. Maalouf NM, Cameron MA, Moe OW, et al. Novel insights into the pathogenesis of uric acid nephrolithiasis. Curr Opin Nephrol Hypertens 2004;13: 181–9.
43. Goldfarb DS. A woman with recurrent calcium phosphate kidney stones. Clin J Am Soc Nephrol 2012;7: 1172–8.
44. Zuckerman JM, Assimos DG. Hypocitraturia: pathophysiology and medical management. Rev Urol 2009;11:134–44.
45. Hyams ES, Shah O. Evaluation and follow-up of patients with urinary lithiasis: minimizing radiation exposure. Curr Urol Rep 2010;11:80–6.
46. Gambaro G, Feltrin GP, Lupo A, et al. Medullary sponge kidney (Lenarduzzi-Cacchi-Ricci disease): a Padua Medical School discovery in the 1930s. Kidney Int 2006;69:663–70.
47. Heilberg IP, Weisinger JR. Bone disease in idiopathic hypercalciuria. Curr Opin Nephrol Hypertens 2006;15:394–402.
48. Lauderdale DS, Thisted RA, Wen M, et al. Bone mineral density and fracture among prevalent kidney stone cases in the Third National Health and Nutrition Examination Survey. J Bone Miner Res 2001;16: 1893–8.
49. Schoofs MW, van der KM, Hofman A, et al. Thiazide diuretics and the risk for hip fracture. Ann Intern Med 2003;139:476–82.
50. Weisinger JR. New insights into the pathogenesis of idiopathic hypercalciuria: the role of bone. Kidney Int 1996;49:1507–18.
51. Beara-Lasic L, Edvardsson VO, Palsson R, et al. Genetic causes of kidney stones and kidney failure. Clin Rev Bone Miner Metab 2012;10:2–18.

Pharmacologic Treatment of Kidney Stone Disease

Brian H. Eisner, MD[a,*], David S. Goldfarb, MD[b], Gyan Pareek, MD[c]

KEYWORDS

• Allopurinol • Citrate • Medication • Nephrolithiasis • Prevention • Thiazides • Uric acid

KEY POINTS

- Thiazide diuretics, alkali citrate, and allopurinol have been shown in randomized controlled trials to decrease recurrent calcium stone formation in patients with hypercalciuria, hypocitraturia, or hyperuricosuria, respectively.
- Thiazides and alkali citrate have been shown in randomized controlled trials to decrease recurrent stone formation in unselected stone formers.
- Urease inhibitors have been shown in randomized controlled trials to decrease struvite stone formation but side effects are common and are a major concern for these medications. Urologic surgical intervention is critical for struvite stones whenever feasible.
- There are no randomized controlled trials for uric acid stones, but alkali citrate to alkalinize urine is highly effective.
- Medical expulsive therapy has been shown in randomized controlled trials to increase spontaneous stone passage and is recommended for all ureteral stones less than 10 mm if surgical intervention is not immediately indicated.

INTRODUCTION

Nephrolithiasis is a common cause of morbidity worldwide, with lifetime prevalence reported at 5% to 10%.[1–4] In addition, recent evidence suggests that kidney stones are becoming more common.[5,6] In the absence of pharmacologic prophylaxis, recurrence rates are high, and may be in excess of 50% within 10 years of an initial stone event.[7,8] In general, prevention of stone recurrence is best directed at the underlying pathophysiology of stone formation and the appropriate regimen differs based on stone composition. Among patients with calcium stones, five major urinary risk factors increase the individual's propensity: (1) hypercalciuria, (2) hyperoxaluria, (3) hyperuricosuria, (4) hypocitraturia, and (5) low urine volume.[9,10] In addition, hypomagnesuria has also been identified as a potential contributor to calcium stone formation, although this association is less certain.[11,12] Stone prevention in patients with calcium stones is based on treatment of these urinary abnormalities. Uric acid stones are commonly treated by increasing urine pH to increase the solubility of uric acid in urine, whereas cystine stones are treated with alkalinization and thiol-binding medications to accomplish the same goal.[13–15] Finally, urease inhibitors and antibiotics may be used as prophylaxis against struvite or infection stones.[16] This

Disclosure: Dr Goldfarb: consultant, Takeda, Keryx. Research: Amgen.

[a] Department of Urology, GRB 1102, Harvard Medical School, Massachusetts General Hospital, 55 Fruit Street, Boston, MA 02114, USA; [b] Nephrology Section, New York Harbor VA Healthcare System, NYU School of Medicine, New York, NY 10010, USA; [c] Department of Urology, Warren Alpert Medical School of Brown University, Providence, RI 02903, USA

* Corresponding author. Department of Urology, GRB 1102, Massachusetts General Hospital, 55 Fruit Street, Boston, MA 02114.
E-mail address: beisner@partners.org

Urol Clin N Am 40 (2013) 21–30
http://dx.doi.org/10.1016/j.ucl.2012.09.013
0094-0143/13/$ – see front matter

article reviews the data on pharmacologic treatment of stone disease, with a focus on prophylaxis against stone recurrence. One of the most effective and important therapies for stone prevention, an increase in urine volume, is not reviewed because this is a dietary, not pharmacologic intervention.[17] Also review are medical expulsive therapy (MET) used to improve the spontaneous passage of ureteral stones and pharmacologic treatment of symptoms associated with ureteral stents. The goal is to review the literature with a focus on the highest level of evidence (ie, randomized controlled trials [RCT]).

CALCIUM STONES

Hypercalciuria and Thiazides

Hypercalciuria is considered an idiopathic disease, with several abnormalities of calcium balance present, including increased intestinal absorption of calcium, reduced bone mineralization, and impaired renal tubular calcium reabsorption. Primary hyperparathyroidism causes resorptive hypercalciuria. Prevention of stone recurrence in patients with idiopathic hypercalciuria is commonly accomplished with thiazide or thiazide-like diuretics, whereas resorptive hypercalcuria is best treated with parathyroid surgery.

Thiazide diuretics enhance renal calcium absorption in the proximal and distal renal tubule, and thus have been the mainstay of treatment of hypercalciuric calcium nephrolithiasis. Multiple RCTs have demonstrated the benefits of thiazide and thiazide-like diuretics in the prevention of recurrent stone disease.[12,18–22] Interestingly, only two of these trials limited their participants to those with hypercalciuria,[18,19] whereas the remainder enrolled calcium stone formers not selected based on urinary calcium excretion. All studies that followed patients for a minimum of 2 years demonstrated a benefit of thiazide treatment. These trials all examined patients with calcium oxalate stones or unspecified calcium stones. Although there are no RCTs that studied calcium phosphate stones per se, thiazides are often used for patients with calcium phosphate stones who also demonstrate hypercalciuria. A Cochrane database review that analyzed five studies (316 patients) using thiazides or thiazide-like diuretics noted a 60% decrease in the number of new stone recurrences in patients treated with thiazides compared with placebo.[23]

Potential side-effects of thiazides and thiazide-like diuretics include hypokalemia, glucose intolerance, dyslipidemia, and hyperuricemia.[24] A review of the RCTs of thiazide therapy for nephrolithiasis noted that serum glucose and lipids were evaluated in two of the studies and were unchanged by therapy, serum uric acid was increased in each of the three studies that examined it, and three of four studies that measured serum potassium noted hypokalemia. Because of this latter potential side effect, potassium supplementation should usually accompany thiazide therapy to avert hypokalemia and resultant thiazide-induced hypocitraturia.[24] Potassium is usually administered as the citrate salt but potassium chloride can also be effective. Amiloride or spironolactone are alternatives to reduce potassium loss, but the poorly soluble triamterene should be avoided.

For patients with idiopathic hypercalciuria, typical doses of these medications are as follows: hydrochlorothiazide, 50 mg daily or 25 mg twice daily; chlorthalidone, 25 to 50 mg daily; indapamide, 1.25 to 2.5 mg daily; amiloride, 5 mg daily; and amiloride/hydrochlorothiazide, 5/50 mg daily.[25] There are several common strategies to avert thiazide-induced hypokalemia, which include the addition of potassium citrate or potassium chloride (10–20 mEq orally daily to twice daily, useful in patients who also have hypocitraturia) or the use of a combination thiazide/potassium-sparing diuretic, such as amiloride/hydrochlorothiazide in patients who do not require citrate repletion. Monitoring of urine pH is also critical because elevation of the urine pH greater than 6.5 can lead to supersaturation of calcium phosphate and possible change in stone recurrence composition.

Hyperoxaluria, Magnesium, Pyridoxine, and Oxalobacter

Hyperoxaluria has often been treated with dietary rather than pharmacologic intervention. Historically, patients have been advised to restrict dietary oxalate, and some have advised a calcium-rich diet in which ingested calcium binds oxalate in the stomach and gastrointestinal tract, limiting its availability for intestinal absorption and for urinary excretion.[26] Two pharmacologic agents that may lower urinary oxalate are magnesium and pyridoxine. In both cases, however, the data are far less compelling than those that favor thiazides.

Magnesium, a cation, forms complexes with oxalate anions in the urine, reducing the oxalate available to bind calcium and form calcium oxalate calculi. Dietary magnesium may reduce intestinal oxalate absorption in a manner similar to dietary calcium, as described previously.[27] There are several noncontrolled trials in the literature evaluating magnesium oxide and magnesium hydroxide preparations that reported decreases in stone recurrence rates on these medications.[28–30] However, the single RCT that examined magnesium hydroxide versus placebo reported no difference between treatment and placebo arms in prevention of stone recurrence.[12] Magnesium supplementation is most often used in patients with hypomagnesiuria, most of whom have bowel disease. Potential side effects of magnesium therapy include diarrhea and gastrointestinal discomfort. Although less well-studied than magnesium supplementation, calcium supplementation (calcium carbonate, calcium citrate) is another potential therapeutic target for hyperoxaluria that functions by the same mechanism, complexing with oxalate anions. Supplementation of calcium is a strategy commonly used to lower stone risk for patients with a history of Roux-en-Y gastric bypass surgery, in whom hyperoxaluria is the most common urine abnormality found on metabolic stone evaluation.[31]

The rationale for use of vitamin B_6 is that deficiencies may lead to excess urine oxalate.[32] The literature is lacking in RCTs regarding this use of pyridoxine for prevention of recurrent stone disease, but uncontrolled studies have shown that vitamin B_6 may decrease urine oxalate or stone recurrence in patients with calcium oxalate stones.[33,34] Epidemiologic studies have failed to demonstrate a benefit of vitamin B_6 supplementation in men,[35] but did show that in women, high daily doses of vitamin B_6 (>40 mg/day) may decrease risk of stone formation compared with those who ingest little or no vitamin B_6.[36] A retrospective study of pyridoxine in addition to dietary counseling in patients with hyperoxaluria noted an approximately 30% decrease in urine oxalate on follow-up 24-hour urine studies.[37]

Another potential therapy is the bacterium *Oxalobacter formigenes*, which colonizes the intestinal tract. Studies have shown that lack of colonization of this bacterium, the sole substrate of which is oxalate, may be associated with an increased incidence of calcium oxalate stone disease.[38] Early evidence demonstrated that oral *Oxalobacter* formulations could decrease urine oxalate excretion.[39] However, a recent RCT of orally administered *Oxalobacter* in patients with primary hyperoxaluria, a rare genetic calcium oxalate stone disease characterized by abnormal hepatic oxalate synthesis, failed to show differences in urine oxalate between the oral *Oxalobacter* group and placebo.[40] This potential therapy might be more successful if targeted toward patients with enteric hyperoxaluria, related to excessive absorption in the setting of inflammatory bowel disease and other causes of short bowel syndrome.

Hypocitraturia, Alkali Citrate, and Fruit Juices

Citrate is a known endogenous inhibitor of calcium oxalate stone formation; it forms soluble complexes with calcium and reduces urinary supersaturation of calcium oxalate.[41] In some cohort studies of stone formers, the incidence of hypocitraturia is in excess of 50%.[42] Several RCTs have been performed, each using a different alkali-citrate preparation.[43–45] Potassium citrate[45] and potassium-magnesium citrate[43] were both shown to significantly decrease recurrent stone formation in patients with hypocitraturia and unselected stone formers, respectively, whereas sodium-potassium citrate[44] failed to show a benefit. Potassium citrate is commercially available in tablet, liquid, and powder forms (to be mixed with water), whereas potassium-magnesium-citrate remains an investigational drug.[46] A typical starting dose of potassium citrate is 40 to 60 mEq daily in divided doses, increasing until the desired level of citraturia is reached.[46] Many clinicians monitor serum potassium 7 to 10 days after starting or changing doses of this medication. A theoretical risk of hyperkalemia exists when using potassium-based preparations, and patients with decreased glomerular filtration rate should be monitored closely when administering this medication. In addition, some patients report gastrointestinal side effects when taking potassium citrate and it is contraindicated in patients with active peptic ulcer disease. For patients with renal insufficiency or others with increased risk of hyperkalemia, sodium citrate or sodium bicarbonate may be used to increase urine citrate; however, excess sodium is another driving force in stone formation, and sodium can lead to exacerbations of congestive heart failure, hypertension, and lower extremity edema or fluid retention.

Urine citrate may also be significantly increased by ingesting beverages that are high in citrate content. In 1996, a retrospective study reported significant increases in urine citrate seen in patients who are hypocitraturic treated with a "homemade lemonade" formula (7.5 cups of water mixed with 0.5 cup of concentrated lemon juice, sweetened to taste with artificial sweetener and consumed daily).[47] Since then, several studies have tested various beverages, including other lemonade-based preparations, orange juice, pomegranate juice, lime juices, melon juice, diet sodas, and others, with equivocal results.[48,49] In addition, a single retrospective study noted that patients on lemonade therapy demonstrated a decreased stone recurrence rate.[50] Although the potential for beverage-based therapies remains of interest to patients who prefer nonpharmacologic interventions, lemonade-based therapies have been the most well-studied and some follow-up studies have produced similar results to the initial report.[48]

Hyperuricosuria and Allopurinol

Urine uric acid is thought to promote the formation of calcium oxalate stones. Uric acid reduces the solubility of calcium, called "salting out," and promotes the formation of calcium oxalate calculi.[51] Thus, hyperuricosuric calcium oxalate nephrolithiasis has traditionally been treated with allopurinol, a xanthine oxidase inhibitor that reduces endogenous uric acid production and urinary uric acid excretion. A single RCT examined stone recurrence in patients who are hyperuricosuric treated with either allopurinol or placebo and noted that the allopurinol arm demonstrated a significant decrease in stone recurrence of more than 50%.[52] This trial excluded patients with hypercalciuria and the effectiveness of xanthine oxidase inhibition in patients with hypercalciuria has not been established. Allopurinol is typically prescribed at a dose of 100 to 300 mg daily for treatment of hyperuricosuric calcium nephrolithiasis and is often used if dietary measures to reduce urine uric acid excretion (ie, dietary protein moderation) are not successful.[46] Rare side effects of this medication include Stevens-Johnson syndrome and elevated liver enzymes. For this reason, liver function tests should be monitored several months after initiation of allopurinol therapy.[53] An uncontrolled trial also demonstrated that potassium citrate is effective in decreasing stone recurrence in patients with hyperuricosuric calcium oxalate nephrolithaisis.[54]

Interesting recent research in uric acid metabolism may lead to novel therapies for hyperuricosuric nephrolithiasis and uric acid nephrolithiasis (see later) in the future. Specifically, recent reports of a new xanthine oxidase inhibitor (febuxostat) and a recombinant form of the enzyme uricase (Rasburicase) have demonstrated superiority to allopurinol in lowering serum uric acid and may also be more potent at reducing the frequency of gouty attacks.[55,56] These medications represent potential therapeutic agents for stone disease but have not been tested to date.[57]

URIC ACID STONES

At urine pH less than 5.5, uric acid has poor solubility in urine and the consequence of such acid urine may be formation of uric acid calculi. Some patients, despite having "normal" 24-hour urine uric acid levels, continue to precipitate uric acid stones if they have persistent "unduly acidic" urine. If urine pH is not increased, xanthine oxidase inhibition of uricosuria may be ineffective; at high urine pH, xanthine oxidase inhibition is redundant in addressing recurrent uric acid stones.

Urinary alkalinization is the main strategy in the treatment of uric acid calculi and is of much greater importance than reduction of uricosuria. There are no RCTs evaluating therapies for prevention of uric acid stones but alkalinization with alkali citrate is clearly so effective that randomized trials are not necessary to establish efficacy.[13,58] A common strategy for treating uric acid calculi is to alkalinize the urine as a first-line treatment and reserve the addition of allopurinol to those patients with persistently acidic urine who do not alkalinize easily, such as in the presence of bowel disease, morbid obesity, or those with hyperuricemia (eg, gout and myeloproliferative disorders). Typical starting doses include potassium citrate, 4 to 60 mEq in divided doses, or sodium bicarbonate, 1300 mg twice daily, with goal urine pH between 6.5 and 7.[46] As described previously for the treatment of hypocitraturia, sodium bicarbonate is a reasonable alternative to potassium citrate for patients with renal insufficiency or other risk for hyperkalemia. Dose titration for either medication may be done by monitoring urine pH in the physician's office or by patients at home using nitrazine paper.

STRUVITE STONES

Infection or struvite stones are those that occur as a result of chronic infection of the genitourinary tract with urease-producing bacteria, most often *Proteus*, *Pseudomonas*, *Klebsiella*, or yeast, and form at relatively high pH (typically >7). Composition of these stones is generally calcium magnesium ammonium phosphate alone, although many struvite stones also have a component of calcium phosphate (carbonate apatite or hydroxyapatite). For these stones in particular, surgical treatment is of paramount importance because it is often quite difficult to sterilize the urine and prevent recurrence if stones colonized with bacteria remain in the kidneys.

Pharmacologic prevention studies have focused on urease inhibitors and chronic suppressive antibiotics. Several RCTs have studied the urease inhibitor acetohydroxamic acid (AHA). This medication neutralizes urease, the enzyme that is central to formation of struvite stones.[16,59,60] Hydroxyurea, another potential urease inhibitor, has not been studied in a randomized trial. Each of these studies showed a significant benefit in terms of stone prevention on this agent. It should be stressed that these trials were done before the availability of the flexible ureteroscopes that today allow the endourologist access to all calyces. The role of these drugs is not well defined in an era in which stones can be more thoroughly evacuated with ureteroscopy. AHA administration was associated with significant side effects, and the rate of severe side effects in these studies from patients on treatment ranged from 22% to 62%.[16,59,60] Known potential side effects include deep vein thrombosis, pulmonary embolism, headache, and tremulousness.[60] Chronic antibiotic suppression has been suggested in these patients, and there are retrospective data, but no randomized data, to support its use.[61] The regimen of AHA and antibiotic suppression is typically reserved for patients who are poor surgical candidates for whom the significant side effect profile of AHA may be an acceptable risk.

For patients with struvite calculi undergoing endourologic procedures, preoperative antibiotics are commonly used. Two prospective studies of antibiotics before percutaneous nephrolithotomy versus placebo in prevention of sepsis after percutaneous nephrolithotomy noted a significant reduction in patients treated with either ciprofloxacin or nitrofurantoin.[62,63] In addition, it is recommended for patients undergoing percutaneous nephrolithotomy to obtain intraoperative renal pelvis and stone culture, because these are the most accurate methods to identify causative bacteria should these patients develop fevers or sepsis postoperatively.[64]

CYSTINE STONES

Cystinuria is an autosomal-recessive condition in which those afflicted excrete cystine in large amounts in the urine. Cystine solubility is reported at 250 mg/L, but many homozygotes with the disease may excrete in excess of 1500 mg per 24 hours, leading to chronic recurrent stone formation. Mainstays of treatment are combination therapy with urinary alkalinization and thiol-binding medications. Because of the relatively high pKa of cystine (8.5), these medications may be more effective in combination than when used alone.[25]

There are no RCTs comparing any treatment with placebo for the prevention of recurrent cystine nephrolithiasis. Four noncontrolled trials have demonstrated that d-penicillamine and α-mercaptopropionylglycine (tiopronin) were effective in decreasing the number of recurrent stone events in patients who are cystinuric.[65–68] Although often well-tolerated, infrequent side effects include the following: bone marrow suppression, proteinuria with nephropathy, hepatotoxicity, aplastic anemia, drug-induced lupus, abdominal pain, diarrhea, nausea and vomiting, and anorexia. A typical starting dose of tiopronin is 200 to 300 mg three times daily (in addition to potassium citrate or sodium bicarbonate with goal urine pH 7.5), with close follow-up of 24-hour urine composition to monitor the efficacy of treatment. It is recommended to check liver function tests, complete blood counts, and urine protein/creatinine ratios at least twice a year in patients taking these drugs. A single study that compared the two medications suggested that side effects may be less frequent for tiopronin than for d-penicillamine.[25]

Captopril, a commonly used antihypertensive that contains a thiol-group, is another theoretical pharmacologic target for cystinuria. However, it does not appear in the urine in sufficient quantities to affect cysteine solubility and several small studies have yielded equivocal data on its ability to decrease urinary cystine levels.[25]

MEDICAL EXPULSIVE THERAPY

MET refers to the use of pharmacotherapy to facilitate the spontaneous passage of ureteral stones. MET is based on the principal of ureteral relaxation and the increase of hydrostatic pressure proximal to the stone.[69] Clinically, the data are most compelling for the use of α-adrenergic antagonists and calcium channel blockers. Since the original description, multiple studies have revealed the efficacy of MET in increasing stone passage rage and decreasing time to passage of stones. In 2006, a meta-analysis of RCTs reported on pooled data from nine trials (N = 693).[70] The main outcome was the proportion of patients who passed stones. The authors concluded that patients given calcium-channel blockers or α-blockers had a 65% greater likelihood of stone passage than those not given these treatments. Additionally, the addition of steroids to the various regimens led to a minor benefit. After this report, other studies demonstrated the efficacy of MET for ureteral stones.[71,72] Overall, efficacy comparing different α-blockers (tamsulosin, doxazosin, terazosin) or α-blockers with a calcium channel blocker (nifedipine) could not be determined. In another large review by Singh and colleagues,[71] MET was established as a cost-effective and well-tolerated therapy. The latter was reported in a systemic review of 16 articles on medical therapy and concluded MET was safe and efficacious for moderately sized ureteral stones. A single RCT comparing alfuzosin with placebo noted that patient discomfort was significantly decreased in the treatment arm compared with placebo.[73]

Because MET is most commonly used in the emergency department setting, Itano and colleagues[74] recently assessed the use of MET in their tertiary-care emergency department.

Of 119 patients evaluated by emergency department physicians, only 14% of patients received MET. The researchers concluded MET was underused and recommended educational interventions in the emergency department setting. The compelling evidence for the use of MET led the American Urological Association guidelines committee to recommend that patients with ureteral stones less than 10 mm in the appropriate clinical setting (without indications for surgical intervention), should be put on a MET regimen.[75] Major trials involving the use of MET are shown in **Table 1**.

PHARMACOLOGIC THERAPY FOR URETERAL STENT SYMPTOMS

Ureteral stents are commonly used to promote healing and decrease obstruction and pain after treatment of ureteral or renal stones.[76] Commonly associated side effects include lower urinary tract

Table 1
Trials of medical expulsive therapy for ureteral stones

Author/Year	Regimen	Mean Stone Size (mm)	Observation Time (d)	Mean Expulsion Time (d)	Stone Expulsion Rate (%)
1. Cha et al,[82] 2012	Tamsulosin, 0.4 mg	5.49 ± 1.31	28	7.82 ± 5.08	23/30 (76.6)
	Tamsulosin, 0.2 mg	5.73 ± 1.57		7.82 ± 5.08	23/30 (76.7)
	Alfuzosin	5.81 ± 1.26		8.22 ± 5.96	27/36 (75)
	Trospium	5.59 ± 1.44		13.56 ± 6.49	16/34 (47.1)
2. Al-Ansari et al,[83] 2010	Tamsulosin	NA	28	6.4 ± 2.77	41/50 (82)
	Placebo			9.87 ± 5.4	28/46 (61)
3. Griwan et al,[84] 2010	Tamsulosin	6.70 ± 1.60	28		27/30 (90)
	watchful waiting	6.33 ± 1.47			21/30 (70)
4. Pedro et al,[73] 2008	Alfuzosin	3.83 ± 0.95	28	5.19 ± 4.82	(73.5)
	Control	4.08 ± 0.17		8.54 ± 6.99	(77.1)
5. Vincendeau et al,[85] 2010	Tamsulosin	2.9	42		47/61 (77)
	Placebo	3.2			43/61 (70.5)
6. Ahmed and Al-Sayed,[86] 2010	Tamsulosin	4.97 ± 2.24	30	7.52 ± 7.06	25/29 (86.2)
	Alfuzosin	5.47 ± 2.13		8.26 ± 7.34	23/30 (76.6)
	Placebo	5.39 ± 1.8		13.90 ± 6.99	14/28 (50)
7. Agrawal et al,[87] 2009	Tamsulosin	6.17	28	12.3	28/34 (82.3)
	Alfuzosin	6.70		14.5	24/34 (70.5)
	Placebo	6.35		24.5	12/34 (35.2)
8. Wang et al,[88] 2008	Tamsulosin	6.5	28	6.3	26/32 (81)
	Terazosin	6.5		6.3	25/32 (78)
	Control	6.5		10.1	17/31 (55)
9. Gurbuz et al,[89] 2011	Hyoscine *N*-butyl bromide	6.13	14	10.55 ± 6.21	11%
	Alfuzosin	5.83		7.38 ± 5.55	52.9%
	Doxazosin	5.59		7.85 ± 5.11	62%
	Terazosin	5.48		7.45 ± 5.32	46%
10. Resorlu et al,[90] 2011	Doxazosin males	6.5	21		29/40 (72.5)
	Doxazosin female	7.5			28/40 (70)
11. Porpiglia et al,[91] 2000	Nifedipine + Deflazacort	5.8	28	7	38/48 (79)
	watchful waiting	5.5		20	17/48 (35)
12. Cooper et al,[92] 2000	Nifedipine	3.9	48	12.6	31/35 (89)
	Control	3.9		11.2	19/35 (54)
13. Dellabella et al,[93] 2005	Phloroglucinol		28	6.2	45/70 (64.3)
	Tamsulosin			7.2	68/70 (97.1)
	Nifedipine			6.2	54/70 (77.1)
14. Dellabella et al,[94] 2005	Tamsulosin + steroid	6.9	28	3	29/30 (96.7)
	Tamsulosin + no steroids	6.4		5	27/30 (90)

symptoms, such as urinary frequency and urgency, pain, and decreased quality of life. Multiple pharmacologic agents have been studied whose purpose is to reduce stent-related symptoms. The most common class of medications is α-blockers.[77,78] Two recent meta-analyses noted that the α-blockers tamsulosin and alfuzosin are each associated with significant decreases in stent-related lower urinary tract symptoms and pain and significant improvements in general health.[77,78] The larger of these two studies examined RCTs that included 946 patients.[78]

Two RCTs have also reported significant benefits from anticholinergic medications (extended release tolterodine[79] and solifenacin[80]). A third RCT failed to show a beneficial effect of extended release oxybutnin, although the authors noted that their sample size was small.[81]

A single study placebo-controlled study examining the use of α-blockers and anticholinergic medications alone or in combination noted that combination therapy (tamsulosin with solifenacin) was associated with the greatest reduction in stent-related symptoms.[80]

REFERENCES

1. Stamatelou KK, Francis ME, Jones CA, et al. Time trends in reported prevalence of kidney stones in the United States: 1976-1994. Kidney Int 2003;63:1817.
2. Soucie JM, Thun MJ, Coates RJ, et al. Demographic and geographic variability of kidney stones in the United States. Kidney Int 1994;46:893.
3. Lee YH, Huang WC, Tsai JY, et al. Epidemiological studies on the prevalence of upper urinary calculi in Taiwan. Urol Int 2002;68:172.
4. Safarinejad MR. Adult urolithiasis in a population-based study in Iran: prevalence, incidence, and associated risk factors. Urol Res 2007;35:73.
5. Scales CD Jr, Smith AC, Hanley JM, et al. Prevalence of kidney stones in the United States. Eur Urol 2012;62:160.
6. Trinchieri A, Coppi F, Montanari E, et al. Increase in the prevalence of symptomatic upper urinary tract stones during the last ten years. Eur Urol 2000; 37:23.
7. Ljunghall S, Danielson BG. A prospective study of renal stone recurrences. Br J Urol 1984;56:122.
8. Trinchieri A, Ostini F, Nespoli R, et al. A prospective study of recurrence rate and risk factors for recurrence after a first renal stone. J Urol 1999;162:27.
9. Levy FL, Adams-Huet B, Pak CY. Ambulatory evaluation of nephrolithiasis: an update of a 1980 protocol. Am J Med 1995;98:50.
10. Pak CY, Britton F, Peterson R, et al. Ambulatory evaluation of nephrolithiasis. Classification, clinical presentation and diagnostic criteria. Am J Med 1980;69:19.
11. Su CJ, Shevock PN, Khan SR, et al. Effect of magnesium on calcium oxalate urolithiasis. J Urol 1991; 145:1092.
12. Ettinger B, Citron JT, Livermore B, et al. Chlorthalidone reduces calcium oxalate calculous recurrence but magnesium hydroxide does not. J Urol 1988; 139:679.
13. Pak CY, Sakhaee K, Fuller C. Successful management of uric acid nephrolithiasis with potassium citrate. Kidney Int 1986;30:422.
14. Coe FL, Clark C, Parks JH, et al. Solid phase assay of urine cystine supersaturation in the presence of cystine binding drugs. J Urol 2001;166:688.
15. Dolin DJ, Asplin JR, Flagel L, et al. Effect of cystine-binding thiol drugs on urinary cystine capacity in patients with cystinuria. J Endourol 2005;19:429.
16. Griffith DP, Khonsari F, Skurnick JH, et al. A randomized trial of acetohydroxamic acid for the treatment and prevention of infection-induced urinary stones in spinal cord injury patients. J Urol 1988;140:318.
17. Borghi L, Meschi T, Schianchi T, et al. Urine volume: stone risk factor and preventive measure. Nephron 1999;81(Suppl 1):31.
18. Borghi L, Meschi T, Guerra A, et al. Randomized prospective study of a nonthiazide diuretic, indapamide, in preventing calcium stone recurrences. J Cardiovasc Pharmacol 1993;22(Suppl 6):S78.
19. Ohkawa M, Tokunaga S, Nakashima T, et al. Thiazide treatment for calcium urolithiasis in patients with idiopathic hypercalciuria. Br J Urol 1992; 69:571.
20. Brocks P, Dahl C, Wolf H, et al. Do thiazides prevent recurrent idiopathic renal calcium stones? Lancet 1981;2:124.
21. Mortensen JT, Schultz A, Ostergaard AH. Thiazides in the prophylactic treatment of recurrent idiopathic kidney stones. Int Urol Nephrol 1986;18:265.
22. Laerum E, Larsen S. Thiazide prophylaxis of urolithiasis. A double-blind study in general practice. Acta Med Scand 1984;215:383.
23. Escribano J, Balaguer A, Pagone F, et al. Pharmacological interventions for preventing complications in idiopathic hypercalciuria. Cochrane Database Syst Rev 2009;(1):CD004754.
24. Huen SC, Goldfarb DS. Adverse metabolic side effects of thiazides: implications for patients with calcium nephrolithiasis. J Urol 2007;177:1238.
25. Moe OW, Pearle MS, Sakhaee K. Pharmacotherapy of urolithiasis: evidence from clinical trials. Kidney Int 2011;79:385.
26. Hess B, Jost C, Zipperle L, et al. High-calcium intake abolishes hyperoxaluria and reduces urinary crystallization during a 20-fold normal oxalate load in humans. Nephrol Dial Transplant 1998;13:2241.

27. Liebman M, Costa G. Effects of calcium and magnesium on urinary oxalate excretion after oxalate loads. J Urol 2000;163:1565.
28. Moore CA, Bunce GE. Reduction in frequency of renal calculus formation by oral magnesium administration. A preliminary report. Invest Urol 1964;2:7.
29. Johansson G, Backman U, Danielson BG, et al. Biochemical and clinical effects of the prophylactic treatment of renal calcium stones with magnesium hydroxide. J Urol 1980;124:770.
30. Vagelli G, Calabrese G, Pratesi G, et al. Magnesium hydroxide in idiopathic calcium nephrolithiasis. Minerva Urol Nefrol 1998;50:113 [in Italian].
31. Kleinman JG. Bariatric surgery, hyperoxaluria, and nephrolithiasis: a plea for close postoperative management of risk factors. Kidney Int 2007;72:8.
32. Williams HE, Smith LH Jr. Disorders of oxalate metabolism. Am J Med 1968;45:715.
33. Mitwalli A, Ayiomamitis A, Grass L, et al. Control of hyperoxaluria with large doses of pyridoxine in patients with kidney stones. Int Urol Nephrol 1988; 20:353.
34. Balcke P, Schmidt P, Zazgornik J, et al. Pyridoxine therapy in patients with renal calcium oxalate calculi. Proc Eur Dial Transplant Assoc 1983;20:417.
35. Curhan GC, Willett WC, Rimm EB, et al. A prospective study of the intake of vitamins C and B6, and the risk of kidney stones in men. J Urol 1996;155:1847.
36. Curhan GC, Willett WC, Speizer FE, et al. Intake of vitamins B6 and C and the risk of kidney stones in women. J Am Soc Nephrol 1999;10:840.
37. Ortiz-Alvarado O, Miyaoka R, Kriedberg C, et al. Pyridoxine and dietary counseling for the management of idiopathic hyperoxaluria in stone-forming patients. Urology 2011;77:1054.
38. Kaufman DW, Kelly JP, Curhan GC, et al. *Oxalobacter formigenes* may reduce the risk of calcium oxalate kidney stones. J Am Soc Nephrol 2008;19:1197.
39. Sidhu H, Allison MJ, Chow JM, et al. Rapid reversal of hyperoxaluria in a rat model after probiotic administration of *Oxalobacter formigenes*. J Urol 2001; 166:1487.
40. Hoppe B, Groothoff JW, Hulton SA, et al. Efficacy and safety of *Oxalobacter formigenes* to reduce urinary oxalate in primary hyperoxaluria. Nephrol Dial Transplant 2011;26:3609.
41. Kok DJ, Papapoulos SE, Bijvoet OL. Excessive crystal agglomeration with low citrate excretion in recurrent stone-formers. Lancet 1986;1:1056.
42. Tracy CR, Pearle MS. Update on the medical management of stone disease. Curr Opin Urol 2009;19:200.
43. Ettinger B, Pak CY, Citron JT, et al. Potassium-magnesium citrate is an effective prophylaxis against recurrent calcium oxalate nephrolithiasis. J Urol 1997;158:2069.
44. Hofbauer J, Hobarth K, Szabo N, et al. Alkali citrate prophylaxis in idiopathic recurrent calcium oxalate urolithiasis–a prospective randomized study. Br J Urol 1994;73:362.
45. Barcelo P, Wuhl O, Servitge E, et al. Randomized double-blind study of potassium citrate in idiopathic hypocitraturic calcium nephrolithiasis. J Urol 1993; 150:1761.
46. Pearle MS, Asplin JR, Coe FL, et al. Medical management of urolithiasis. In: Denstedt JD, Khoury S, editors. 2nd International Consultation on Stone Disease. Paris (France): Health Publications; 2008. p. 57–84.
47. Seltzer MA, Low RK, McDonald M, et al. Dietary manipulation with lemonade to treat hypocitraturic calcium nephrolithiasis. J Urol 1996;156:907.
48. Kurtz MP, Eisner BH. Dietary therapy for patients with hypocitraturic nephrolithiasis. Nat Rev Urol 2011;8:146.
49. Sumorok NT, Asplin JR, Eisner BH, et al. Effect of diet orange soda on urinary lithogenicity. Urol Res 2012;40:237.
50. Kang DE, Sur RL, Haleblian GE, et al. Long-term lemonade based dietary manipulation in patients with hypocitraturic nephrolithiasis. J Urol 2007; 177:1358.
51. Grover PK, Ryall RL. Urate and calcium oxalate stones: from repute to rhetoric to reality. Miner Electrolyte Metab 1994;20:361.
52. Ettinger B, Tang A, Citron JT, et al. Randomized trial of allopurinol in the prevention of calcium oxalate calculi. N Engl J Med 1986;315:1386.
53. Fritsch PO, Sidoroff A. Drug-induced Stevens-Johnson syndrome/toxic epidermal necrolysis. Am J Clin Dermatol 2000;1:349.
54. Pak CY, Peterson R. Successful treatment of hyperuricosuric calcium oxalate nephrolithiasis with potassium citrate. Arch Intern Med 1986;146:863.
55. Becker MA, Schumacher HR Jr, Wortmann RL, et al. Febuxostat compared with allopurinol in patients with hyperuricemia and gout. N Engl J Med 2005; 353:2450.
56. Coutsouvelis J, Wiseman M, Hui L, et al. Effectiveness of a single fixed dose of rasburicase 3 mg in the management of tumour lysis syndrome. Br J Clin Pharmacol 2012, in press.
57. Goldfarb DS. Potential pharmacologic treatments for cystinuria and for calcium stones associated with hyperuricosuria. Clin J Am Soc Nephrol 2011;6: 2093.
58. Rodman JS. Intermittent versus continuous alkaline therapy for uric acid stones and ureteral stones of uncertain composition. Urology 2002;60:378.
59. Griffith DP, Gleeson MJ, Lee H, et al. Randomized, double-blind trial of Lithostat (acetohydroxamic acid) in the palliative treatment of infection-induced urinary calculi. Eur Urol 1991;20:243.

60. Williams JJ, Rodman JS, Peterson CM. A randomized double-blind study of acetohydroxamic acid in struvite nephrolithiasis. N Engl J Med 1984;311:760.
61. Martinez-Pineiro JA, de Iriarte EG, Armero AH. The problem of recurrences and infection after surgical removal of staghorn calculi. Eur Urol 1982;8:94.
62. Bag S, Kumar S, Taneja N, et al. One week of nitrofurantoin before percutaneous nephrolithotomy significantly reduces upper tract infection and urosepsis: a prospective controlled study. Urology 2011;77:45.
63. Mariappan P, Smith G, Moussa SA, et al. One week of ciprofloxacin before percutaneous nephrolithotomy significantly reduces upper tract infection and urosepsis: a prospective controlled study. BJU Int 2006;98:1075.
64. Korets R, Graversen JA, Kates M, et al. Post-percutaneous nephrolithotomy systemic inflammatory response: a prospective analysis of preoperative urine, renal pelvic urine and stone cultures. J Urol 2011;186:1899.
65. Chow GK, Streem SB. Medical treatment of cystinuria: results of contemporary clinical practice. J Urol 1996;156:1576.
66. Dahlberg PJ, van den B, Kurtz SB, et al. Clinical features and management of cystinuria. Mayo Clin Proc 1977;52:533.
67. Pak CY, Fuller C, Sakhaee K, et al. Management of cystine nephrolithiasis with alpha-mercaptopropionylglycine. J Urol 1986;136:1003.
68. Barbey F, Joly D, Rieu P, et al. Medical treatment of cystinuria: critical reappraisal of long-term results. J Urol 2000;163:1419.
69. Sivula A, Lehtonen T. Spontaneous passage of artificial concretions applied in the rabbit ureter. Scand J Urol Nephrol 1967;1:259.
70. Hollingsworth JM, Rogers MA, Kaufman SR, et al. Medical therapy to facilitate urinary stone passage: a meta-analysis. Lancet 2006;368:1171.
71. Singh A, Alter HJ, Littlepage A. A systematic review of medical therapy to facilitate passage of ureteral calculi. Ann Emerg Med 2007;50:552.
72. Seitz C, Liatsikos E, Porpiglia F, et al. Medical therapy to facilitate the passage of stones: what is the evidence? Eur Urol 2009;56:455.
73. Pedro RN, Hinck B, Hendlin K, et al. Alfuzosin stone expulsion therapy for distal ureteral calculi: a double-blind, placebo controlled study. J Urol 2008;179:2244.
74. Itano N, Ferlic E, Nunez-Nateras R, et al. Medical expulsive therapy in a tertiary care emergency department. Urology 2012;79:1242.
75. Preminger GM, Tiselius HG, Assimos DG, et al. 2007 Guideline for the management of ureteral calculi. Eur Urol 2007;52:1610.
76. Bader MJ, Eisner B, Porpiglia F, et al. Contemporary management of ureteral stones. Eur Urol 2012;61:764.
77. Lamb AD, Vowler SL, Johnston R, et al. Meta-analysis showing the beneficial effect of alpha-blockers on ureteric stent discomfort. BJU Int 2011;108:1894.
78. Yakoubi R, Lemdani M, Monga M, et al. Is there a role for alpha-blockers in ureteral stent related symptoms? A systematic review and meta-analysis. J Urol 2011;186:928.
79. Park SC, Jung SW, Lee JW, et al. The effects of tolterodine extended release and alfuzosin for the treatment of double-j stent-related symptoms. J Endourol 2009;23:1913.
80. Lim KT, Kim YT, Lee TY, et al. Effects of tamsulosin, solifenacin, and combination therapy for the treatment of ureteral stent related discomforts. Korean J Urol 2011;52:485.
81. Norris RD, Sur RL, Springhart WP, et al. A prospective, randomized, double-blinded placebo-controlled comparison of extended release oxybutynin versus phenazopyridine for the management of postoperative ureteral stent discomfort. Urology 2008;71:792.
82. Cha WH, Choi JD, Kim KH, et al. Comparison and efficacy of low-dose and standard-dose tamsulosin and alfuzosin in medical expulsive therapy for lower ureteral calculi: prospective, randomized, comparative study. Korean J Urol 2012;53:349.
83. Al-Ansari A, Al-Naimi A, Alobaidy A, et al. Efficacy of tamsulosin in the management of lower ureteral stones: a randomized double-blind placebo-controlled study of 100 patients. Urology 2010;75:4.
84. Griwan MS, Singh SK, Paul H, et al. The efficacy of tamsulosin in lower ureteral calculi. Urol Ann 2010; 2:63.
85. Vincendeau S, Bellissant E, Houlgatte A, et al. Tamsulosin hydrochloride vs placebo for management of distal ureteral stones: a multicentric, randomized, double-blind trial. Arch Intern Med 2010;170:2021.
86. Ahmed AF, Al-Sayed AY. Tamsulosin versus alfuzosin in the treatment of patients with distal ureteral stones: prospective, randomized, comparative study. Korean J Urol 2010;51:193.
87. Agrawal M, Gupta M, Gupta A, et al. Prospective randomized trial comparing efficacy of alfuzosin and tamsulosin in management of lower ureteral stones. Urology 2009;73:706.
88. Wang CJ, Huang SW, Chang CH. Efficacy of an alpha1 blocker in expulsive therapy of lower ureteral stones. J Endourol 2008;22:41.
89. Gurbuz MC, Polat H, Canat L, et al. Efficacy of three different alpha 1-adrenergic blockers and hyoscine N-butylbromide for distal ureteral stones. Int Braz J Urol 2011;37:195.
90. Resorlu B, Bozkurt OF, Senocak C, et al. Effectiveness of doxazosin in the management of lower

ureteral stones in male and female patients. Int Urol Nephrol 2011;43:645.

91. Porpiglia F, Destefanis P, Fiori C, et al. Effectiveness of nifedipine and deflazacort in the management of distal ureter stones. Urology 2000;56:579.
92. Cooper JT, Stack GM, Cooper TP. Intensive medical management of ureteral calculi. Urology 2000;56:575.
93. Dellabella M, Milanese G, Muzzonigro G. Randomized trial of the efficacy of tamsulosin, nifedipine and phloroglucinol in medical expulsive therapy for distal ureteral calculi. J Urol 2005;174:167.
94. Dellabella M, Milanese G, Muzzonigro G. Medical-expulsive therapy for distal ureterolithiasis: randomized prospective study on role of corticosteroids used in combination with tamsulosin-simplified treatment regimen and health-related quality of life. Urology 2005;66:712.

Diet and Alternative Therapies in the Management of Stone Disease

Kristina L. Penniston, PhD, RD*, Stephen Y. Nakada, MD

KEYWORDS

• Urolithiasis • Diet • Nutrition • Prevention • Therapy

KEY POINTS

- Nutrition therapy, widely used for secondary prevention of urolithiasis, is the application of nutritional assessment, diagnosis, intervention, and counseling to prevent or manage disease.
- Nutrition therapy for prevention of kidney stone recurrence is based primarily on the idea that the reduction of known lithogenic risk factors reduces or prevents calculus formation and growth.
- After assessment of the nutritional intake of the patient, urinary and other risk factors are evaluated with respect to their cause and whether or not nutrition intervention is likely to address them.

INTRODUCTION

Therapeutic nutrition recommendations for the secondary prevention of urolithiasis are widely used. General nutrition guidelines are useful in promoting public health and for developing nutrition plans that reduce the risk for or attenuate the effects of diseases that are affected by nutrition. Examples of such guidelines are the dietary reference intake values[1] (which include the recommended dietary allowance (RDA), adequate intake, and the tolerable upper intake level for individual nutrients) and the dietary guidelines for Americans.[2] However, general guidelines are insufficient in developing interventions to address specific disease conditions in individual patients. Nutrition therapy is the application of nutritional assessment, diagnosis, intervention, and counseling to prevent or manage disease.[3]

Food and nutrition are inherently complex. Plants grow in different soils and conditions throughout the world and therefore have variations with respect to their nutrient and molecular profiles. Animalia of all types eat different foods and are subject to different management techniques, rendering their nutrient profiles variable. People from different cultures and backgrounds may derive the same essential nutrients but from vastly different foods and preparation methods. Conversely, the intake of certain nutrients and biologically active nonnutrients is also known to vary between cultures, between individuals, and even within individuals over time. The intake of individual nutrients or food components rarely, if ever, occurs in isolation; a single food item may contain hundreds of biologically active compounds. In the context of an entire meal, thousands of nutrients and nonnutrients are consumed. Certain micronutrients and other food constituents interact in antagonistic, synergistic, or benign ways. Individuals vary with respect to their consumption, digestion, and absorption of foods and their components, even within an individual over the course of the life span. Moreover, a single food-derived compound may affect hundreds of molecular systems and even cause epigenomic changes.[4]

Disclosures: The authors have no disclosures to report.
Department of Urology, University of Wisconsin School of Medicine and Public Health, 1685 Highland Avenue, UW Medical Foundation Centennial Building, Madison, WI 53705-2281, USA
* Corresponding author.
E-mail address: penn@urology.wisc.edu

Urol Clin N Am 40 (2013) 31–46
http://dx.doi.org/10.1016/j.ucl.2012.09.011

General nutritional influences on stone disease are difficult to characterize. Although interest for nutrition interventions is high among patients, evidence-based data from well-designed research studies to support specific recommendations are lacking. A recent systematic review of published randomized trials on nutritional prevention of urolithiasis collectively identified 8 trials with reasonable but variable quality, all but one reporting reduced stone recurrence (**Table 1**).[13] Few studies have been designed to assess the effects of a whole diet intervention or of multiple, simultaneous nutrition interventions. Many more studies have evaluated the effects of single nutrients or individual food components, but most of these have assessed effects on stone risk factors, not stone formation. The use of stone risk factors as outcomes is attractive because it is accomplished in a shorter time frame than assessment of stone formation and growth and may be evaluated with a single diagnostic test, such as a 24-hour urine analysis. Although risk reduction alone has not been definitively tied to reduced recurrence, much of what we believe and practice about nutrition interventions to prevent recurrence comes from this assumption.

Table 1
Published randomized trials involving nutrition intervention for urolithiasis

Author, Year, Journal	Intervention	Duration
Borghi et al,[5] 1996, J Urol	Increased fluids vs no treatment	5 y
Sarica et al,[6] 2006, Urol Res	Increased fluids vs no treatment	2–3 y
Di Silverio et al,[7] 2000, Eur Urol	Mineral vs tap water	19 mo
Shuster et al,[8] 1992, J Clin Epidemiol	Decreased soft drinks vs no treatment	3 y
Dussol et al,[9] 2008, Nephron	Increased fiber vs decreased animal protein	4 y
Hiatt et al,[10] 1996, Am J Epidemiol	Whole diet approach (vs control diet)	2 y
Borghi et al,[11] 2002, N Engl J Med	Whole diet approach (vs self-select diet)	5 y
Kocvara et al,[12] 1999, BJU Int	Whole diet approach (tailored vs empiric diet)	3 y

NUTRITION THERAPY: THE APPROACH

Nutrition therapy for prevention of kidney stone recurrence is based primarily on the idea that the reduction of known lithogenic risk factors, such as urine supersaturation and the relative urinary excretion of lithogenic promoters versus inhibitors, reduces or prevents calculus formation and growth. In concert with pharmacologic therapy, or as monotherapy, nutrition therapy seems useful. Nutrition therapy includes the assessment of a patient's nutritional status and intake, the diagnosis of the nutritional risk factor(s), and the development and application of the nutrition intervention.[3]

Role of Registered Dietitian

A registered dietitian is helpful as a member of the health care team because the application of nutrition therapy requires detailed nutrition knowledge and expertise in delivering individualized patient education. Education that is not tailored appropriately to the individual patient's learning style, education background and nutrition knowledge, economic capacity, food preferences, and motivation to change is likely to be unsuccessful.[14] Moreover, unless it is integrated into their individual regimen, patients with diabetes, Crohn disease, and cardiovascular disease likely have received specific nutrition recommendations for those conditions and thus may not embrace nutrition therapy for stone prevention. These scenarios may confound the true impact of nutrition intervention on the course of urolithiasis and might lead to the false conclusion that "dietary changes don't work" or that "patients won't comply."

Empiric Versus Tailored

There are 2 approaches for applying nutrition therapy. The first is an empiric approach, applied to all patients. This approach might involve a general discussion of various nutritional strategies that address multiple risk factors and could be provided to a patient without knowing their specific urinary risk factors. If the stone composition of the patient is known, this approach could be modified by developing multiple versions of a stone prevention diet based on the patient's previous stone composition. The second is a tailored approach that is continually monitored and altered as needed based on the disappearance or emergence of a patient's specific risk factors. Both approaches could be termed whole diet approaches because both include recommendations about multiple foods and nutrients. One study that compared the empiric versus tailored nutrition therapy approach reported reduced stone recurrence with the latter.[11] Two other studies in calcium stone formers found reduced stone recurrence with an empiric whole diet approach, but this was not directly compared with a tailored approach.[10,12]

In practice, because of time constraints or for simplicity, urologists and other urology providers may rely more on empiric approaches such as general handouts or standardized patient instructions. Shortcomings of this approach include:

- It potentially addresses risk factors that the patient does not show, and thus may impose unnecessary recommendations.
- It does not prioritize the recommendations, which could lead to patients' confusion about what is most important for them.
- Patient compliance with nutrition and other therapies may hinge on the number of recommendations provided, with greater compliance more achievable with a short list of modifications.
- Unless otherwise addressed, it may conflict with other nutrition information that the patient has received for a different comorbidity.
- Unless otherwise addressed, specific strategies to aid the patient in achieving the stated goals are lacking. These include, for example, behavioral modifications, recommendations for alternative food choices or different food preparation methods, changes in grocery shopping habits, education on estimating portion sizes, tips for adherence when eating out, strategies and resources for economically disadvantaged patients, and motivational techniques to encourage patients' movement along the stages of change toward action.[15]

Attention to these potential barriers to success of the nutrition intervention is strongly encouraged if an empiric approach is used.

Clearly, a tailored nutrition therapy approach is favorable and may avoid some of the pitfalls. In this approach, nutrition therapy is targeted to the patient's individual risk factors (**Fig. 1**), which may be different than another patient's, even if they both form the same type of calculi. Risk factors that are manifest are addressed foremost, and secondary focus is given, if appropriate, to nonexistent potential risk factors. A tailored or individual approach also allows for the integration of stone prevention strategies with nutritional therapy that the patient may have received for other conditions. By focusing on the most salient risk factors rather than discussing all potential

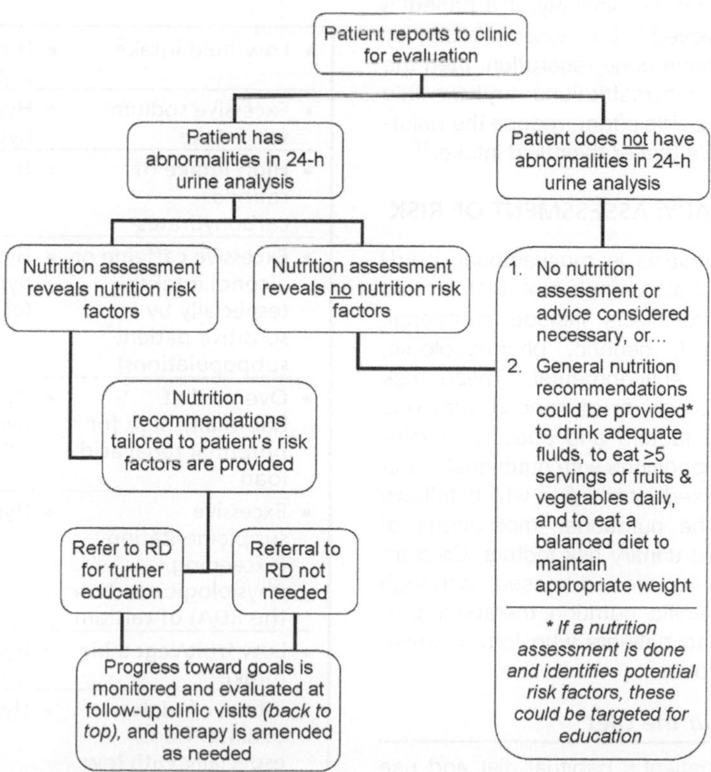

Fig. 1. Tailored nutrition therapy.

risk factors, there may be time to provide patients with pragmatic solutions to specific problems. These solutions might include how to read nutrition labels to monitor sodium intake, making appropriate food choices when eating out or during frequent travel, and titrating calcium supplementation for patients with hyperoxaluria, if needed, with a patient's usual food calcium intake.

Lithogenic risk factors should be assessed first for nutrition influences. If nutrition is determined to be contributory, then identifying the nutrition risk is necessary in order to apply the appropriate nutrition therapy. Some risk factors have an obvious cause and solution. Low urine output, for example, is usually safely assumed as originating from a fluid intake too low to produce the target urine volume. Although it may mean compensating for extraordinary dermal, fecal, or other losses, the cause and solution remain the same, the solution being to drink more fluids. Examples of conditions without obvious cause include hyperoxaluria and hypercalciuria, each of which may manifest but for multiple different reasons. If a patient's hyperoxaluria is caused primarily by a suboptimal calcium intake or one that is not timed with meals, then admonishing them to avoid spinach, rhubarb, beets, and chocolate without addressing their calcium intake is not likely to result in reduced urinary oxalate excretion. Similarly, if a patient's hypercalciuria is believed to be caused primarily by acidosis and excessive bone resorption, then the most stringent of sodium restrictions may have little effect and may, as a side effect, reduce the palatability of the patient's diet or their fluid intake.[16]

NUTRITION THERAPY: ASSESSMENT OF RISK

The cause of urolithiasis is multifactorial; nutritional factors are not always relevant. Risk factors associated with urolithiasis include nutritional, physiologic, medical, genetic, pharmacologic, and nonnutritional environmental. These risk factors may exist singly or in concert with one another. Nutritional factors and specific physiologic and medical conditions with nutritional implications are addressed later, after which follows a description of the nutritional implications of commonly assessed urinary risk factors. Calcium and uric acid stones are addressed, although aspects of the specific nutrition therapies presented may apply to patients who form cystine, struvite, or other stones.

Nutritional Risks in the Diet

Assessment of a patient's habitual diet and use of over-the-counter supplements is useful in determining where there may be excesses, deficiencies, or imbalances of nutrients and other food constituents that are not nutrients but that are relevant to kidney stones. Techniques used by a registered dietitian could include a 24-hour diet recall conducted one-on-one with the patient (either with or without the use of nutrient analysis software), a multiple-day diet record kept by the patient and returned to the dietitian for analysis, or a targeted assessment that evaluates the most relevant nutritional factors. In the nutrition assessment, the dietitian considers a combination of general age-specific and gender-specific nutrition guidelines as well as accepted therapeutic nutritional recommendations for certain medical conditions[17] (see next section). The nutrition diagnosis should focus on the nutrition-related cause for or contributor to the patient's risk for urolithiasis. In the case of hyperoxaluria, an example of the nutrition diagnosis is "Increased nutritional lithogenic risk related to suboptimal calcium intake not timed with meals, contributing to low oxalate binding potential in gastrointestinal tract and resulting in hyperoxaluria."

The following may be considered the major nutritional factors that contribute to increased lithogenic risk:

Nutritional factor	Risk
• Low fluid intake	• High urine supersaturation
• Excessive sodium salt intake	• Hypercalciuria, hypocitraturia
• High intake of refined carbohydrates	• Hypercalciuria
• Excessive caffeine or alcohol intake (especially by sensitive patient subpopulations)	• Hypercalciuria, hyperuricosuria (alcohol)
• Overall diet habitually high for potential renal acid load	• Hypercalciuria, hypocitraturia, acid urine
• Excessive supplementation (exceeding physiologic needs or the RDA) of calcium	• Hypercalciuria
• Low fruit/vegetable intake	• Hypocitraturia, acid urine
• Intake of high-oxalate foods, especially with low calcium intake	• Hyperoxaluria

• Suboptimal calcium intake	• Hyperoxaluria
• Excessive intake of some over-the-counter supplements such as vitamin C, and possibly some herbal or plant-derived concentrates (eg, cinnamon, cranberry, turmeric)	• Hyperoxaluria
• Excessive calorie intake resulting in overweight	• Acid urine, hypocitraturia

Aside from single foods or food groups, overall dietary patterns seem to be more or less risk-conferring than others.[18] For example, data confirm that the Atkins diet for weight loss[19] or the ketogenic diet for seizure disorders[20] can both increase risk for stone formation. Disordered eating patterns, by people with pica or other eating disorders, may also result in increased risk for urinary tract stones.[21] Vegetarian diets, despite typically being higher in oxalate, are associated with reduced risk,[22] as was a low-salt, adequate-calcium, moderate-protein diet (not unlike the dietary pattern known as the dietary approaches to stop hypertension [DASH] diet).[12] Recently, specific gastrointestinal microbiotic profiles have been identified, containing discrete combinations of bacterial species, and these seem to be regulated in large part by dietary patterns.[23] For example, people who consume high-fiber diets have a different microbiotic profile than those who do not.[24] Another study showed that people whose diets are rich in meats have a different bacterial enterotype than those whose diets are rich in carbohydrates.[25] As research progresses, it is possible that certain dietary patterns could results in changes in the gut microbiome that could be linked with antilithogenic effects, such as a more favorable concentration of oxalate-degrading bacteria.

Nutritional Risks Related to Specific Physiologic and Medical Factors

Diabetes confers known risks for urinary tract stones.[26] It is not clear whether good control of diabetes with prescribed diabetic nutrition interventions results in reduced stone risk. However, it seems intuitive that appropriate control of insulin and blood glucose through nutrition and pharmacologic therapy would be helpful, especially with the integration of specific nutrition strategies to reduce stone risk factors. Malabsorptive conditions, including Crohn disease, celiac sprue, short bowel, postgastric bypass or duodenal switch, and chronic diarrhea, confer well-known risks for urinary tract stones.[27] Multiple nutritional strategies to attenuate the malabsorptive effects of these conditions may be used that could have antilithogenic effects. Although not a nutritional problem per se, chronic or frequent antibiotic use could reduce gastrointestinal bacteria capable of degrading oxalate.[28] Every course of antibiotics tends to deplete beneficial bacteria, and in the months required to recover these, pathogenic bacteria may grow.[29] Nutritional and supplemental means, such as probiotic foods and supplements and foods rich in prebiotic components, are capable of altering and optimizing gut bacterial profiles; nutrition therapy may thus play an important role in addressing urolithiasis risk in the setting of antibiotic exposure.[23–25]

Nutritional Implications of Urinary Risk Factors

The analysis of a 24-hour urine versus a spot urine collection is necessary to account for diurnal and other rhythmical excretion patterns of various products of metabolism. Multiple analyses over time are most useful in establishing risk and in monitoring changes.[30] Parameters commonly measured and monitored to predict risk of lithogenesis are: calcium, oxalate, uric acid, urine pH, urine volume, phosphate, citrate, magnesium, and supersaturation indices for specific crystalloids. Where cystinuria is suspected or known, cystine is measured. Urinary phytate could be measured, because it is a potent inhibitor of calcium lithogenesis, but it is not currently assessed by major commercial laboratories.[31]

Many of the urinary parameters monitored for stone risk are related to nutritional intake but are not necessarily surrogates for intake. For example, calcium is under tight homeostatic control, and its excretion in urine is not always related to intake.[32] Sulfate, although commonly used as a surrogate for meat intake, may also reflect the intake of soy beans and foods made from soy (eg, tofu, tempeh), because soy is rich in methionine. Frequently, more than 1 parameter in the 24-hour urine collection must be viewed together and, in addition to the nutrition assessment, may provide a good picture of what is going on in the diet.

Other parameters frequently measured in urine may not be risk factors for renal stone formation per se but may (1) contribute indirectly to lithogenesis by altering renal handling of other excretory products, (2) be used for calculation of urine supersaturation, or (3) provide information to corroborate or rule out underlying disorders or nutritional contributors. These parameters include sodium, potassium, sulfate, ammonium, chloride, urine urea nitrogen, and protein catabolic rate (calculated from the product of urine urea nitrogen and a factor accounting for the average nitrogen content of dietary proteins, divided by the patient's body weight). Although this latter group of urine parameters may be useful in estimating nutritional potentiates of stone formation and growth, many may be altered in the setting of underlying disorders, and none are perfect biomarkers for intake; nutritional assessment of the patient's diet is thus imperative.

NUTRITION THERAPY: IN PRACTICE

After assessment of the nutritional intake of the patient, urinary risk factors for urolithiasis are evaluated with respect to their cause and whether or not nutrition intervention is likely to address them. Frequently, multiple risk factors are present in a patient's 24-hour urine analysis. If nutrition therapy to address multiple risk factors is applied, the need to integrate them into a whole diet, addressing any contradictions between recommendations, is important. This strategy includes the need to integrate stone prevention strategies with nutrition strategies that the patient is following for any other health condition.

Hypercalciuria

Assess for nutrition contributors (**Fig. 2**). Sodium, acid load of diet, gastrointestinal and renal calcium handling, and omega-3 fatty acids are addressed.

Sodium

Sodium exerts a potent hypercalciuric influence because of expansion of extracellular volume and competition between sodium and calcium ions in the renal tubule.[33] If dietary sodium seems contributory to hypercalciuria, assess food source(s), focusing not only on notoriously high-sodium foods but also on foods that are not necessarily high in sodium but, when consumed in large quantity, confer a high sodium load (**Table 2**). Foods at the top of the list for sodium content include miso, table salt, canned sauerkraut and tomato sauce, cured ham, and baking soda, all of which provide more than 1000 mg sodium in a single serving.[34] However, these are not necessarily foods that patients might eat every day or in large quantity. On the other hand, foods that are far lower on the sodium content scale

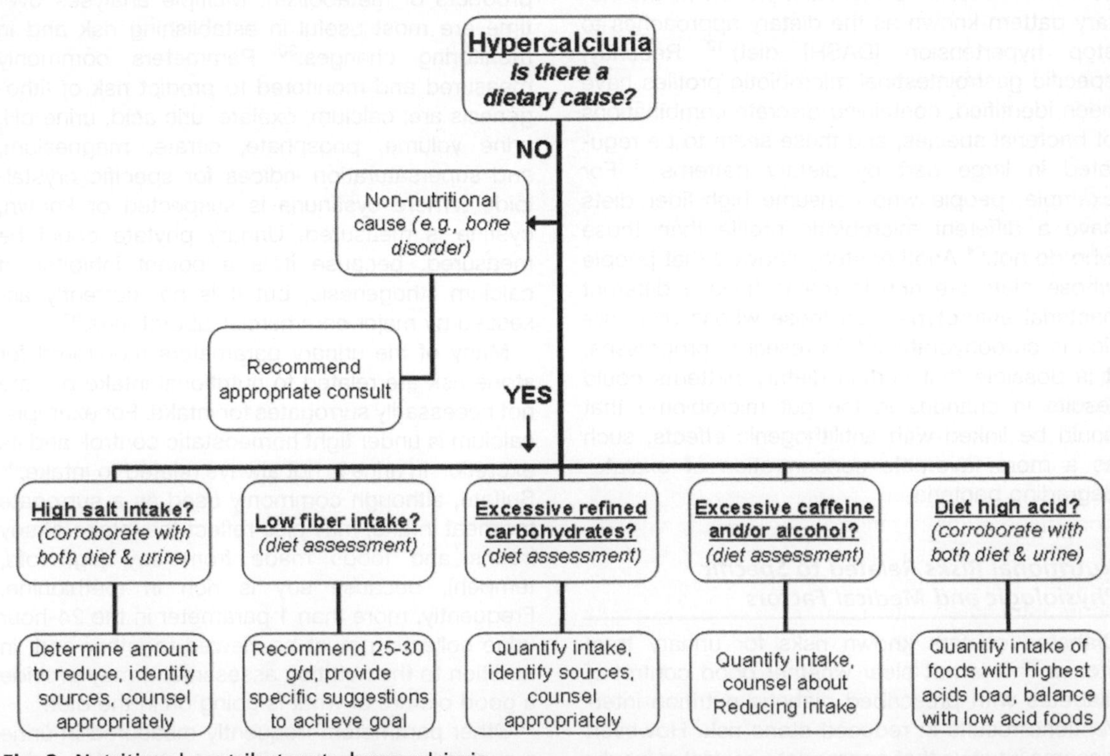

Fig. 2. Nutritional contributors to hypercalciuria.

Table 2
Nutritional sodium sources identified from multiple-day weighed-diet records of stone-forming patients at a stone clinic

Food Group	Contribution to Total Sodium Intake (%)	Cumulative Percentage Toward Total Sodium Intake
Luncheon meats and other processed meats	14	–
Breads and baked goods (bagels, buns, muffins, rolls, tortillas)	14	28
Added salt (NaCl) and spices containing salt	14	42
Canned soups/vegetables and pickled goods	9	51
Salad dressings, condiments, spreads, sauces	8	59
Salty snacks (chips, pretzels, popcorn, candy)	7	73
Homemade casseroles, soups, and other mixed dishes	7	80
Cheese and cheese products	7	66
Pizza and prepared sandwiches (including fast food)	6	86
Meal starters and helpers (eg, pasta and rice mixes)	5	91
Breakfast cereals	5	96
Milk, yogurt, frozen dairy	3	99
Miscellaneous	1	100

Data from Penniston KL, Wojciechowski KF, Nakada SY. The salt shaker provides less than 15% of total sodium intake in stone formers: food strategies to reduce sodium are needed. J Urol 2011;185:e861.

are sometimes items that are eaten daily in high quantity.[35] For example, 5 servings of bread, which is easily achievable with 2 pieces of toast in the morning, a sandwich at lunch, and a roll at dinner, could provide as much or more than 1000 mg sodium. These foods and their intake patterns must be identified when providing nutrition therapy if sodium intake is determined to be a nutritional risk factor.

Acid load of diet

Dietary acid load has a well-known effect on urinary calcium excretion, believed to be caused by reduced renal tubular calcium reabsorption, increased glomerular filtration rate, increased bone mineral mobilization to buffer the acid load, or increased intestinal calcium absorption.[36] To address the acid load of diet if it is a suspected contributor, intervention aims to balance the intake of high-acid foods with low-acid or alkaline foods. A scale has been developed to estimate the potential renal acid load (PRAL) of foods.[37] It accounts for the anion/cation ratio of a food and has been suggested as a reasonable model for estimating the effects of the diet on renal net acid excretion. Foods conferring an acid load caused by the amount of sulfur in their amino acid structure include:

- All foods of flesh origin, including those from land and water
- Cheese, all types
- Eggs, largely from the yolk
- Grains, nearly all types, especially when consumed in high quantity

Milk, yogurt, and fats are neutral on the PRAL scale. Foods conferring an alkaline load (negative numbers on the PRAL scale) include nearly all fruits and vegetables. The few fruits and vegetables that have a slight acid load, and these include cranberries and lentils, need not be restricted, because the magnitude of their acid load is so much lower than that of the high-acid foods so as to be negligible. Moreover, fruits and vegetables are usually recommended to be increased, and the unnecessary restriction of some is a frequent source of frustration and confusion for patients.

Gastrointestinal and renal calcium handling

Reducing the gastrointestinal absorption of calcium in an effort to reduce the renal filtered load could be considered in those who are not at risk for calcium deficiency. Fiber may reduce the amount of gastrointestinal calcium absorbed.[38] If fiber intake is not at recommended levels (25–30 g/d for most adults), and if calcium and bone status seems normal, then it is appropriate to recommend increased fiber intake from foods or in combination with over-the-counter fiber supplements. Because of a high binding affinity, oxalate is also capable of reducing gastrointestinal calcium absorption, and its intake has been correlated inversely with urinary calcium excretion.[39] A high intake of carbohydrates may contribute to hypercalciuria, although it may be a transient effect.[40,41] If nutritional assessment suggests that a high carbohydrate intake is contributory, especially of refined carbohydrates (eg, sweetened beverages and juices, candy, refined grains, and foods made from them), intake should be reduced by suggesting whole-grain alternatives, whole fruits instead of juices, and nonsweetened beverages and foods. Caffeine and alcohol may contribute to urinary calcium excretion, but the need to limit or restrict these compounds should be individually assessed based on the amount typically consumed and on patient preferences.[42,43]

Omega-3 fatty acids

Some reports suggest efficacy of omega-3 fatty acids in reducing urinary calcium excretion,[44–46] and these may be supplemented using commercially available, over-the-counter formulations. However, the dosages required to achieve reduced urinary calcium excretion are unclear.

Hyperoxaluria

Assess for nutrition contributors (**Fig. 3**). Calcium intake, food oxalate, and over-the-counter supplements are addressed.

Calcium intake

If the nutrition assessment reveals a low calcium intake, or one that is not timed with meals, there could be a lack of oxalate-binding potential in the gastrointestinal tract.[47] For most patients, it might be sufficient to recommend consuming something containing around 300 mg of calcium at each meal daily. Assuming 3 meals daily, this figure would provide 900 mg of calcium from calcium-rich foods or beverages alone. Considering that other foods in a generally balanced diet collectively provide, on average, around 300 to 400 mg calcium, there is no need to supplement in this scenario. Special strategies for calcium intake that meets both physiologic needs and enhances binding potential for oxalate must be devised for: (1) patients who are

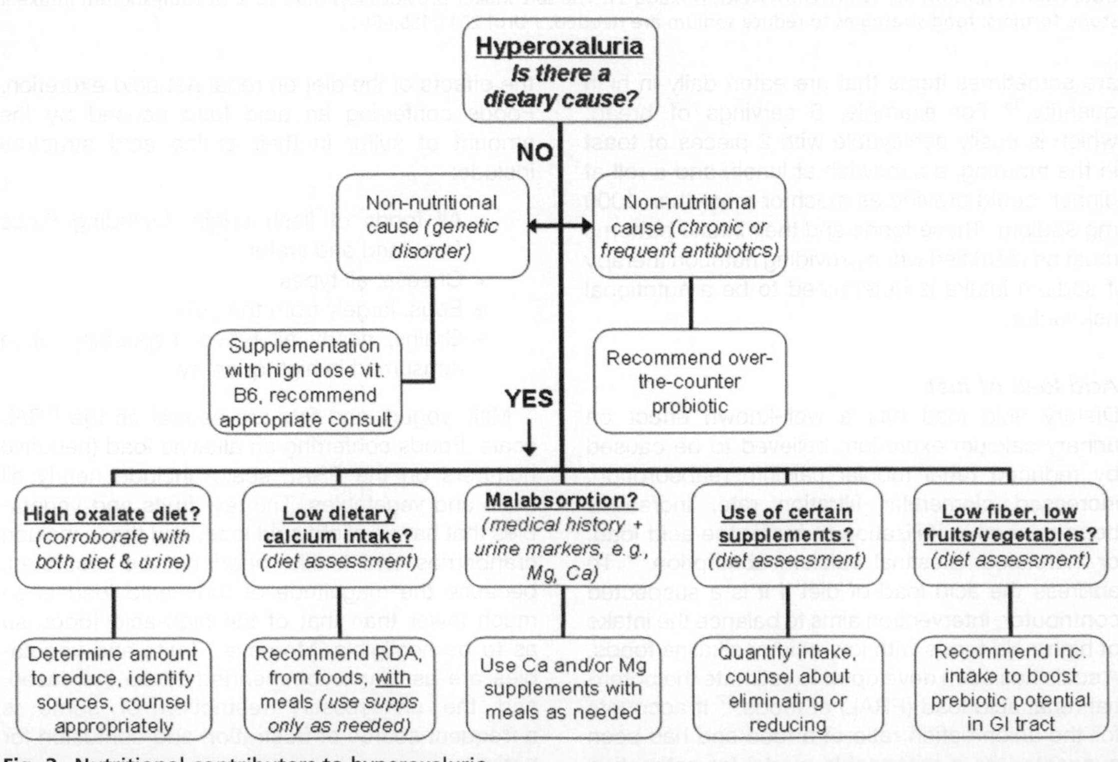

Fig. 3. Nutritional contributors to hyperoxaluria.

lactose intolerant or otherwise do not use dairy foods, which are among those highest in calcium per serving, (2) those who do not eat regular meals daily, (3) those who snack or graze frequently throughout the day instead of eating discrete meals, and (4) those who have altered gut physiology or any other condition resulting in malabsorption, because the extraordinary fecal calcium in these individuals is bound to fatty acids, resulting in less calcium available to bind to oxalate. A combination of foods and supplements, frequently large doses but always timed with meals, is usually required in these cases. Magnesium is also known to bind oxalate in the gut and thereby reduce its absorption[48] and could also be incorporated into nutrition therapy.

Food oxalate

The restriction of food-derived oxalate is controversial. For the most part, foods that contain oxalate are healthy foods and, moreover, are frequently those conferring general health benefits and specific nutrients that are often underconsumed, including fiber, potassium, magnesium, and antioxidants. Elimination or restriction of such foods may do more harm than good, especially if other strategies could be used, such as appropriate calcium (and magnesium) intake timed with meals and snacks. A reduction of dietary oxalate also requires a simultaneous reduction in dietary calcium in order to maintain an appropriately low calcium/oxalate ratio in urine, and some have questioned the value of the low-oxalate strategy for this reason.

The relative bioavailability of oxalate in foods is another topic of interest, because foods high in oxalate might not necessarily be those from which oxalate is readily absorbed.[49] Although more research is needed on the different forms of dietary oxalate, it is assumed that the less water soluble the oxalate, the lower its bioavailability. Thus, restricting high-oxalate foods based on their oxalate concentration without accounting for bioavailability could result in unnecessary restriction. Research to confirm and identify foods with high oxalate bioavailability is needed. Oxalate is a prebiotic for oxalate-degrading bacteria.[50] Although there may be no need for oxalate-degrading bacteria in the gut in a setting of a low oxalate intake, bacteria capable of degrading oxalate may also provide other biological benefits and serve as part of the microbiome required for optimum health status. (**Table 3** provides definitions for and examples of food probiotics and prebiotics.)

Therefore, if dietary oxalate seems contributory to hyperoxaluria, focus not only on foods that are known to be high in oxalate but also on foods that are not necessarily high-oxalate but, when consumed in large quantity, confer a high oxalate load (**Table 4**). Several of the oft-cited high-oxalate foods are not necessarily those that are consumed daily or in high amounts. Rather than focusing on the few pieces of rhubarb pie a patient might have in a year, a better strategy is to identify foods with appreciable oxalate that are eaten habitually and in high amounts. Depending on the individual, these foods might include chocolate, nuts and seeds, spinach, potatoes, and potato chips. In addition, because whole grains are frequently ample for oxalate but not necessarily identified as high in oxalate, and because grains are frequently eaten multiple times in a day, these can be a source for oxalate (see **Table 4**).[51] Discretion in recommending reduced oxalate intake must be used and individual plans developed for patients who rely on nuts and seeds as a protein source or as a low-carbohydrate snack and for those who are vegetarian and who enjoy ample fruits, vegetables, and whole grains. Recommendations to avoid all oxalate in these situations might reduce the nutritional quality and diversity of the diet, not to mention risking diminished compliance.

Over-the-counter supplements

Over-the-counter supplements have been implicated in increased urinary oxalate excretion, and these include cinnamon, turmeric,[52] and cranberry.[53] Others are associated with reduced oxalate excretion, and these include omega-3 fatty acids[46,54] and pyridoxine (vitamin B_6).[44] The dosages required to achieve reduced urinary oxalate excretion with omega-3 fatty acids are unclear and its success in practice is not well characterized. Similarly, although supraphysiologic supplementation with pyridoxine is used in patients with primary hyperoxaluria to address enzyme deficiencies, its effectiveness and practice in patients with idiopathic or enteric hyperoxaluria are not well characterized.

Hyperuricosuria

Assess for nutrition contributors. Purine intake, alcohol and fructose, and acid load of diet are addressed.

Purine intake

Some foods that are rich in nucleoproteins known as purines may contribute to hyperuricosuria, because uric acid is an end-product of purine metabolism.[55] The average daily intake of purines seems to range between 500 and 1500 mg.[56] Virtually all foods have some purines, but those

Table 3
Definitions for and examples of probiotics and prebiotics

Definition	Mechanism	Examples	Food Sources
Probiotics			
Live, nonpathogenic microorganisms in the gastrointestinal tract that confer a health benefit on the host when administered in adequate amounts	Effects are strain specific (not species or genus specific) and include immune modulation, production of antimicrobial compounds, and maintenance of gut integrity and function	Certain variants of: Lactobacilli Bifidobacteria Streptococci Bacilli Yeasts	Cultured yogurts and fermented dairy products, aged cheeses, some nondairy products (eg, soy milk), fermented foods, over-the-counter supplements, chewing gum, lozenges, infant formulas
Prebiotics			
Nondigestible food component or ingredient that beneficially affects the host through effects on the microbiome	Must reach the large intestine intact, where overall effect is to selectively stimulate growth or activity of 1 or a limited number of bacteria or to directly stimulate immunity, protect against pathogens, and facilitate host metabolism and mineral absorption	Certain nondigestible carbohydrates, including: Inulin Various oligosaccharides Pyrodextrins Fructan Lactulose Lactitol	Fruits (especially bananas, berries, kiwi), vegetables (especially onions, garlic, leeks, artichokes), whole grains (especially oats, barley), and whole-grain foods, honey, over-the-counter supplements, powders, commercial extraction of chicory root, fortified foods

Data from Saulnier DM, Spinler JK, Gibson GR, et al. Mechanisms of probiosis and prebiosis: considerations for enhanced functional foods. Curr Opin Biotechnol 2009;20:135–41; and Figueroa-Gonzalez I, Quijano G, Ramirez G, et al. Probiotics and prebiotics–perspectives and challenges. J Sci Food Agric 2011;91:1341–8.

most concentrated (providing up to 1000 mg per serving of 85–113 g [3–4 ounces]) include anchovies, sardines, organ meats (eg, brain, liver, kidney), and glandular tissue, commonly referred to as sweetbreads. Appreciable amounts of purines, up to 100 mg per serving of 85 g to 113 g (3–4 ounces), are provided by shellfish, game meats, water fowl, mutton, beef, pork, poultry, and fish.[57] As with other nutrition recommendations, the patient who does not typically eat purine-rich foods does not benefit from advice to limit or eliminate them from their diet. If nutrition assessment documents a high intake of purine-rich foods, education about lowering dietary purines is appropriate. Avoiding the foods highest in purine concentration and reducing recurrent intake of those with lower concentrations would be recommended. Foods of plant and dairy origins contain purines, but the impact of these on uric acid synthesis is different. A recent study in men with gout concluded that vegetable-derived purines did not increase risk and dairy foods lowered risk.[58] Thus, patients are unlikely to benefit from avoiding plant and dairy foods that contain purines because they might compromise their vegetable intake, calcium intake, and the diversity of their overall diet.

Another potential concern is the tendency to refer only to red meat as the major culprit with respect to uric acid synthesis. Recently, fish and chicken were reported to increase both serum and urine uric acid to the same degree as or higher than red meat.[59] Recommending reduced red meat intake may cause the patient with hyperuricosuria to substitute with more chicken and fish, when a reduction of all of these foods may be necessary to achieve favorable results. The amount of reduction should be individually titrated based on the current amount of these foods the patient eats. Reduction could occur with reduced portion sizes, reduced frequency of intake throughout the week, or both. Patients usually

Table 4
Nutritional oxalate sources identified from multiple-day weighed-diet records of stone-forming patients at a stone clinic

Food Group	Contribution to Total Oxalate Intake (%)	Cumulative Percentage Toward Total Oxalate Intake
Nuts, seeds, nut butters	26	–
Spinach	12	38
Breads, flours, baked goods	12	50
Cereals	7	57
Potatoes (includes sweet potatoes), French fries	7	64
Leafy vegetables, nonspinach	6	70
Mixed dishes, casseroles, meats	6	76
Nonleafy vegetables	5	81
Chips, crackers	5	86
Chocolate	5	91
Soymilk, kefir, cheese	4	95
Tea, spices	2	97
Fruit	2	99
Pasta, rice	1	100

Data from Penniston KL, Wojciechowski KF, Nakada SY. Dietary oxalate: what's important and what isn't for patients with calcium oxalate stones? J Urol 2011;185:e824–5.

require assistance conceiving of alternate means for obtaining protein, especially if their protein intake is compromised by compliance with the recommendation.

Alcohol and fructose

Alcohol is a contributor to uric acid biosynthesis, because it enhances purine degradation and increases xanthine oxidase expression, which is the enzyme that catalyzes the final step in uric acid production.[60] Fructose, a monosaccharide found naturally in sucrose (table sugar) and fruits and also used ubiquitously in food manufacture and production as a sweetener, has also been suggested to increase serum uric acid and potentially urinary uric acid excretion.[61,62] The nutrition assessment should quantify the intake of both alcohol and fructose in the patient with hyperuricosuria and discuss ways to reduce intake if it is believed to be contributing to stone risk.

Acid load of diet

Although not a contributor to uric acid biosynthesis and the urinary excretion of uric acid, the acid load of the diet can reduce urine pH such that urinary uric acid is less soluble. Refer to elsewhere in the text for addressing and correcting acid load of diet if the nutrition assessment identifies it as a risk factor.

Hypocitraturia

Assess for nutrition contributors (**Fig. 4**). The acid load of the diet, dietary citrate, chronic or frequent diarrhea, and sodium are addressed.

Acid load of diet

If the diet is assessed as high for acid load, which exerts a hypocitraturic effect because of enhanced renal citrate reabsorption,[63] reducing the acid load with smaller amounts of cheese, meats, and other flesh foods would be advised.[37] Specific strategies to achieve this goal could be tailored to patients' needs. For example, for the patient unable or unwilling to give up meat or some other flesh food at both lunch and dinner, a specific recommendation for smaller portions at each of these meals could have the same effect as eating those foods at only 1 meal of the day. If a patient's calorie load is not a concern, simply balancing their present intake of high-acid foods with an appropriate quantity of low-acid or alkaline foods (ie, most fruits and vegetables) could be suggested.

Dietary citrate

Although citric acid does not fit the definition for a nutrient and thus does not have a recommended intake or RDA, increased intake from foods and beverages may enhance urinary citrate excretion.[64–67] This goal could be achieved with specific

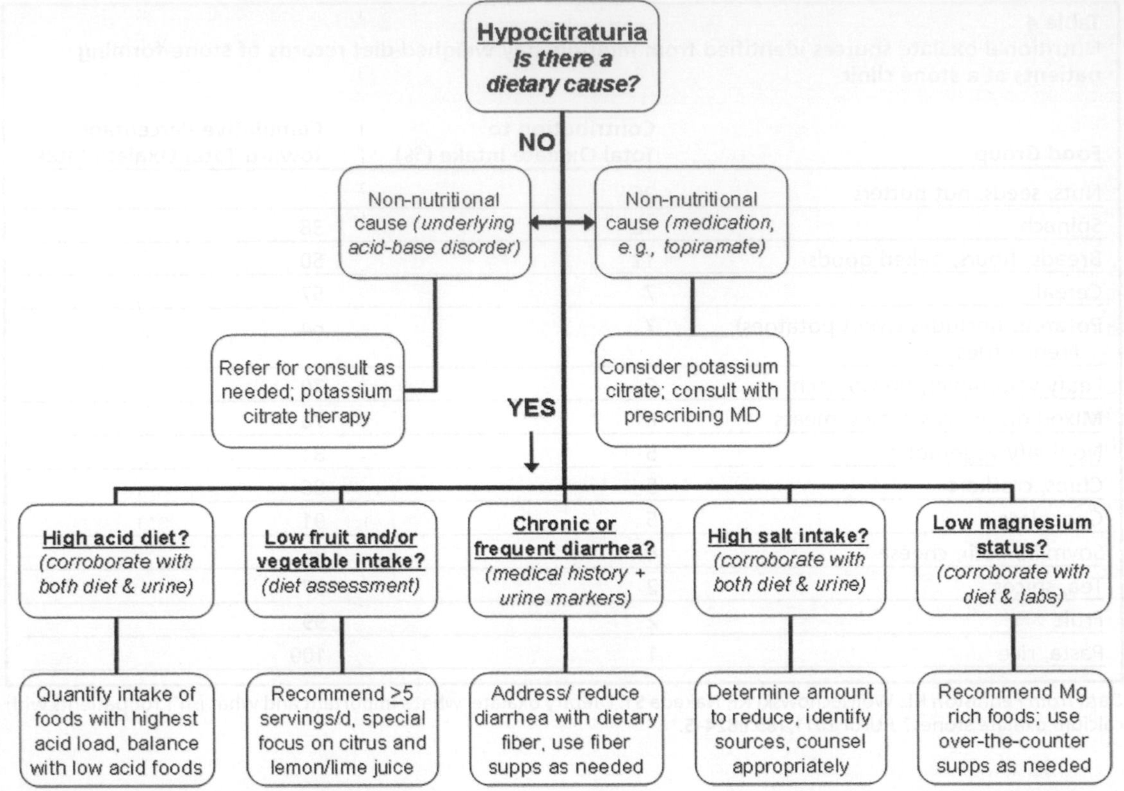

Fig. 4. Nutritional contributors to hypocitraturia.

recommendations about using lemon or lime juice, which are particularly concentrated with citric acid, diluted in water or another beverage to prevent degeneration of tooth enamel. Recommendations to use commercially available, ready-to-consume lemonade preparations, especially if they are not sugar-free, are rarely if ever indicated, because they contain a minimal amount of lemon juice and provide ample carbohydrates and food calories. Recommendations for increased citrus fruit intake might be incorporated and would provide beneficial nutrients as well, such as fiber, potassium, antioxidants, and prebiotics.

Recently, low-sugar, low-calorie beverage drinks flavored with citrate and other organic acids were suggested as agents capable of enhancing urinary citrate.[68] Depending on the urinary citrate level targeted as therapeutic for an individual patient, specific volumes of these beverages could be recommended and may also have a side benefit of increasing overall fluid intake. However, the ability of diet-derived citrate to fully correct severe hypocitraturia is questionable, but this may depend on the magnitude of the patient's hypocitraturia and on other nutritional and physiologic factors.

Chronic or frequent diarrhea

If frequent diarrhea is believed to be contributory to hypocitraturia, because of excessive bicarbonate losses in stool resulting in enhanced renal citrate reabsorption, nutrition strategies to correct diarrhea can be used.[69] Increased dietary fiber, with a specific focus on insoluble versus soluble as determined by the specific situation, could be recommended and specific strategies provided to achieve the goal. Over-the-counter fiber supplements, of which there are multiple varieties, may be beneficial in addressing and stemming diarrhea, and this could result in correction of hypocitraturia.[70] A growing body of literature supports probiotic supplementation for correcting diarrhea, and multiple probiotic formulations are commercially available and could be tried.[71,72]

Sodium

If a high sodium salt intake is considered contributory to hypocitraturia, refer to the section on sodium under hypercalciuria earlier in the text.[73]

Low Fluid Intake

Fluids of any kind help promote urine output and may be the single most useful way to reduce recurrence risk.[5] Low-sugar, low-calorie beverages are most desired, but it is acceptable to count other beverages toward one's fluid intake; a diversity of different fluids, most of which are noncaloric, should be encouraged.

Fluid intake may be considered low when urine output does not meet the target volume. It may help to explain to a patient that they may require more fluids than another patient to produce a target amount of urine given variable extrarenal fluid losses between individuals depending on such factors as how much a person sweats or how much they lose in stool. It may also be helpful to identify the day of the week that the person carried out the 24-hour urine collection on which the assessment of low urine volume is made. Some people have ample fluid intakes during the workweek, when they are eating and drinking in more or less a similar pattern, and may even be conscious of drinking a certain volume of fluids, but on a weekend or nonwork day, schedules and dietary patterns are frequently different. Knowledge of how a patient drinks throughout the week, accounting for workday versus nonworkday differences, helps to address specific days when fluid intake is suboptimal.

Some patients benefit from more specific advice than to simply increase fluid intake. In these situations, a fluid intake schedule can be devised. By breaking the day into 3 equal sections (eg, of 5 hours each depending on the patient's lifestyle), with advice to drink about 1200 mL of fluids in each section, a person could consume approximately 4 L (120 ounces) of fluids. It may be helpful to ask the patient to use a fluid container with visible volume measurements to make meeting the specific goal easier. Carrying a fluid container was identified as an important cue to action in a recent analysis of factors influencing fluid intake in stone formers.[74] As necessary, fluid recommendations should compensate for excessive dermal or fecal losses, and patients may need to be educated as appropriate to their lifestyle and comorbid conditions.

Those at particular risk for low fluid intake for other reasons may require special attention. These at-risk groups include those with occupations requiring self-censorship of fluid intake because of lack of access for long periods to restrooms[75] (eg, truck drivers, elementary school teachers, airplane pilots) and those who live or work in hot conditions. Recently, armed services personnel stationed and working in a desert environment had low urine output despite intakes of fluids exceeding 17 L per day.[76] Individuals with urinary incontinence may limit their fluid intake in an effort to avoid publicly embarrassing situations. In these situations, fluid goals and fluid intake schedules should be amended on a patient-by-patient basis. In the case of urinary incontinence, special attention in developing a plan may be required with respect to patients' emotional concerns and quality of life. There are a growing number of community-based or hospital-based urinary incontinence support groups, and providing information about these to the patient may be helpful. Collaboration with a health psychologist who could work with the patient to identify ways to achieve fluid goals might also be useful in this situation.

Hyperphosphaturia

As with calcium, urinary phosphorus excretion is not always related to nutritional intake because it is subject to homeostatic regulation involving parathyroid hormone, vitamin D, bone status, calcium status, and renal reabsorptive mechanisms.[77] Phosphorus is widely distributed in foods of both plant and animal origin. Patients with chronic kidney disease and whose circulating phosphorus concentrations are increased are managed multifactorially to reduce serum phosphorus, and this may include dietary restriction. However, the reduction of dietary phosphorus in stone formers to reduce risk for calcium phosphate stone formation is not widely practiced. In these patients, the control of urinary citrate, calcium, urine pH, and volume are of most importance.

Overweight/obesity are associated independently with increased risk for lithogenesis.[78] Because both are conditions of malnutrition, with or without concomitant genetic or metabolic contributors, nutrition therapy should address weight loss. Nutrition interventions can be highly successful in motivated individuals, and patients should be referred as needed to nutritionists with expertise and experience in weight-loss counseling.[79]

SUMMARY

A tailored nutritional approach, targeted to patients' lithogenic risk factors, is recommended. There are some risk factors, observed in the 24-hour urine analysis, for example, which may not have a nutritional input and may not therefore be amenable to nutrition intervention. In part because of the complexity of studying nutrition and disease, evidence from appropriately designed studies may be lacking; yet nutrition therapy for kidney stone prevention is widely practiced. This article synthesizes best practice scenarios, most of which are evidence-based, for successful nutrition therapy against stone recurrence. An important concept stressed throughout is the need to

determine the cause of the observed risk factor(s) and to apply nutrition therapy accordingly.

REFERENCES

1. Food and Nutrition Board, Institute of Medicine. Dietary reference intakes: applications in dietary assessment. Washington, DC: National Academies Press; Available at: http://www.iom.edu/. Accessed July 29, 2012.
2. US Department of Agriculture, US Department of Health and Human Services. Dietary guidelines for Americans. 7th edition. Washington, DC: US Government Printing Office; 2010. Available at: http://www.health.gov. Accessed July 29, 2012.
3. Smith RE, Patrick S, Michael P, et al. Medical nutrition therapy: the core of ADA's advocacy efforts (part 1). J Am Diet Assoc 2005;105:825–34.
4. Jones DP, Park Y, Ziegler TR. Nutritional metabolomics: progress in addressing complexity in diet and health. Annu Rev Nutr 2012;32:183–202.
5. Borghi L, Meschi T, Amato F, et al. Urinary volume, water and recurrence in idiopathic calcium nephrolithiasis: a 5-year randomized prospective study. J Urol 1996;155:839–43.
6. Sarica K, Inal Y, Erturhan S, et al. The effect of calcium channel blockers on stone regrowth and recurrence after shock wave lithotripsy. Urol Res 2006;34:184–9.
7. Di Silverio F, Ricciuti GP, D'Angelo AR, et al. Stone recurrence after lithotripsy in patients with recurrent idiopathic calcium urolithiasis: efficacy of treatment with Fiuggi water. Eur Urol 2000;37:145–8.
8. Shuster J, Jenkins A, Logan C, et al. Soft drink consumption and urinary stone recurrence: a randomized prevention trial. J Clin Epidemiol 1992;45:911–6.
9. Dussol B, Iovanna C, Rotily M, et al. A randomized trial of low-animal-protein or high-fiber diets for secondary prevention of calcium nephrolithiasis. Nephron 2008;110:185–94.
10. Hiatt RA, Ettinger B, Caan B, et al. Randomized controlled trial of a low animal protein, high fiber diet in the prevention of recurrent calcium oxalate kidney stones. Am J Epidemiol 1996;144:25–33.
11. Borghi L, Schianchi T, Meschi T, et al. Comparison of two diets for the prevention of recurrent stones in idiopathic hypercalciuria. N Engl J Med 2002;346:77–84.
12. Kocvara R, Plasqura P, Petrik A, et al. A prospective study of nonmedical prophylaxis after a first kidney stone. BJU Int 1999;84:393–8.
13. Fink HA, Akornor JW, Garimella PS, et al. Diet, fluid, or supplements for secondary prevention of nephrolithiasis: a systematic review and meta-analysis of randomized trials. Eur Urol 2009;56:72–80.
14. Spahn JM, Reeves RS, Keim KS, et al. State of the evidence regarding behavior change theories and strategies in nutrition counseling to facilitate health and food behavior change. J Am Diet Assoc 2010;110:879–91.
15. Fappa E, Yannakoulia M, Pitsavos C, et al. Lifestyle intervention in the management of metabolic syndrome: could we improve adherence issues? Nutrition 2008;24:286–91.
16. Stoller ML, Chi T, Eisner BH, et al. Changes in urinary stone risk factors in hypocitraturia calcium oxalate stone formers treated with dietary sodium supplementation. J Urol 2009;181:1140–4.
17. Hampl JS, Anderson JV, Mullis R, et al. Position of the American Dietetic Association: the role of dietetics professionals in health promotion and disease prevention. J Am Diet Assoc 2002;102:1680–7.
18. Meschi T, Nouvenne A, Borghi L. Lifestyle recommendations to reduce the risk of kidney stones. Urol Clin North Am 2011;38:313–20.
19. Reddy ST, Wang CY, Sakhaee K, et al. Effect of low-carbohydrate high-protein diets on acid base balance, stone-forming propensity, and calcium metabolism. Am J Kidney Dis 2002;40:265–74.
20. Kielb S, Koo HP, Bloom DA, et al. Nephrolithiasis associated with the ketogenic diet. J Urol 2000;164:464–6.
21. Leaf DE, Bukberg PR, Goldfarb DS. Laxative abuse, eating disorders, and kidney stones: a case report and review of the literature. Am J Kidney Dis 2012;60:295–8.
22. Robertson WG, Peacock M, Marshall DH. Prevalence of urinary stone disease in vegetarians. Eur Urol 1982;8:334–9.
23. Arumugam M, Raes J, Pelletier E, et al. Enterotypes of the human gut microbiome. Nature 2011;473:174–80.
24. Claesson MJ, Jeffery IB, Conde S, et al. Gut microbiota composition correlates with diet and health in the elderly. Nature 2012. http://dx.doi.org/10.1038/nature11319. [Epub ahead of print].
25. Wu GD, Chen J, Hoffmann C, et al. Linking long-term dietary patterns with gut microbial enterotypes. Science 2011;334:105–8.
26. Bell DS. Beware the low urine pH–the major cause of the increased prevalence of nephrolithiasis in the patient with type 2 diabetes. Diabetes Obes Metab 2012;14(4):299–303.
27. Worcester EM. Stones from bowel disease. Endocrinol Metab Clin North Am 2002;31:979–99.
28. Siva S, Barrack ER, Reddy GP, et al. A critical analysis of the role of gut *Oxalobacter formigenes* in oxalate stone disease. BJU Int 2009;103:18–21.
29. Dethlefsen L, Huse S, Sogin ML, et al. The pervasive effects of an antibiotic on the human gut microbiota, as revealed by deep 16S rRNA sequencing. PLoS Biol 2008;6:e280.

30. Parks JH, Goldfisher E, Asplin JR, et al. A single 24-hour urine collection is inadequate for the medical evaluation of nephrolithiasis. J Urol 2002; 167:1607–12.
31. Grases F, Isern B, Sanchis P, et al. Phytate acts as an inhibitor in formation of renal calculi. Front Biosci 2007;12:2580–7.
32. Worcester EM, Coe FL. New insights into the pathogenesis of idiopathic hypercalciuria. Semin Nephrol 2008;28:120–32.
33. Sakhaee K, Harvey JA, Padalino PK, et al. The potential role of salt abuse on the risk for kidney stone formation. J Urol 1993;150:310–2.
34. United States Department of Agriculture, Agricultural Research Service. USDA national nutrient database for standard reference, release 24. Nutrient data laboratory home page. 2011. Available at: http://www.ars.usda.gov/ba/bhnrc/ndl. Accessed July 29, 2012.
35. Penniston KL, Wojciechowski KF, Nakada SY. The salt shaker provides less than 15% of total sodium intake in stone formers: food strategies to reduce sodium are needed. J Urol 2011;185:e861.
36. Remer T. Influence of diet on acid-base balance. Semin Dial 2000;13:221–6.
37. Remer T, Manz F. Potential renal acid load of foods and its influence on urine pH. J Am Diet Assoc 1995;95:791–7.
38. Jahnen A, Heynck H, Gertz B, et al. Dietary fibre: the effectiveness of a high bran intake in reducing renal calcium excretion. Urol Res 1992;20:3–6.
39. Penniston KL, Jones AN, Nakada SY, et al. Vitamin D repletion does not alter urinary calcium excretion in healthy postmenopausal women. BJU Int 2009; 104:1512–6.
40. Iguchi M, Umekawa T, Takamura C, et al. Glucose metabolism in renal stone patients. Urol Int 1993; 51:185–90.
41. Garg A, Bonanome A, Grundy SM, et al. Effects of dietary carbohydrates on metabolism of calcium and other minerals in normal subjects and patients with noninsulin-dependent diabetes mellitus. J Clin Endocrinol Metab 1990;70:1007–13.
42. Weaver CM, Rothwell AP, Wood KV. Measuring calcium absorption and utilization in humans. Curr Opin Clin Nutr Metab Care 2006;9:568–74.
43. Siener R, Schade N, Niccolay C, et al. The efficacy of dietary intervention on urinary risk factors for stone formation in recurrent calcium oxalate stone patients. J Urol 2005;173:1601–5.
44. Ortiz-Alvarado O, Miyaoka R, Kriedberg C, et al. Pyridoxine and dietary counseling for the management of idiopathic hyperoxaluria in stone-forming patients. Urology 2011;77:1054–8.
45. Yasui T, Tanaka H, Fujita K, et al. Effects of eicosapentaenoic acid on urinary calcium excretion in calcium stone formers. Eur Urol 2001;39:580–5.
46. Buck AC, Davies RL, Harrison T. The protective role of eicosapentaenoic acid (EPA) in the pathogenesis of nephrolithiasis. J Urol 1992;146:188–94.
47. Hess B, Jost C, Zipperle L, et al. High-calcium intake abolishes hyperoxaluria and reduced urinary crystallization during a 20-fold normal oxalate load in humans. Nephrol Dial Transplant 1998;13:2241–7.
48. Zimmermann DJ, Voss S, von Unruh GE, et al. Importance of magnesium in absorption and excretion of oxalate. Urol Int 2005;74:262–7.
49. Massey LK. Food oxalate: factors affecting measurement, biological variation, and bioavailability. J Am Diet Assoc 2007;107:1191–4.
50. Yadav S, Gite S, Nilegaonkar S, et al. Effect of supplementation of micronutrients and phytochemicals to fructooligosaccharides on growth response of probiotics and *E. coli*. Biofactors 2011;37:58–64.
51. Penniston KL, Wojciechowski KF, Nakada SY. Dietary oxalate: what's important and what isn't for patients with calcium oxalate stones? J Urol 2011; 185:e824–5.
52. Tang M, Larson-Meyer DE, Liebman M. Effect of cinnamon and turmeric on urinary oxalate excretion, plasma lipids, and plasma glucose in healthy subjects. Am J Clin Nutr 2008;87:1262–7.
53. Terris MK, Issa MM, Tacker JR. Dietary supplementation with cranberry concentrate tablets may increase the risk of nephrolithiasis. Urology 2001;57:26–9.
54. Ortiz-Alvarado O, Miyaoka R, Kriedberg C, et al. Omega-3 fatty acids eicosapentaenoic acid and docosahexaenoic acid in the management of hypercalciuric stone formers. Urology 2012;79:282–6.
55. Moran ME. Uric acid stone disease. Front Biosci 2003;8:s1339–55.
56. Zhang Y, Chen C, Choi H, et al. Purine-rich foods intake and recurrent gout attacks. Ann Rheum Dis 2012;71(9):1448–53.
57. de Oliveira EP, Burini RC. High plasma uric acid concentration: causes and consequences. Diabetol Metab Syndr 2012;4:12.
58. Choi HK, Atkinson K, Karlson EW, et al. Purine-rich foods, dairy and protein intake, and the risk of gout in men. N Engl J Med 2004;350:1093–103.
59. Best S, Tracy C, Bagrodia A, et al. Effect of various animal protein sources on urinary stone risk factors. J Urol 2011;185:e859–60.
60. Yamamoto T, Moriwaki Y, Takahashi S. Effect of ethanol on metabolism of purine bases (hypoxanthine, xanthine, and uric acid). Clin Chim Acta 2005;356:35–57.
61. Lanaspa MA, Tapia E, Soto V, et al. Uric acid and fructose: potential biological mechanisms. Semin Nephrol 2011;31:426–32.
62. Taylor EN, Curhan GC. Fructose consumption and the risk of kidney stones. Kidney Int 2008;73:207–12.
63. Adeva MM, Souto G. Diet-induced metabolic acidosis. Clin Nutr 2011;30:416–21.

64. Seltzer MA, Low RD, McDonald M, et al. Dietary manipulation with lemonade to treat hypocitraturic calcium nephrolithiasis. J Urol 1996;156:907–9.
65. Kang DE, Sur RL, Haleblian GE, et al. Long-term lemonade based dietary manipulation in patients with hypocitraturic nephrolithiasis. J Urol 2007;144: 1358–62.
66. Penniston KL, Steele TH, Nakada SY. Lemonade therapy increases urinary citrate and urine volumes in patients with recurrent calcium oxalate stone formation. Urology 2007;70:856–60.
67. Yilmaz E, Batislam E, Kacmaz M, et al. Citrate, oxalate, sodium, and magnesium levels in fresh juices of three different types of tomatoes: evaluation in the light of the results of studies on orange and lemon juices. Int J Food Sci Nutr 2010;61:339–45.
68. Eisner BH, Asplin JR, Goldfarb DS, et al. Citrate, malate and alkali content in commonly consumed diet sodas: implications for nephrolithiasis treatment. J Urol 2010;183:2419–23.
69. Shenoy C. Hypocitraturia despite potassium citrate tablet supplementation. MedGenMed 2006;8:8.
70. Parisi GC, Zilli M, Miani MP, et al. High-fiber diet supplementation in patients with irritable bowel syndrome (IBS): a multicenter, randomized, open trial comparison between wheat bran diet and partially hydrolyzed guar gum (PHGG). Dig Dis Sci 2002;47:1697–704.
71. Cui S, Hu Y. Multistrain probiotic preparation significantly reduces symptoms of irritable bowel syndrome in a double-blind placebo-controlled study. Int J Clin Exp Med 2012;5:238–44.
72. Ringel Y, Ringel-Kulka T. The rationale and clinical effectiveness of probiotics in irritable bowel syndrome. J Clin Gastroenterol 2011;45:S145–8.
73. Martini LA, Cuppari L, Cunha MA, et al. Potassium and sodium intake and excretion in calcium stone forming patients. J Ren Nutr 1998;8:127–31.
74. McCauley LR, Dyer AJ, Stern K, et al. Factors influencing fluid intake behavior among kidney stone formers. J Urol 2012;187:1282–6.
75. Borghi L, Meschi T, Amato F, et al. Hot occupation and nephrolithiasis. J Urol 1993;150:1757–60.
76. Masterson JH, Jourdain V, Choe C, et al. 24 hour urine collections of men from a temperate climate exposed to a desert environment for one month. J Urol 2012;187:e905.
77. Yucha C, Dungan J. Renal handling of phosphorus and magnesium. Nephrol Nurs J 2004;31:33–7.
78. Obligado SH, Goldfarb DS. The association of nephrolithiasis with hypertension and obesity: a review. Am J Hypertens 2008;21:257–64.
79. Raatz SK, Wimmer JK, Kwong CA, et al. Intensive diet instruction by registered dietitians improves weight-loss success. J Am Diet Assoc 2008;108: 110–3.

Imaging Techniques for Stone Disease and Methods for Reducing Radiation Exposure

Michael E. Lipkin, MD*, Glenn M. Preminger, MD

KEYWORDS

• Imaging • Nephrolithiasis • Computed tomography • Ultrasound • Radiation

KEY POINTS

- Imaging is a key component in the evaluation and management of patients with urolithiasis.
- Non-contrast computed tomography is considered the first line imaging study for the diagnosis of urolithiasis and provides critical information for operative planning.
- Beyond diagnosis, imaging provides important information that allows urologists to determine the most appropriate treatment modality for the patient. This information includes the size, location, and in some cases composition of stones.

INTRODUCTION

Imaging is a key component in the evaluation and management of patients with urolithiasis. Imaging allows for the rapid and definitive diagnosis of stones. Beyond diagnosis, imaging provides important information that allows urologists to determine the most appropriate treatment modality for the patient. This information includes the size, location, and, in some cases, composition of stones.

Historically, plain abdominal radiography (KUB) and excretory radiography (IVP) have been considered the studies of choice for the evaluation of patients with stones. These modalities have been largely supplanted by noncontrast computed tomography of the abdomen and pelvis (NCCT). Ultrasound has also been used in place of traditional radiography. Magnetic resonance imaging (MRI) has a limited role in the evaluation of patients with suspected urolithiasis.

Patients with urolithiasis are at risk for significant radiation exposure from imaging studies. Most of the radiation comes from NCCT. Plain radiography also exposes stone patients to radiation. Once diagnosed with a stone, a significant number of patients will undergo surgical intervention. Fluoroscopy used during shock wave lithotripsy (SWL), ureteroscopy (URS), and percutaneous nephrolithotomy (PNL) contributes to the overall radiation exposure of patients with urolithiasis.

This article reviews currently available imaging modalities for the evaluation of urolithiasis. Methods to reduce radiation exposure to patients with stones are discussed as well.

Computed Tomography

Evaluation of renal colic

NCCT was first reported for the evaluation of urinary stones in the late 1970s.[1,2] The initial indication for NCCT in the workup of urolithiasis was in diagnosing radiolucent stones.[1–3] It was eventually demonstrated that NCCT had improved sensitivity for diagnosing ureteral stones in patients with flank pain compared with IVP.[4] NCCT can be rapidly performed and does not require intravenous contrast. Unlike IVP, NCCT can identify stones of any composition, with the exception of stones formed by protease inhibitors, such as indinavir, which may not be visible on NCCT.[5]

Currently, NCCT is considered the first-line imaging study for the evaluation of the patient with acute flank pain and a suspected stone.[6]

Department of Urology, Duke University Medical Center, DUMC 3167, Durham, NC 27710, USA
* Corresponding author.
E-mail address: michael.lipkin@duke.edu

Urol Clin N Am 40 (2013) 47–57
http://dx.doi.org/10.1016/j.ucl.2012.09.008

NCCT has a reported sensitivity of 95% to 98% and specificity of 96% to 98% for the diagnosis of a ureteral stone in a patient with acute flank pain (**Table 1**).[7–9] Besides identifying the stone, NCCT allows for the evaluation of the signs of obstruction associated with ureteral stones. In patients with ureteral stones, NCCT was able to identify hydroureter in 82.7% of cases, hydronephrosis in 80% of cases, periureteric edema in 59% of cases, and unilateral renal enlargement in 57.2% of cases.[10]

When evaluating patients with acute flank pain, NCCT also has the ability to evaluate the rest of the abdominal and pelvic organs and possibly identify other causes of pain. In a series of 1000 consecutive NCCT performed for the evaluation of renal colic, an alternative diagnosis was made in 10.1% of the cases.[11] In another report reviewing the results of 1500 NCCT performed for the evaluation of flank pain with a suspected stone, 24% of the patients had an alternative CT finding without a urinary calculus.[12] In additional, another 7% had a completely negative CT. A urinary stone was identified in 69% of the patients, and of those patients with a stone, an additional pathologic condition was found in 47%.

Preoperative evaluation

Beyond the diagnosis of stones, NCCT is useful in the preoperative planning for the treatment of stones. Stone size and location are easily evaluated with NCCT. When planning SWL, the skin-to-stone distance can be determined on preoperative NCCT. This has been demonstrated to be an independent predictor of successful treatment with SWL.[13–16] A skin-to-stone distance greater than or equal to 11 cm has been associated with worse stone-free outcomes for SWL when compared with skin-to-stone distances less than 11 cm.[14,15] Prone NCCT can be useful for the preoperative evaluation for planning prone percutaneous nephrolithotomy (PNL). Prone NCCT can determine the anatomic relations of adjacent organs and the pleura with upper pole calyces.[17,18] This information can help determine the feasibility and risk of complication of an upper pole puncture during prone PNL.

Stone composition

Determining the stone composition preoperatively can also aide in deciding the best surgical modality to treat the stone. NCCT can provide information to aide in the determination of different stone types. Hounsfield units or CT attenuation has been frequently used to help identify stone composition.[19] Harder stone types typically have higher attenuations. Calcium oxalate and brushite stones have been shown to have the highest CT attenuations, averaging more than 1400 HU. Uric acid stones typically have the lowest CT attenuation, on average 409 HU.[19] A number of reports have demonstrated that the efficacy of SWL decreases with increasing stone attenuation as measured on NCCT.[13,14,20,21] One series found that the rate of success for stone fragmentation was significantly lower in stones with a CT attenuation greater than 1000 HU when compared with stones with lower attenuation.[20] Another group reported a significantly higher effectiveness coefficient for SWL treating stones with attenuation less than 1200 HU versus those with greater than 1200 HU (80.4% vs 66.2%, $P = .03$).[21] Finally, 2 reports have demonstrated that stone attenuation less than 900 HU is an independent predictor of SWL success.[13,14]

Dual-energy NCCT is a novel technology that can be used to differentiate stones of different compositions more accurately.[22–24] In an in vivo study, dual-energy NCCT was able to determine and differentiate stone compositions accurately,

Table 1
Sensitivity and specificity for identifying urolithiasis with different imaging techniques

Imaging Technique	Sensitivity	Specificity
Noncontrast computed tomography	95%–98%[7–9]	96%–98%[7–9]
"Low-dose" CT	97%[73]	95%[73]
Ultrasound		
Renal stones	29%–81%[25–28]	82%–90%[25–27]
Ureteral stones	11%–93%[26,29–33]	87%–100%[26,29–33]
Plain radiography		
KUB	45%–58%[44–47]	69%–77%[44,45]
IVP	85.2%[53]	90.4%[53]
Magnetic resonance imaging	93%–100%[54–56]	95%–100%[54–56]

including stones of mixed composition.[22] Dual-energy NCCT has also been very effective in determining uric acid stone composition.

Ultrasound

Ultrasound is commonly performed during the evaluation of urolithiasis. The main advantage ultrasound has over other imaging modalities such as NCCT is that it is performed without any radiation exposure to the patient. However, ultrasound is not as sensitive or specific for the detection of renal or ureteral stones. The reported sensitivity of ultrasound for diagnosing renal stones ranges from 29% to 81%.[25–28] The specificity ranges from 82% to 90%.[25–27] The sensitivity of ultrasound for the detection of ureteral stones in patients with acute renal colic ranges from 11% to 93% and the specificity ranges from 87% to 100%.[26,29–33]

Evaluation of renal colic

The sensitivity of ultrasound for the identification of a ureteral stone in a patient with renal colic is less than NCCT; however, it still plays a large role in evaluating patients with renal colic. Ultrasound, like NCCT, can be used to evaluate other abdominal or pelvic organs while concurrently imaging the urinary tract. This allows for identification of alternative diagnoses when evaluating for renal colic. One study comparing the sensitivity of ultrasound and NCCT for the diagnosis of a ureteral stone in patients with renal colic found that ultrasound had a significantly lower sensitivity compared with NCCT, 61% versus 96% (P = .02).[30] However, the sensitivity for ultrasound in determining any cause for the patient's symptoms, including hydronephrosis, stones, or appendicitis, was 85%. Another study comparing ultrasound and NCCT for the evaluation of renal colic found a 93% sensitivity for the diagnosis of a ureteral stone with ultrasound.[31] In 6 of the 62 patients included in this study, ultrasound was able to find an alternative diagnosis: appendicitis, cholecystitis, cholelithiasis, adnexal mass, and torsed ovary.

When patients with renal colic are diagnosed with a distal ureteral stone with an NCCT, ultrasound can be effective at identifying the stone in the distal ureter during follow-up. One prospective study looked at the utility of ultrasound to follow up patients diagnosed with distal ureteral stones on an initial NCCT.[34] After their initial diagnosis, during follow-up the patients were imaged with ultrasound in addition to either repeat NCCT or radiography. The sensitivity of ultrasound on follow-up was 94.3% and the specificity was 99.1%.

Color Doppler ultrasound can be useful to improve the ability of ultrasound to detect ureteral stones. The "twinkling sign" on Doppler ultrasound appears as random color encoding in the area behind the stone where shadowing would be seen in traditional B-mode ultrasound. Doppler ultrasound using the "twinkling sign" has been shown to detect a higher percentage of stones than traditional gray-scale ultrasonography, 97% versus 66%.[35]

Evaluation for obstruction

In patients with renal colic, ultrasound is excellent at identifying signs of ureteral obstruction. The sensitivity and specificity of ultrasound for the diagnosis of obstruction have been reported to be as high as 100%.[33] In 1 study looking at ultrasound for the evaluation of patients with confirmed renal colic, hydronephrosis was identified in 95% of cases, ureteral dilation in 89% of cases, and perirenal fluid in 23% of cases.[33]

In addition to these signs of obstruction, the resistive index (RI) is a measure on color Doppler ultrasound that can improve the detection of ureteral obstruction in patients with renal colic.[36–41] Ultrasound-determined RI has been shown to have a sensitivity of 88% and a specificity of 98% for ureteral obstruction, using IVP as the standard.[36] In this report, the RI in the obstructed kidneys were significantly greater than the RI in nonobstructed kidneys, 0.73 versus 0.64 (P<.001). In a prospective study, Doppler ultrasound with RI performed equally well when compared with NCCT for the detection of ureteral obstruction.[37] With IVP being the standard, the sensitivity and specificity for NCCT were 96% and 96% compared with 90% and 100% for Doppler ultrasound. Using an RI of 0.70 and a 10% difference in RI between kidneys as diagnostic of obstruction improves the sensitivity and specificity of ultrasound for the diagnosis of ureteral obstruction from 94.8% and 55.5% to 98.9% and 90.9%.[38] Doppler ultrasound can also identify ureteral jets, which can further aide in ruling out obstruction.[40,41]

Limitations of ultrasound in the evaluation of urolithiasis

Ultrasound has limitations in the evaluation of urolithiasis and these are to stone location, size, and patient size. Ultrasound is not as sensitive at identifying stones in the ureter as it is in identifying stones in the kidney.[25–33] One study evaluated 228 patients who underwent ultrasound for renal colic and suspected renal colic before ureteroscopy and found the sensitivity of ultrasound was 86.4% for identifying ureteral stones.[42] Patients in whom ultrasound failed to diagnose the stone had significantly smaller mean stone size (4 mm vs 6 mm, $P<.001$). In addition to being less sensitive at identifying smaller stones, ultrasound has been shown to overestimate stone size compared with NCCT.[43] In 1 report, ultrasound overestimated stone size by nearly 2 mm compared with NCCT.[43] The mean stone size on NCCT was 7.4 ± 4 mm versus 9.2 ± 5 mm on ultrasound ($P = .018$). Patient body habitus and body mass index (BMI) are other factors that can influence the accuracy of ultrasound. As the skin-to-stone distance increases, the discordance between ultrasound and NCCT for the measurement of stone size increases.[43] The ability of ultrasound to detect stones has been shown to be lower in patients with higher BMI.[42]

Plain Radiography

Plain radiography of the abdomen/pelvis

Historically, KUB was the imaging modality of choice for the evaluation of urolithiasis. This was because most stones contained calcium and therefore would be expected to be visible on KUB. However, compared with NCCT and ultrasound, the sensitivity and specificity of KUB for detecting stones are poor. The sensitivity of KUB is reported to be 45 to 58%; the specificity is reported to be 69 to 77%.[44–47] There are a number of factors that contribute to the reduced sensitivity and specificity of KUB, such as overlying bowel gas, extrarenal and extra-ureteral calcifications, and patient body habitus.[48]

The use of tomography can improve the diagnostic accuracy of KUB for the evaluation of nephrolithiasis.[49] In 1 study evaluating KUB versus KUB with tomograms, 46% of patients had additional stones identified on tomograms. In 8% of patients, stones were only seen on tomograms.[49] The use of tomograms increases the amount of radiation the patient is exposed to. The effective doses for a KUB and each tomogram have been estimated to be 0.67 mSv and 1.1 mSv, respectively.[50] Therefore, if a KUB is performed with 3 tomograms, the total radiation exposure would be 3.97 mSv, greater than a low-dose NCCT.

KUB with ultrasound

KUB is useful as an adjunct to ultrasound in the evaluation of patients with renal colic. The sensitivity of ultrasound combined with KUB for the diagnosis of a ureteral calculus in a patient with renal colic has been reported to be as high as 96% with a specificity of 91%.[51] When performed together, it is recommended that KUB be performed first to identify calcifications. Ultrasound can then be used to confirm that these calcifications are in the urinary tract and therefore are stones.

Preoperative evaluation

KUB is useful in the preoperative evaluation before SWL. It can determine if a stone is radio-opaque and thereby seen with fluoroscopy. Obtaining a KUB can change the decision on how a stone is managed. One study reported that when a KUB is obtained after NCCT, the surgical management was changed in 17 of 100 patients based on information from the KUB.[52] An NCCT scout image is not as sensitive for identifying stones compared with a KUB.[46,47] Therefore, scout images from NCCT cannot be used as a surrogate for a KUB, and if SWL using fluoroscopy is planned, a KUB should be obtained preoperatively to determine if the stone will be visible on fluoroscopy during SWL.

Intravenous Pyelography

Before the advent of NCCT, IVP was considered the standard imaging technique for the evaluation of patients with renal colic. Currently, NCCT has largely supplanted IVP because of its superior sensitivity for detecting stones in these patients.[4,53] In a prospective randomized trial comparing NCCT with IVP for the evaluation of acute flank pain, NCCT was demonstrated to have a sensitivity and specificity of 94.1% and 94.2% for identifying a stone compared with a sensitivity and specificity of 85.2% and 90.4% for IVP.[53]

There are still some advantages of IVP in the evaluation of patients with urolithiasis. Because it is performed with contrast, IVP can provide information about renal function and whether a kidney is obstructed. Delayed images can be useful in evaluating ureteral anatomy for filling defects or strictures. It also provides detailed pelvicalyceal anatomy, which can be useful in planning surgical interventions, especially in those individuals with urinary tract anomalies. However, for these indications, IVP has largely been supplanted by CT with intravenous contrast or CT urograms.

Magnetic Resonance Imaging

There are limited indications for the use of MRI in the evaluation of urolithiasis. Although stones cannot be directly visualized using MRI, when evaluating patients with renal colic, MRI can detect signs of obstruction and can evaluate for alternative diagnoses. A number of different techniques and sequences have been reported for the evaluation of stones. The most common technique is to evaluate the T2-weighted images and assess for signs of obstruction or look for filling defects, which may be stones.[54–57] Using T2-weighted images, the findings of perirenal fluid and ureteral dilation had a sensitivity and specificity of 93% and 95% for the diagnosis of ureteral calculi in patients with renal colic.[56] Another group reported using a 3-dimensional fast low-angle shot (3D FLASH) sequence that requires the administration of gadolinium.[54] The sensitivity and specificity for the 3D FLASH sequence was 96.2% to 100% and 100% for the diagnosis of a ureteral stone. The 3D FLASH sequence combined with T2-weighted images has been shown to be as sensitive and specific for the diagnosis of ureteral stones as NCCT.[55] The addition of gadolinium for the 3D FLASH sequence can aide in the determination of stone size on MRI.[55]

New Technology

Digital tomosynthesis

Digital tomosynthesis (DT) is a new imaging technology similar to KUB with tomograms. When DT is performed, a scout KUB is taken and then a single tomographic sweep over approximately 60° arc is done. A digital flat-panel detector records the data from the sweep and then software reconstructs the information to provide high-resolution "slice" or coronal images at varying depths (**Fig. 1**). This reconstruction removes overlying structures such as bowel gas from slices, improving the resolution and visualization of stones. It also provides depth information. The depth information is useful in differentiating a calcification in the ureter versus an overlying transverse process from the spine (see **Fig. 1**).

There have been reports of the use of DT for the evaluation of urolithiasis.[58,59] In 1 report, DT was compared with KUB with an additional plain film of the pelvis.[58] All patients underwent DT, KUB with the additional image of the pelvis, and NCCT, which was used as the standard. DT was superior to KUB for identifying intrarenal stones. The technology for DT can be used to perform an IVP, improving the image quality.[59] Two uroradiologists reviewed both traditional IVP and IVP performed with DT. They evaluated the subjective diagnostic quality and found that 95.5% of the IVP with DT were of diagnostic quality versus 46.5% of the traditional IVPs. In addition, the dose of radiation was lower for the IVP with DT and they took less time. The dose of radiation from DT has been shown to be lower than that of a "low-dose" NCCT.[50,58]

RADIATION REDUCTION

Radiation exposure from medical sources has been steadily increasing over the past 3 decades. In 1980, the per capita radiation exposure in the

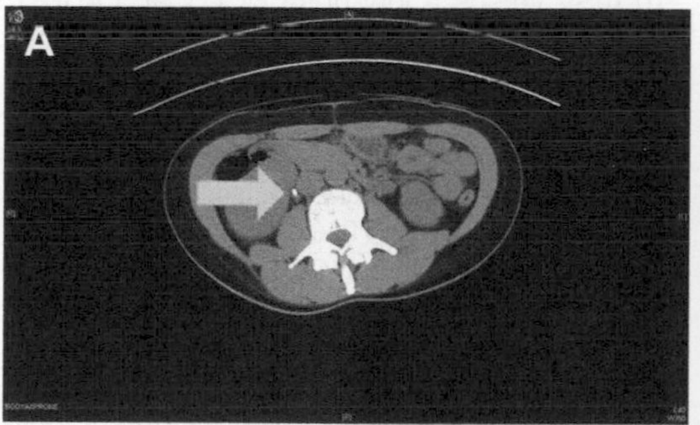

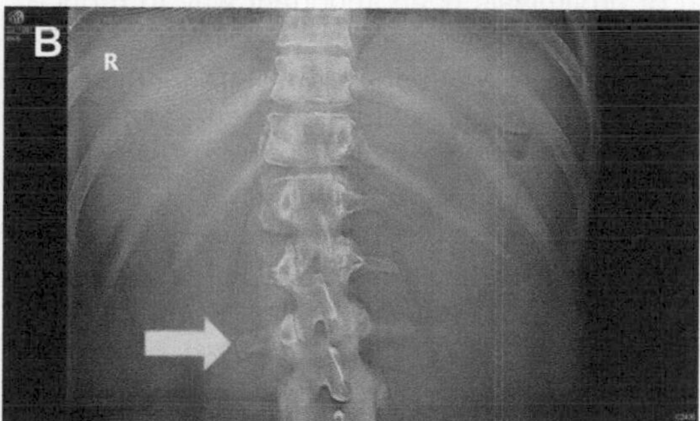

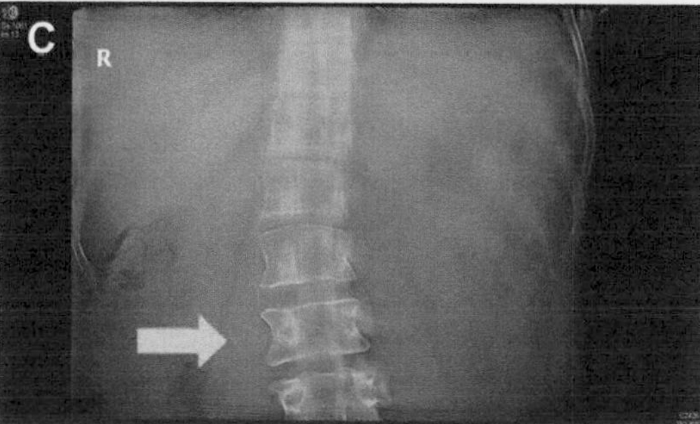

Fig. 1. (*A*) NCCT demonstrated a right mid ureteral stone. *Arrow* points to the stone. (*B*) Coronal "slice" from digital tomosynthesis demonstrated a spinal transverse process. *Arrow* points to spinal transverse process (*C*) Anterior coronal "slice" from digital tomosynthesis demonstrating the ureteral stone. *Arrow* points to the ureteral stone.

United States from medical sources was 0.54 mSv.[60] In 2006, this increased nearly 600% to 3.0 mSv. Most of this increase was from the use of CT scans. In 2006, there were an estimated 62 million CT scans performed in the United States.[61] It is estimated that an additional 29,000 cancers could be related to CT scans performed in the United States in 2007.[62]

Patients with urolithiasis are at increased risk for significant radiation exposure from diagnostic imaging, specifically NCCT. From 1996 to 2007, the use of NCCT to assess patients with suspected stones increased significantly from 4% to 42.5%.[6] The use of NCCT for the evaluation of flank pain in the emergency room has increased significantly from 19.6% to 45.5% of patient visits over the past decade.[63] It has been reported that patients undergo a median of 1.7 NCCT in a 1-year period following an acute stone episode.[64] Of the 108 patients included in this study, 94 (87) went on to have a surgical intervention. Fluoroscopy used during these surgical interventions also contributes to these patients' overall radiation exposure. Given that patients with urolithiasis constitute a high-risk population, measures to reduce the amount of radiation these patients are exposed to are extremely important.

Study Selection

Proper selection of imaging studies for the evaluation of urolithiasis is an important way to reduce radiation. Whenever possible, radiation-free techniques such as ultrasound or MRI should be used. Ultrasound should be considered the first-line imaging study for the evaluation of stones or renal colic in pediatric patients and pregnant women. The use of MRI has also been reported for the evaluation of renal colic in pregnant women.[65] Both of these modalities have high sensitivity for diagnosing ureteral obstruction.[33,36–41,54–57] The combination of ultrasound and KUB has been shown to have high sensitivity for the diagnosis of ureteral stones and exposes patients to less radiation than an NCCT.[51]

The American Urological Association recently submitted guidelines regarding appropriate imaging selection for the evaluation of ureteral calculi.[66] The authors recommend "low-dose" NCCT as the initial imaging modality for a patient with flank pain and a suspected ureteral stone if the BMI is less than 30 kg/m^2 and a standard-dose NCCT if the patient is obese. They recommend a KUB concurrently with the NCCT if the stone is not seen on the scout image. For follow-up of radio-opaque stones, they recommend ultrasound along with KUB. In cases of radiolucent stones, they recommend follow-up imaging with NCCT.

Low-dose computed tomography

Although ultrasound and MRI can be used for the evaluation of patients with urolithiasis, NCCT has the highest sensitivity and specificity for the diagnosis of stones. NCCT also is very valuable for preoperative planning. The amount of radiation a patient is exposed to from an NCCT of the abdomen and pelvis is dependent on the protocol and machine used, as well as patient characteristics. For a standard NCCT of the abdomen and pelvis performed for the evaluation of stones, the effective dose has been reported to be as high as 9.6 mSv for men and 12.6 mSv for women.[67]

With the advent of new CT scanner technology and new software, NCCT for the evaluation of urolithiasis can be performed with lower radiation doses while maintaining diagnostic accuracy. These "low-dose" CT scans can greatly reduce the amount of radiation patients are exposed to. There is no standard definition for "low-dose" CT. A recent meta-analysis evaluating the performance of low-dose CT for the diagnosis of urolithiasis defined low-dose CT as applying an effective dose less than 3 mSv for the entire examination.

There have been a number of reports assessing the effectiveness of low-dose CT for the evaluation of stones and renal colic.[67–72] One report compared a standard NCCT at a dose of 7.3 to 10 mSv versus a low-dose NCCT at 1.4 to 1.97 mSv for the evaluation of acute renal colic.[71] Low-dose NCCT had equivalent sensitivities to standard NCCT for the diagnosis of ureteral stones with the exception of ureteral stones less than 2 mm. In these cases, the sensitivity of low-dose NCCT was 68% to 79% versus 95% sensitivity for the standard-dose NCCT.[71]

In another evaluation of low-dose versus standard-dose NCCT for the evaluation of acute renal colic, low-dose NCCT achieved sensitivities and specificities for diagnosing a stone or indirect signs of a stone approaching standard-dose NCCT.[67] Compared to standard-dose CT, low-dose NCCT had a sensitivity of 97% and a specificity of 98% for identifying at least 1 direct or indirect sign of a ureteral stone. The authors in this trial did report decreased sensitivity and specificity for the diagnosis of ureteral calculi with patient BMI greater than 30 kg/m^2, 50% and 89%, respectively, compared with 95% and 97% in non-obese patients.[67] A recent meta-analysis of studies evaluating low-dose NCCT demonstrated a pooled sensitivity of 97% and a specificity of 95%.[73]

Low-dose NCCT has been shown to be useful for the follow-up of recurrent stone formers to evaluate for new stone formation or stone growth.[70] Even at a dose reduction of 56%, the authors reported no significant intraobserver or interobserver differences for the detection of urolithiasis. Low-dose CT has also been reported for the evaluation of renal colic and flank pain in pregnant patients with high sensitivity and specificity.[74]

Low-dose NCCT appears to perform as well as standard NCCT for the evaluation of urolithiasis and, in cases where NCCT is to be performed; low-dose NCCT should be considered the first-line imaging study.

FLUOROSCOPY

Fluoroscopy is commonly used during surgical procedures to treat patients with urolithiasis including SWL, URS, and PNL. Therefore, patients who undergo treatment of stones are exposed to even more radiation. The amounts of radiation patients are exposed to during PNL and URS have been quantified using a validated model.[75,76] At 1 institution, nonobese patients undergoing PNL were exposed to a median 9.34 mSv for a left-sided procedure and 7.11 mSv for a right-sided procedure.[75] Nonobese patients undergoing URS were exposed to a median of 1.13 mSv.[76] There are a number of methods to reduce the amount of radiation patients are exposed to in the operating room.

As Low as Reasonably Achievable

The principle of *As Low As Reasonably Achievable* (ALARA) should always be applied when using fluoroscopy. This includes collimating the image as much as possible and placing the image intensifier as close to the patient as possible.[77] Pulsed fluoroscopy should be used at the lowest possible frames per second that provides usable image quality to perform the procedure. Last image hold should be used to save and transfer images to an adjacent screen to be used as a reference during the procedure. Close adherence to the principles of ALARA has been demonstrated to reduce radiation dose during pediatric interventional radiology procedures.[78]

Radiation Reduction During PNL

When performing a retrograde pyelogram to aide in fluoroscopic access during PNL, the use of air instead of iodinated contrast may reduce radiation exposure. A retrospective review of 96 PNL procedures demonstrated that the use of air reduced radiation exposure nearly 50% when compared with contrast, 4.45 mSv versus 7.67 mSv ($P = .001$).[79]

The use of ultrasound to obtain access also can reduce radiation exposure by reducing or eliminating the need for fluoroscopy. There have been a number of reports on the use of ultrasound to aide in access during PNL.[80–85] Two randomized controlled trials have been performed comparing PNL with ultrasound combined with fluoroscopy versus fluoroscopy alone.[83,84] In the first trial, the authors report that access took significantly longer with ultrasound, 11 minutes versus 5.5 minutes ($P<.0001$). However, the fluoroscopy time was significantly longer in the patients who had their entire procedure performed with fluoroscopy (41.4 seconds vs 57.0 seconds, $P = .0001$). The second trial demonstrated shorter time to successful puncture in the ultrasound group (1.8 minutes vs 3.2 minutes, $P<.01$) and significantly shorter fluoroscopy time with the use of ultrasound (14.4 seconds vs 28.6 seconds, $P<.01$).[84]

Although these trials demonstrated a reduction in fluoroscopy time with ultrasound, the patients were still exposed to a small amount of radiation from fluoroscopy.[83,84] The ideal situation to reduce radiation exposure would be to eliminate fluoroscopy altogether. Studies have demonstrated the feasibility and safety of performing PNL with ultrasound alone in a select patient population.[80,81] In 1 series, 47 patients with a solitary stone located in the renal pelvic associated with mild-to-moderate hydronephosis were treated with PNL using ultrasound alone.[80] The mean stone size was 31.5 mm and the stone-free rate was 83%. In 2 morbidly obese patients, fluoroscopy was needed to aide in access. The second series reported on 34 patients with a solitary renal pelvic stone.[81] The mean stone size was 24 mm and a single lower pole puncture was obtained in all cases. The stone-free rate was 94%. The use of ultrasound to perform PNL without fluoroscopy seems to be safe and efficacious in a select group of patients.

Radiation Reduction During URS

The same principles of ALARA apply to fluoroscopy use during URS. In addition, there have been reports on methods to reduce fluoroscopy time for URS. One group of investigators demonstrated a 24% reduction in fluoroscopy time when surgeons were given periodic reports documenting their mean fluoroscopy time compared with that of their peers.[86] In addition, intraoperative techniques have been reported to reduce fluoroscopy time during URS.[87] These measures include the use of a laser-guided C-arm, tactile cues for the placement of guidewires, stent placement under direct vision through a cystoscope, use of a designated fluoroscopy technician, and single pulse fluoroscopy mode for portions of the case. When these measures were implemented, the authors reported a reduction in the mean fluoroscopy time during URS from 86.1 seconds to 15.5 seconds.

Radiation Reduction During SWL

The principles of ALARA apply to the use of fluoroscopy during SWL as well. In addition, ultrasound can be used to target the stone instead of fluoroscopy with good success.[88]

SUMMARY

Imaging plays an important role in the evaluation of patients with urolithiasis. NCCT of the abdomen and pelvis is the most sensitive and specific imaging modality for diagnosing stones. Images from NCCT also play an important role in determining the best surgical approach to treat a stone. When NCCT is performed for the evaluation of stones, a "low-dose" protocol should be used to reduce the amount of radiation these patients are exposed to whenever possible. Ultrasound is also useful in the evaluation of urolithiasis. Ultrasound should be considered first-line imaging for stones in pediatric and pregnant patients. Ultrasound has decreased sensitivity and specificity for identifying stones compared with NCCT; however, it has nearly equivalent sensitivities and specificities for diagnosing obstruction. Plain abdominal radiography is mostly useful for preoperative planning before SWL and as an adjunct to ultrasound. The role of MRI in the evaluation of urolithiasis is limited.

Stone patients are exposed to significant amounts of radiation from diagnostic imaging, primarily NCCT, and fluoroscopy in the operating room. Proper imaging modality selection helps to minimize radiation exposure. Following the principles of ALARA in the operating room can help reduce the amount of radiation patients are exposed to from fluoroscopy.

REFERENCES

1. Segal AJ, Spataro RF, Linke CA, et al. Diagnosis of nonopaque calculi by computed tomography. Radiology 1978;129(2):447–50.
2. Tessler AN, Ghazi MR. Case profile: computerized tomographic assistance in diagnosis of radiolucent calculi. Urology 1979;13(6):672–3.
3. Federle MP, McAninch JW, Kaiser JA, et al. Computed tomography of urinary calculi. AJR Am J Roentgenol 1981;136(2):255–8.
4. Smith RC, Rosenfield AT, Choe KA, et al. Acute flank pain: comparison of non-contrast-enhanced CT and intravenous urography. Radiology 1995;194(3):789–94.
5. Sundaram CP, Saltzman B. Urolithiasis associated with protease inhibitors. J Endourol 1999;13(4):309–12.
6. Westphalen AC, Hsia RY, Maselli JH, et al. Radiological imaging of patients with suspected urinary tract stones: national trends, diagnoses, and predictors. Acad Emerg Med 2011;18(7):699–707.
7. Dalrymple NC, Verga M, Anderson KR, et al. The value of unenhanced helical computerized tomography in the management of acute flank pain. J Urol 1998;159(3):735–40.
8. Smith RC, Verga M, McCarthy S, et al. Diagnosis of acute flank pain: value of unenhanced helical CT. AJR Am J Roentgenol 1996;166(1):97–101.
9. Vieweg J, Teh C, Freed K, et al. Unenhanced helical computerized tomography for the evaluation of patients with acute flank pain. J Urol 1998;160(3 Pt 1):679–84.
10. Ege G, Akman H, Kuzucu K, et al. Acute ureterolithiasis: incidence of secondary signs on unenhanced helical CT and influence on patient management. Clin Radiol 2003;58(12):990–4.
11. Katz DS, Scheer M, Lumerman JH, et al. Alternative or additional diagnoses on unenhanced helical computed tomography for suspected renal colic: experience with 1000 consecutive examinations. Urology 2000;56(1):53–7.
12. Hoppe H, Studer R, Kessler TM, et al. Alternate or additional findings to stone disease on unenhanced computerized tomography for acute flank pain can impact management. J Urol 2006;175(5):1725–30 [discussion: 1730].
13. Perks AE, Schuler TD, Lee J, et al. Stone attenuation and skin-to-stone distance on computed tomography predicts for stone fragmentation by shock wave lithotripsy. Urology 2008;72(4):765–9.
14. Wiesenthal JD, Ghiculete D, D'A Honey RJ, et al. Evaluating the importance of mean stone density and skin-to-stone distance in predicting successful shock wave lithotripsy of renal and ureteric calculi. Urol Res 2010;38(4):307–13.
15. Patel T, Kozakowski K, Hruby G, et al. Skin to stone distance is an independent predictor of stone-free status following shockwave lithotripsy. J Endourol 2009;23(9):1383–5.
16. Pareek G, Hedican SP, Lee FT Jr, et al. Shock wave lithotripsy success determined by skin-to-stone distance on computed tomography. Urology 2005;66(5):941–4.
17. Ng CS, Herts BR, Streem SB. Percutaneous access to upper pole renal stones: role of prone 3-dimensional computerized tomography in inspiratory and expiratory phases. J Urol 2005;173(1):124–6.

18. Hopper KD, Yakes WF. The posterior intercostal approach for percutaneous renal procedures: risk of puncturing the lung, spleen, and liver as determined by CT. AJR Am J Roentgenol 1990;154(1): 115–7.
19. Mostafavi MR, Ernst RD, Saltzman B. Accurate determination of chemical composition of urinary calculi by spiral computerized tomography. J Urol 1998;159(3):673–5.
20. Joseph P, Mandal AK, Singh SK, et al. Computerized tomography attenuation value of renal calculus: can it predict successful fragmentation of the calculus by extracorporeal shock wave lithotripsy? A preliminary study. J Urol 2002;167(5):1968–71.
21. Shah K, Kurien A, Mishra S, et al. Predicting effectiveness of extracorporeal shockwave lithotripsy by stone attenuation value. J Endourol 2010;24(7): 1169–73.
22. Zilberman DE, Ferrandino MN, Preminger GM, et al. In vivo determination of urinary stone composition using dual energy computerized tomography with advanced post-acquisition processing. J Urol 2010;184(6):2354–9.
23. Manglaviti G, Tresoldi S, Guerrer CS, et al. In vivo evaluation of the chemical composition of urinary stones using dual-energy CT. AJR Am J Roentgenol 2011;197(1):W76–83.
24. Ferrandino MN, Pierre SA, Simmons WN, et al. Dual-energy computed tomography with advanced postimage acquisition data processing: improved determination of urinary stone composition. J Endourol 2010;24(3):347–54.
25. Fowler KA, Locken JA, Duchesne JH, et al. US for detecting renal calculi with nonenhanced CT as a reference standard. Radiology 2002;222(1): 109–13.
26. Unal D, Yeni E, Karaoglanoglu M, et al. Can conventional examinations contribute to the diagnostic power of unenhanced helical computed tomography in urolithiasis? Urol Int 2003;70(1):31–5.
27. Ulusan S, Koc Z, Tokmak N. Accuracy of sonography for detecting renal stone: comparison with CT. J Clin Ultrasound 2007;35(5):256–61.
28. Viprakasit DP, Sawyer MD, Herrell SD, et al. Limitations of ultrasonography in the evaluation of urolithiasis: a correlation with computed tomography. J Endourol 2012;26(3):209–13.
29. Yilmaz S, Sindel T, Arslan G, et al. Renal colic: comparison of spiral CT, US and IVU in the detection of ureteral calculi. Eur Radiol 1998;8(2):212–7.
30. Sheafor DH, Hertzberg BS, Freed KS, et al. Nonenhanced helical CT and US in the emergency evaluation of patients with renal colic: prospective comparison. Radiology 2000;217(3):792–7.
31. Patlas M, Farkas A, Fisher D, et al. Ultrasound vs CT for the detection of ureteric stones in patients with renal colic. Br J Radiol 2001;74(886):901–4.
32. Hamm M, Wawroschek F, Weckermann D, et al. Unenhanced helical computed tomography in the evaluation of acute flank pain. Eur Urol 2001;39(4): 460–5.
33. Ripolles T, Agramunt M, Errando J, et al. Suspected ureteral colic: plain film and sonography vs unenhanced helical CT. A prospective study in 66 patients. Eur Radiol 2004;14(1):129–36.
34. Moesbergen TC, de Ryke RJ, Dunbar S, et al. Distal ureteral calculi: US follow-up. Radiology 2011; 260(2):575–80.
35. Mitterberger M, Aigner F, Pallwein L, et al. Sonographic detection of renal and ureteral stones. Value of the twinkling sign. Int Braz J Urol 2009;35(5): 532–9 [discussion: 540–1].
36. Shokeir AA, Abdulmaaboud M. Resistive index in renal colic: a prospective study. BJU Int 1999; 83(4):378–82.
37. Shokeir AA, Abdulmaaboud M. Prospective comparison of nonenhanced helical computerized tomography and Doppler ultrasonography for the diagnosis of renal colic. J Urol 2001;165(4):1082–4.
38. Pepe P, Motta L, Pennisi M, et al. Functional evaluation of the urinary tract by color-Doppler ultrasonography (CDU) in 100 patients with renal colic. Eur J Radiol 2005;53(1):131–5.
39. Kavakli I IS, Koktener A, Yilmaz A. Diagnostic value of renal resistive index for the assessment of renal colic. Singapore Med J 2011;52(4):271–3.
40. Gandolpho L, Sevillano M, Barbieri A, et al. Scintigraphy and Doppler ultrasonography for the evaluation of obstructive urinary calculi. Braz J Med Biol Res 2001;34(6):745–51.
41. Andreoiu M, MacMahon R. Renal colic in pregnancy: lithiasis or physiological hydronephrosis? Urology 2009;74(4):757–61.
42. Pichler R, Skradski V, Aigner F, et al. In young adults with a low body mass index ultrasonography is sufficient as a diagnostic tool for ureteric stones. BJU Int 2012;109(5):770–4.
43. Ray AA, Ghiculete D, Pace KT, et al. Limitations to ultrasound in the detection and measurement of urinary tract calculi. Urology 2010;76(2):295–300.
44. Mutgi A, Williams JW, Nettleman M. Renal colic. Utility of the plain abdominal roentgenogram. Arch Intern Med 1991;151(8):1589–92.
45. Levine JA, Neitlich J, Verga M, et al. Ureteral calculi in patients with flank pain: correlation of plain radiography with unenhanced helical CT. Radiology 1997; 204(1):27–31.
46. Jackman SV, Potter SR, Regan F, et al. Plain abdominal x-ray versus computerized tomography screening: sensitivity for stone localization after nonenhanced spiral computerized tomography. J Urol 2000;164(2):308–10.
47. Johnston R, Lin A, Du J, et al. Comparison of kidney-ureter-bladder abdominal radiography and

computed tomography scout films for identifying renal calculi. BJU Int 2009;104(5):670–3.

48. Sandhu C, Anson KM, Patel U. Urinary tract stones–Part I: role of radiological imaging in diagnosis and treatment planning. Clin Radiol 2003;58(6):415–21.
49. Goldwasser B, Cohan RH, Dunnick NR, et al. Role of linear tomography in evaluation of patients with nephrolithiasis. Urology 1989;33(3):253–6.
50. Wang AJ, Nguyen G, Toncheva G, et al. Radiation exposure from non-contrast CT, digital tomosynthesis, and standard KUB and tomograms. J Endourol 2011;25(S1):A304–5.
51. Mitterberger M, Pinggera GM, Pallwein L, et al. Plain abdominal radiography with transabdominal native tissue harmonic imaging ultrasonography vs unenhanced computed tomography in renal colic. BJU Int 2007;100(4):887–90.
52. Lamb AD, Wines MD, Mousa S, et al. Plain radiography still is required in the planning of treatment for urolithiasis. J Endourol 2008;22(10):2201–5.
53. Pfister SA, Deckart A, Laschke S, et al. Unenhanced helical computed tomography vs intravenous urography in patients with acute flank pain: accuracy and economic impact in a randomized prospective trial. Eur Radiol 2003;13(11):2513–20.
54. Sudah M, Vanninen R, Partanen K, et al. MR urography in evaluation of acute flank pain: T2-weighted sequences and gadolinium-enhanced three-dimensional FLASH compared with urography. Fast low-angle shot. AJR Am J Roentgenol 2001;176(1):105–12.
55. Sudah M, Vanninen RL, Partanen K, et al. Patients with acute flank pain: comparison of MR urography with unenhanced helical CT. Radiology 2002;223(1):98–105.
56. Regan F, Kuszyk B, Bohlman ME, et al. Acute ureteric calculus obstruction: unenhanced spiral CT versus HASTE MR urography and abdominal radiograph. Br J Radiol 2005;78(930):506–11.
57. Kalb B, Sharma P, Salman K, et al. Acute abdominal pain: is there a potential role for MRI in the setting of the emergency department in a patient with renal calculi? J Magn Reson Imaging 2010;32(5):1012–23.
58. Mermuys K, De Geeter F, Bacher K, et al. Digital tomosynthesis in the detection of urolithiasis: diagnostic performance and dosimetry compared with digital radiography with MDCT as the reference standard. AJR Am J Roentgenol 2010;195(1):161–7.
59. Wells IT, Raju VM, Rowberry BK, et al. Digital tomosynthesis–a new lease of life for the intravenous urogram? Br J Radiol 2011;84(1001):464–8.
60. Mettler FA Jr, Thomadsen BR, Bhargavan M, et al. Medical radiation exposure in the U.S. in 2006: preliminary results. Health Phys 2008;95(5):502–7.
61. Brenner DJ, Hall EJ. Computed tomography–an increasing source of radiation exposure. N Engl J Med 2007;357(22):2277–84.
62. Berrington de Gonzalez A, Mahesh M, Kim KP, et al. Projected cancer risks from computed tomographic scans performed in the United States in 2007. Arch Intern Med 2009;169(22):2071–7.
63. Hyams ES, Korley FK, Pham JC, et al. Trends in imaging use during the emergency department evaluation of flank pain. J Urol 2011;186(6):2270–4.
64. Ferrandino MN, Bagrodia A, Pierre SA, et al. Radiation exposure in the acute and short-term management of urolithiasis at 2 academic centers. J Urol 2009;181(2):668–72 [discussion: 673].
65. Mullins JK, Semins MJ, Hyams ES, et al. Half Fourier single-shot turbo spin-echo magnetic resonance urography for the evaluation of suspected renal colic in pregnancy. Urology 2012;79(6):1252–5.
66. Fulgham PF, Assimos DG, Pearle MS, et al. Clinical effectiveness protocol for imaging in the management of ureteral calculous disease: AUA technology assessment. 2012. Available at: http://www.auanet.org/content/media/imaging_assessment.pdf. Accessed August 1, 2012.
67. Poletti PA, Platon A, Rutschmann OT, et al. Low-dose versus standard-dose CT protocol in patients with clinically suspected renal colic. AJR Am J Roentgenol 2007;188(4):927–33.
68. Jellison FC, Smith JC, Heldt JP, et al. Effect of low dose radiation computerized tomography protocols on distal ureteral calculus detection. J Urol 2009;182(6):2762–7.
69. Jin DH, Lamberton GR, Broome DR, et al. Effect of reduced radiation CT protocols on the detection of renal calculi. Radiology 2010;255(1):100–7.
70. Zilberman DE, Tsivian M, Lipkin ME, et al. Low dose computerized tomography for detection of urolithiasis–its effectiveness in the setting of the urology clinic. J Urol 2011;185(3):910–4.
71. Kim BS, Hwang IK, Choi YW, et al. Low-dose and standard-dose unenhanced helical computed tomography for the assessment of acute renal colic: prospective comparative study. Acta Radiol 2005;46(7):756–63.
72. Kluner C, Hein PA, Gralla O, et al. Does ultra-low-dose CT with a radiation dose equivalent to that of KUB suffice to detect renal and ureteral calculi? J Comput Assist Tomogr 2006;30(1):44–50.
73. Niemann T, Kollmann T, Bongartz G. Diagnostic performance of low-dose CT for the detection of urolithiasis: a meta-analysis. AJR Am J Roentgenol 2008;191(2):396–401.
74. White WM, Zite NB, Gash J, et al. Low-dose computed tomography for the evaluation of flank pain in the pregnant population. J Endourol 2007;21(11):1255–60.
75. Lipkin ME, Mancini JG, Toncheva G, et al. Organ-specific radiation dose rates and effective dose rates during percutaneous nephrolithotomy. J Endourol 2012;26(5):439–43.

76. Lipkin ME, Wang AJ, Toncheva G, et al. Determination of patient radiation dose during ureteroscopic treatment of urolithiasis using a validated model. J Urol 2012;187(3):920–4.
77. Park S, Pearle MS. Imaging for percutaneous renal access and management of renal calculi. Urol Clin North Am 2006;33(3):353–64.
78. Sheyn DD, Racadio JM, Ying J, et al. Efficacy of a radiation safety education initiative in reducing radiation exposure in the pediatric IR suite. Pediatr Radiol 2008;38(6):669–74.
79. Lipkin ME, Mancini JG, Zilberman DE, et al. Reduced radiation exposure with the use of an air retrograde pyelogram during fluoroscopic access for percutaneous nephrolithotomy. J Endourol 2011;25(4):563–7.
80. Hosseini MM, Hassanpour A, Farzan R, et al. Ultrasonography-guided percutaneous nephrolithotomy. J Endourol 2009;23(4):603–7.
81. Gamal WM, Hussein M, Aldahshoury M, et al. Solo ultrasonography-guided percutanous nephrolithotomy for single stone pelvis. J Endourol 2011;25(4):593–6.
82. Osman M, Wendt-Nordahl G, Heger K, et al. Percutaneous nephrolithotomy with ultrasonography-guided renal access: experience from over 300 cases. BJU Int 2005;96(6):875–8.
83. Basiri A, Ziaee AM, Kianian HR, et al. Ultrasonographic versus fluoroscopic access for percutaneous nephrolithotomy: a randomized clinical trial. J Endourol 2008;22(2):281–4.
84. Agarwal M, Agrawal MS, Jaiswal A, et al. Safety and efficacy of ultrasonography as an adjunct to fluoroscopy for renal access in percutaneous nephrolithotomy (PCNL). BJU Int 2011;108(8):1346–9.
85. Alan C, Kocoglu H, Ates F, et al. Ultrasound-guided X-ray free percutaneous nephrolithotomy for treatment of simple stones in the flank position. Urol Res 2011;39(3):205–12.
86. Ngo TC, Macleod LC, Rosenstein DI, et al. Tracking intraoperative fluoroscopy utilization reduces radiation exposure during ureteroscopy. J Endourol 2011;25(5):763–7.
87. Greene DJ, Tenggadjaja CF, Bowman RJ, et al. Comparison of a reduced radiation fluoroscopy protocol to conventional fluoroscopy during uncomplicated ureteroscopy. Urology 2011;78(2):286–90.
88. Elhilali MM, Stoller ML, McNamara TC, et al. Effectiveness and safety of the Dornier compact lithotriptor: an evaluative multicenter study. J Urol 1996;155(3):834–8.

Shockwave Lithotripsy–New Concepts and Optimizing Treatment Parameters

Naeem Bhojani, MD, James E. Lingeman, MD*

KEYWORDS

• Radiodensity • Lithotripsy • Kidney stones • ESWL • Acoustic coupling and focus zone

KEY POINTS

- Stone radiodensity and skin to stone distance can both be used to optimize extracorporeal shock wave lithotripsy (ESWL) outcomes.
- The importance of acoustic coupling cannot be overemphasized. Air pockets within coupling gel can significantly reduce ESWL efficiency.
- ESWL outcomes are maximized using a frequency of 60 shock waves per minute compared with 120 shock waves per minute.
- Power ramping with a brief pause can not only improve ESWL stone fragmentation outcomes but also decrease renal tissue injury.
- Lithotripters with larger focal zones have superior stone fragmentation rates along with better renal safety profiles.
- Improved acoustic feedback and stone monitoring systems, as well as residual stone fragment clearance techniques, are being developed that will further improve the stone fragmentation outcomes of ESWL.

INTRODUCTION

The treatment of kidney stone disease has changed dramatically over the past 30 years. This change is due in large part to the arrival of ESWL. Before the advent of ESWL in the early 1980's, most kidney stones were treated with open surgery. ESWL along with the advances in ureteroscopic and percutaneous techniques has led to the virtual extinction of open surgical treatments for kidney stone disease.

The first successful ESWL treatment was accomplished in 1980 in Germany by Dr Christian Chaussy using a Dornier HM1 lithotripter. Owing to its effectiveness and its rare side effects, ESWL was quickly approved by the US Food and Drug Administration (FDA) for clinical use. Dr James Lingeman using the unmodified Dornier HM3 lithotripter performed the first ESWL procedure in North America. Since then, ESWL has been used with increasing frequency to treat more and more complex stones. Multiple sources have confirmed that kidney stone disease is on the rise, and as a result, surgical treatments for these kidney stones are also on the rise.[1–5] Turney and colleagues[6] have recently shown that over the past decade, ESWL for upper tract stones has increased by 55%. Most of this increase was caused by ESWL performed on kidney stones (69% increase). ESWL performed on the ureter remained stable. With the increase in stone disease, surgical treatment must not only be effective but also be efficient.

Department of Urology, Indiana University School of Medicine, 1801 Senate Boulevard, Suite 220, Indianapolis, IN 46202, USA

* Corresponding author.

E-mail address: jlingeman@iuhealth.org

Urol Clin N Am 40 (2013) 59–66

http://dx.doi.org/10.1016/j.ucl.2012.09.001

0094-0143/13/$ – see front matter

Initial work with ESWL was very optimistic because it was reported to be extremely effective even when applied to complex stone cases.[7–9] Furthermore, this noninvasive technique was found to have very few side effects. With the increasingly widespread acceptance and use of ESWL, it was discovered that this procedure was associated with a few important limitations. Some urinary stones were found to be resistant, and their fragmentation could not be accomplished consistently using ESWL.[10–12] Also, some renal stones that could be fragmented would not fragment completely and secondary treatments were necessary. In addition, renal anatomy (calyceal diverticulum or acute infundibulopelvic angles) and location (lower pole calyx) of the stone were crucial to ESWL stone-free outcomes.[13] Finally, many reports have demonstrated the frequent minor complications and the rare major complications.[14,15]

For the reasons stated above, much research has gone into understanding how ESWL can be made more efficient and safe. This article discusses the parameters that can be used to optimize ESWL outcomes as well as the new concepts that are affecting the efficacy and efficiency of ESWL.

OPTIMIZING PARAMETERS

Numerous parameters can be used to optimize ESWL outcomes. These parameters include stone characterization, acoustic coupling, and shock wave rate and sequence.

Stone Characterization

One of the main drawbacks of ESWL is its inability to fragment certain types of stones. This drawback is extremely important because patients who harbor these types of stones will be subjected to ESWL and will thus be exposed to its complications (minor and major) without the achievable benefit of fragmentation. In addition, failure of stone fragmentation will lead to secondary treatments, which will increase medical costs. The stones most resistant to ESWL include brushite, calcium oxalate monohydrate, and cystine.[10–12] Therefore, if one could predict the type of stone, then the likelihood of that stone being fragmented by ESWL could be predicted. Numerous studies have demonstrated that noncontrast computed tomography (NCCT) can be used to measure differences in radiodensity, which can be used to distinguish between different types of stones.[16–20] More recently, studies have shown that preoperative NCCT can be used to predict the likelihood of stone fragmentation.[21–26] El-Assmy and colleagues[21] demonstrated that stones with Hounsfield units (HU) greater than 1000 required a statistically significant higher number of shock waves to be fragmented. Also, Wang and colleagues[23] concluded that stone densities greater than 900 HU were a significant predictor of ESWL failure.

Along with the type of stone, the distance of the stone from the patient's skin can have a significant impact on the likelihood of stone fragmentation. Numerous studies have shown that the distance of the stone from the skin, also known as the skin to stone distance (SSD) can be used as an indicator of the likelihood of stone fragmentation.[27–29] SSD is measured by averaging 3 fixed distances from the stone to the skin. These 3 measurements include 1 horizontal, 1 vertical, and 1 diagonal measurement from the stone to the skin. Pareek and colleagues[27] found SSD to be a statistically significant predictor of ESWL failure when it was greater than 10 cm. In 2009, Patel and colleagues[29] found that patients with an average SSD of 10.7 cm had a statistically significant higher rate of residual stone after ESWL compared with those who had an average SSD of 8.3 cm.

As both SSD and stone radiodensity have been demonstrated to be independent predictors of stone fragmentation by ESWL, Perks and colleagues[28] used both these factors to evaluate their combined ability to predict stone fragmentation by ESWL. In this retrospective study on 111 patients, Perks and colleagues[28] found that stones with a radiodensity of less than 900 HU combined with an SSD of less than 9 cm predicted ESWL success, an observation that was independent of stone size, location, or body mass index.

As mentioned previously, cystine calculi are extremely hard to fragment with ESWL. Kim and colleagues[10] evaluated the hypothesis that cystine stones with specific morphologies might be easier to fragment with ESWL. This study demonstrated that cystine stones with a "rough" morphology contained void regions that are visible on NCCT. The investigators concluded that cystine calculi that appeared homogenous on NCCT required 61% more shock waves for fragmentation than did stones that appeared heterogeneous.

In summary, careful attention to stone characterization, including SSD and stone radiodensity, can be used to accurately select patients who have a greater possibility of having their stones fragmented using ESWL. This ability will translate into fewer secondary treatments, which will cut down on medical costs.

Acoustic Coupling

Over the past 30 years, ESWL has gone through numerous changes with the ultimate goal of complete and universal stone fragmentation with minimal side effects. Much research has gone into the achievement of this goal. One parameter that has recently undergone reevaluation is acoustic coupling. The HM3 uses water as a medium for coupling, which has been found to be ideal. This is because body tissue has an acoustic impedance very close to that of water, and therefore, a shock wave generated in water will pass into the body with minimal reflection or absorption of energy at the water–skin interface. Unlike the Dornier HM3, modern lithotripters have incorporated dry head energy sources that have treatment heads that are brought into contact with the patient. At present, the only machine that does not have a "dry head" is the Storz SLX (Storz Medical AG, Tägerwilen, Switzerland), which uses a partial water bath for coupling. Typically, gel is used to couple the dry head lithotripters to the skin of the patients. Once the gel is applied, the head of the lithotripter is brought into contact with the patient's skin. An important potential problem of gel coupling is the introduction of air pockets into the gel. These air pockets, which are often abundant, have a deleterious effect on shock wave propagation. Shock waves travel well through water and coupling gels, but not through air.

In 2006, Pishchalnikov and colleagues[30] demonstrated a negative relationship between increasing air pockets and ESWL efficiency. More specifically, using a Dornier DoLi-50 electromagnetic lithotripter, this in vitro study established that with as little as 2% of the coupling area covered with air pockets, there was a reduction in stone breakage by 20% to 40%. Jain and colleagues[31] found that optimal fragmentation was obtained using bubble-free ultrasound gel. In addition, Bergsdorf and colleagues[32] demonstrated in a clinical study that gel with lower viscosity and better quality provided significantly better stone fragmentation. Finally, in a study by Neucks and colleagues[33] it was discovered that the quality of coupling can be improved by the way the gel is handled and applied. The most effective way to apply coupling gel is to place it directly from the container as a mound to the center of the treatment head. Then, without spreading it around, the treatment head should be pressed against the patient.

The importance of acoustic coupling through gel application cannot be overemphasized. It is paramount that air pockets be limited so that shock waves can be delivered with the greatest efficiency. If coupling is overlooked, ESWL becomes less effective, leading to inferior outcomes and the need for increased secondary treatments.

Shock Wave Rate

Another important parameter that has a significant impact on ESWL outcomes is the rate at which shock waves are delivered. In vitro work first reported that slowing the rate at which shock waves are delivered can have a major impact on both stone fragmentation and acute renal tissue damage.[34] Numerous prospective clinical trials have confirmed that ESWL stone fragmentation outcomes are improved at 60 shock waves per minute compared with the standard 120 shock waves per minute.[35–38] Porcine models have also demonstrated that acute renal injury can be reduced at 60 shock waves per minute.[39,40] A meta-analysis by Semins and colleagues[35] showed that a treatment performed at a rate of 60 shocks per minute is associated with a higher rate of treatment success than treatment performed at a rate of 120 shocks per minute. One drawback of slowing the rate of shock wave delivery is the increased time required to break urinary calculi, which may extend the time that the patient is subjected to sedation.

One hypothesis proposed for the decreased stone fragmentation with an increased shock wave rate was an increase in the formation of cavitation bubbles, which would interfere with the transmission of the positive pressure phase of shock waves. However, Pishchalnikov and colleagues[41] proposed an alternative explanation suggesting that the main reason was actually the loss of the negative pressure portion of the shock wave and not the interference with the positive pressure portion.

In summary, many studies have confirmed that ESWL outcomes are maximized using a frequency of 60 shock waves per minute compared with 120 shock waves per minute. These outcomes includes a higher rate of stone fragmentation as well as a decreased rate of renal tissue damage.

Shock Wave Sequence

The last ESWL parameter to consider, which can have a dramatic impact on ESWL outcomes, including stone fragmentation and effect on acute renal tissue injury is the sequence that is used to deliver the shock waves. Sequence refers to the timing of shock waves and the number of shock waves given at a specific power level. Power ramping refers to the delivery of several shock waves at lower power levels before getting to the desired treating power level. Most centers treating under sedation perform some form of power ramping to help the patient get accustomed to the shock waves.

In in vitro studies on pigs, power ramping has been shown to enhance stone breakage.[42–44]

In vitro studies using the Dornier HM3 lithotripter demonstrated that progressively increasing the output voltage can produce superior stone comminution.[42] It has also been confirmed that stepwise power ramping can significantly decrease renal injury.[45–47] In a porcine model, treatment with 100 shocks at 18 kV followed by 2000 shocks at 24 kV significantly decreased acute renal lesion sizes compared with 2000 shocks at 24 kV. It was thought that the key to the protective effect in power ramping was a brief pause (roughly 3 minutes) between the lower and higher power settings.[47] However, more recently Handa and colleagues[48] confirmed that renal protection can be achieved without instituting a pause in ESWL treatment but that a ramping protocol is, however, necessary.

Therefore, power ramping with a brief pause can not only improve ESWL stone fragmentation outcomes but also decrease renal tissue injury and should be incorporated into all ESWL protocols.

In conclusion, optimizing parameters including SSD, stone radiodensity, acoustic coupling, reduced shock wave rate, and power ramping can and should always be applied when performing ESWL. Application of these will not only improve stone fragmentation but also decrease renal tissue injury. These simple yet effective techniques will reduce, if not eliminate, the need for secondary procedures, which will in turn reduce medical costs.

NEW CONCEPTS

With the tremendous amount of research being done in ESWL, more and more new concepts are being investigated. This section concentrates on these newer concepts including small versus large focal zone lithotripters, tandem and dual head lithotripters, acoustic feedback systems, stone monitoring systems, and residual fragment clearance techniques.

Small versus Large Focal Zone Lithotripters

ESWL acoustic energy is focused on to a relatively small zone surrounding the focal point of the lithotripter. The focal point is a geometric point and is usually the location of the kidney stone of interest. The focal zone can be either small or large, and the amount of energy or peak pressure that is applied to it can be manipulated. This relationship is also known as the acoustic output, which is the amplitude and spatial distribution of the acoustic energy delivered to a specific focal volume. The original Dornier HM3 produces peak positive pressures of about 40 MPa on a focal width of about 10 to 12 mm. Most modern lithotripters generate higher pressures between 60 and 160 MPa delivered to a more narrow focal width of 3 to 6 mm. The XX-ES CS-2012A (Xi Xin Medical Instruments Co. Ltd, Suhou, China) and the LithoGold LG-380 (Tissue Regeneration Technologies, Woodstock, GA, USA) produce low pressures (roughly 20 MPa) with broad focal zones (roughly 18–20 mm).

In vitro studies have demonstrated that a larger focal zone can improve stone breakage.[49] Owing to respiratory movements, urinary stones are in continual motion. It is hypothesized that the stone will have a greater chance of staying within the target focal zone if the zone is larger. Pishchalnikov and colleagues[50] demonstrated this hypothesis in an in vitro study. Furthermore, lithotripters with tighter focal zones tend to have fewer shock waves that actually hit the stone and more shock wave energy that is deposited directly into renal tissue.[51] This mechanism is not the only one by which large focal zone lithotripters improve stone breakage. Focal width also seems to have a crucial role in the mechanism of stone comminution. Numerical modeling studies have shown that shear waves necessary to cause large internal stresses are enhanced when the focal width is larger than the diameter of the stone.[52,53]

An important aspect of ESWL is safety, and numerous studies have shown that the use of a tighter focal zone with higher peak pressures is associated with not only a higher retreatment rate but also a higher rate of side effects when compared with a wider focal width.[54–58] Porcine models using treatment protocols recommended by both the XX-ES CS-2012A and the LG-380 broad focal zone lithotripter machines produce minimal renal lesions.[59,60]

Tandem and Dual Head Lithotripters

Tandem head lithotripters

As ESWL progresses, more and more research is being focused on ways of improving the fragmentation of stones. In light of this, efforts have been made to enhance one of the key mechanisms of stone breakage. Cavitation bubbles are an essential part of stone comminution, and a novel idea is to use 2 shock waves in rapid succession to drive the forceful collapse of bubbles against the stone. This method of stone breakage has been achieved by 2 methods. One is to add an auxiliary piezoelectric array to generate a second shock wave along the same axis as the first shock wave.[61–63] This method has led to significant improvements in stone comminution in vitro.[62] The other method is to fit a piezoelectric lithotripter with an additional charging and discharge circuit to produce a second pulse. Fernandez and colleagues[64] found clinically that this technique did not increase the efficiency of fragmentation but that it did significantly decrease the time required to fragment the stone.

Dual head lithotripters

Dual head lithotripters deliver closely timed shock waves from different treatment heads that are aligned to the exact same focal point.[65,66] Initial reports suggest that these machines can be safe and effective.[67,68]

Acoustic Feedback Systems

The main disadvantages of ESWL are the inefficiency side effects associated with it. These disadvantages are interrelated in that excess shock waves are commonly applied in an effort to assure stone breakage and ESWL effects on tissue are related to the shock wave dose. Recent research has demonstrated the possible role for an acoustic feedback system to monitor stone fragmentation.[69] This acoustic feedback system uses a broadband receiver to monitor shock waves and reverberations from the acoustic wave transmitted into the stone. As the stone fragments, reverberations from smaller fragments generate higher frequency signals. In vitro studies have demonstrated the feasibility of this system to discriminate between fragments that differ in size by only 1 to 2 mm.[69] This system allows the urologist to know when the stone is fragmented and therefore reduces excess or unnecessary shock waves to the renal tissue.

Stone Monitoring Systems

Once a stone has been localized, its movement in and out of the focal zone affects fragmentation. The longer the stone remains within the focal zone, the more likely it is to fragment. Maintaining the stone in the focal zone is challenged by respiratory motion. Depending on the patient's respiratory rate, the stone can be outside the focal zone during 50% or more of the administered shock waves.[51] This movement translates to more shock wave energy missing the stone and hitting renal tissue instead.

Several targeting systems have been developed to track stones during ESWL. These systems use ultrasound imagers, tracking algorithms, and piezoelectric lithotripters with built-in systems to continually locate the stone before shock wave firing.[70–72] Although these systems show promise, none of them are currently being used in the clinical setting.

Residual Fragment Clearance Techniques

ESWL has been proved to be an excellent treatment of renal stone disease. However, one of its main limitations is the clearance of residual fragments, which will often lead to secondary treatments. This drawback is especially important for lower pole calculi that are subjected to ESWL. Numerous methods of residual fragment clearance have been proposed including percussion, diuresis, and inversion therapy.[73–75] The success of these methods of residual stone fragment clearance have been limited.

There has been recent research in the domain of focused ultrasound technology directed at residual stone fragment clearance, and it shows great promise.[76] Shah and colleagues[76] recently demonstrated the use of focused ultrasound technology in a study involving live porcine models implanted with human stones. With this technology they were able to expel calculi effectively and safely from the kidney in their animal model. This technology could hold promise in the clearance of residual fragments after ESWL.

SUMMARY

Over the past 30 years, treatment of renal stone disease has changed dramatically. Treatments have become more and more minimally invasive. The only entirely noninvasive treatment remains ESWL. However, limitations to ESWL have been identified and have led to more emphasis on other treatment modalities. In an effort to return to noninvasive therapy, ESWL must improve. Therefore, with the incorporation of optimizing parameters, ESWL can become more efficient and safer. In addition, new concepts, novel ideas, and future research are leading the way toward a brighter future for ESWL.

REFERENCES

1. Romero V, Akpinar H, Assimos DG. Kidney stones: a global picture of prevalence, incidence, and associated risk factors. Rev Urol 2010;12(2–3):e86–96.
2. Stamatelou KK, Francis ME, Jones CA, et al. Time trends in reported prevalence of kidney stones in the United States: 1976-1994. Kidney Int 2003; 63(5):1817–23.
3. Pearle MS, Calhoun EA, Curhan GC. Urologic diseases in America project: urolithiasis. J Urol 2005;173(3):848–57.
4. Amato M, Lusini ML, Nelli F. Epidemiology of nephrolithiasis today. Urol Int 2004;72(Suppl 1):1–5.
5. Trinchieri A, Coppi F, Montanari E, et al. Increase in the prevalence of symptomatic upper urinary tract

stones during the last ten years. Eur Urol 2000;37(1): 23–5.
6. Turney BW, Reynard JM, Noble JG, et al. Trends in urological stone disease. BJU Int 2012;109(7):1082–7.
7. Chaussy C, Schmiedt E, Jocham D, et al. First clinical experience with extracorporeally induced destruction of kidney stones by shock waves. J Urol 1982;127(3):417–20.
8. Chaussy C, Brendel W, Schmiedt E. Extracorporeally induced destruction of kidney stones by shock waves. Lancet 1980;2(8207):1265–8.
9. Chaussy CG, Fuchs GJ. Current state and future developments of noninvasive treatment of human urinary stones with extracorporeal shock wave lithotripsy. J Urol 1989;141(3 Pt 2):782–9.
10. Kim SC, Burns EK, Lingeman JE, et al. Cystine calculi: correlation of CT-visible structure, CT number, and stone morphology with fragmentation by shock wave lithotripsy. Urol Res 2007;35(6):319–24.
11. Dretler SP. Stone fragility–a new therapeutic distinction. J Urol 1988;139(5):1124–7.
12. Klee LW, Brito CG, Lingeman JE. The clinical implications of brushite calculi. J Urol 1991;145(4):715–8.
13. Lingeman J, Matlaga BR, Evan AP. Surgical management of upper urinary tract calculi. In: Wein AJ, Kavoussi LR, Novick AC, et al, editors. Campbell-Walsh urology. Philadelphia: W.B. Sauders; 2007. p. 1431–507.
14. Kaude JV, Williams CM, Millner MR, et al. Renal morphology and function immediately after extracorporeal shock-wave lithotripsy. AJR Am J Roentgenol 1985;145(2):305–13.
15. Mcateer JA, Evan AP. The acute and long-term adverse effects of shock wave lithotripsy. Semin Nephrol 2008;28(2):200–13.
16. Mostafavi MR, Ernst RD, Saltzman B. Accurate determination of chemical composition of urinary calculi by spiral computerized tomography. J Urol 1998;159(3):673–5.
17. Nakada SY, Hoff DG, Attai S, et al. Determination of stone composition by noncontrast spiral computed tomography in the clinical setting. Urology 2000; 55(6):816–9.
18. Deveci S, Coskun M, Tekin MI, et al. Spiral computed tomography: role in determination of chemical compositions of pure and mixed urinary stones–an in vitro study. Urology 2004;64(2):237–40.
19. Sheir KZ, Mansour O, Madbouly K, et al. Determination of the chemical composition of urinary calculi by noncontrast spiral computerized tomography. Urol Res 2005;33(2):99–104.
20. Bellin MF, Renard-Penna R, Conort P, et al. Helical CT evaluation of the chemical composition of urinary tract calculi with a discriminant analysis of CT-attenuation values and density. Eur Radiol 2004; 14(11):2134–40.
21. El-Assmy A, Abou-El-Ghar ME, El-Nahas AR, et al. Multidetector computed tomography: role in determination of urinary stones composition and disintegration with extracorporeal shock wave lithotripsy–an in vitro study. Urology 2011;77(2):286–90.
22. Gupta NP, Ansari MS, Kesarvani P, et al. Role of computed tomography with no contrast medium enhancement in predicting the outcome of extracorporeal shock wave lithotripsy for urinary calculi. BJU Int 2005;95(9):1285–8.
23. Wang LJ, Wong YC, Chuang CK, et al. Predictions of outcomes of renal stones after extracorporeal shock wave lithotripsy from stone characteristics determined by unenhanced helical computed tomography: a multivariate analysis. Eur Radiol 2005; 15(11):2238–43.
24. Garcia Marchinena P, Billordo Peres N, Liyo J, et al. CT SCAN as a predictor of composition and fragility of urinary lithiasis treated with extracorporeal shock wave lithotripsy in vitro. Arch Esp Urol 2009;62(3): 215–22 [discussion: 222] [in Spanish].
25. Wiesenthal JD, Ghiculete D, DaH RJ, et al. Evaluating the importance of mean stone density and skin-to-stone distance in predicting successful shock wave lithotripsy of renal and ureteric calculi. Urol Res 2010;38(4):307–13.
26. El-Nahas AR, El-Assmy AM, Mansour O, et al. A prospective multivariate analysis of factors predicting stone disintegration by extracorporeal shock wave lithotripsy: the value of high-resolution noncontrast computed tomography. Eur Urol 2007;51(6): 1688–93 [discussion: 1693–4].
27. Pareek G, Hedican SP, Lee FT Jr, et al. Shock wave lithotripsy success determined by skin-to-stone distance on computed tomography. Urology 2005; 66(5):941–4.
28. Perks AE, Schuler TD, Lee J, et al. Stone attenuation and skin-to-stone distance on computed tomography predicts for stone fragmentation by shock wave lithotripsy. Urology 2008;72(4):765–9.
29. Patel T, Kozakowski K, Hruby G, et al. Skin to stone distance is an independent predictor of stone-free status following shockwave lithotripsy. J Endourol 2009;23(9):1383–5.
30. Pishchalnikov YA, Neucks JS, Vonderhaar RJ, et al. Air pockets trapped during routine coupling in dry head lithotripsy can significantly decrease the delivery of shock wave energy. J Urol 2006;176(6 Pt 1):2706–10.
31. Jain A, Shah TK. Effect of air bubbles in the coupling medium on efficacy of extracorporeal shock wave lithotripsy. Eur Urol 2007;51(6):1680–6 [discussion: 1686–7].
32. Bergsdorf T, Chaussy C, Turoff S. Energy coupling in extracorporeal shock wave lithotripsy-the impact of coupling quality on disintegration efficacy. J Endourol 2008;22(Suppl):A161.
33. Neucks JS, Pishchalnikov YA, Zancanaro AJ, et al. Improved acoustic coupling for shock wave lithotripsy. Urol Res 2008;36(1):61–6.

34. Paterson RF, Lifshitz DA, Lingeman JE, et al. Stone fragmentation during shock wave lithotripsy is improved by slowing the shock wave rate: studies with a new animal model. J Urol 2002;168(5):2211–5.
35. Semins MJ, Trock BJ, Matlaga BR. The effect of shock wave rate on the outcome of shock wave lithotripsy: a meta-analysis. J Urol 2008;179(1):194–7 [discussion: 197].
36. Pace KT, Ghiculete D, Harju M, et al. Shock wave lithotripsy at 60 or 120 shocks per minute: a randomized, double-blind trial. J Urol 2005;174(2):595–9.
37. Madbouly K, El-Tiraifi AM, Seida M, et al. Slow versus fast shock wave lithotripsy rate for urolithiasis: a prospective randomized study. J Urol 2005;173(1): 127–30.
38. Yilmaz E, Batislam E, Basar M, et al. Optimal frequency in extracorporeal shock wave lithotripsy: prospective randomized study. Urology 2005;66(6): 1160–4.
39. Evan AP, Mcateer JA, Connors BA, et al. Renal injury during shock wave lithotripsy is significantly reduced by slowing the rate of shock wave delivery. BJU Int 2007;100(3):624–7 [discussion: 627–8].
40. Connors BA, Evan AP, Blomgren PM, et al. Extracorporeal shock wave lithotripsy at 60 shock waves/min reduces renal injury in a porcine model. BJU Int 2009;104(7):1004–8.
41. Pishchalnikov YA, Mcateer JA, Williams JC Jr. Effect of firing rate on the performance of shock wave lithotriptors. BJU Int 2008;102(11):1681–6.
42. Zhou Y, Cocks FH, Preminger GM, et al. The effect of treatment strategy on stone comminution efficiency in shock wave lithotripsy. J Urol 2004;172(1):349–54.
43. Maloney ME, Marguet CG, Zhou Y, et al. Progressive increase of lithotripter output produces better in-vivo stone comminution. J Endourol 2006;20(9):603–6.
44. Demirci D, Sofikerim M, Yalcin E, et al. Comparison of conventional and step-wise shockwave lithotripsy in management of urinary calculi. J Endourol 2007; 21(12):1407–10.
45. Willis LR, Evan AP, Connors BA, et al. Prevention of lithotripsy-induced renal injury by pretreating kidneys with low-energy shock waves. J Am Soc Nephrol 2006;17(3):663–73.
46. Handa RK, Bailey MR, Paun M, et al. Pretreatment with low-energy shock waves induces renal vasoconstriction during standard shock wave lithotripsy (SWL): a treatment protocol known to reduce SWL-induced renal injury. BJU Int 2009; 103(9):1270–4.
47. Connors BA, Evan AP, Blomgren PM, et al. Effect of initial shock wave voltage on shock wave lithotripsy-induced lesion size during step-wise voltage ramping. BJU Int 2009;103(1):104–7.
48. Handa RK, Mcateer JA, Connors BA, et al. Optimising an escalating shockwave amplitude treatment strategy to protect the kidney from injury during shockwave lithotripsy. BJU Int 2012. http://dx.doi.org/10.1111/j.1464-410X.2012.11207.x.
49. Pishchalnikov YA, Vonderhaar RJ, Williams JC Jr, et al. The advantage of a broad focal zone in SWL: in vitro stone breakage comparing two electromagnetic lithotripters. J Urol 2008;179:464–5.
50. Cleveland RO, Mcateer JA. The physics of shock wave lithotripsy. In: Smith AD, Badlani GH, Bagley DH, et al, editors. Smith's textbook on endourology. Hamilton (Ontario): BC Decker, Inc; 2007. p. 317–32.
51. Cleveland RO, Anglade R, Babayan RK. Effect of stone motion on in vitro comminution efficiency of Storz Modulith SLX. J Endourol 2004;18(7):629–33.
52. Cleveland RO, Sapozhnikov OA. Modeling elastic wave propagation in kidney stones with application to shock wave lithotripsy. J Acoust Soc Am 2005; 118(4):2667–76.
53. Sapozhnikov OA, Maxwell AD, Macconaghy B, et al. A mechanistic analysis of stone fracture in lithotripsy. J Acoust Soc Am 2007;121(2):1190–202.
54. Tan EC, Tung KH, Foo KT. Comparative studies of extracorporeal shock wave lithotripsy by Dornier HM3, EDAP LT 01 and Sonolith 2000 devices. J Urol 1991;146(2):294–7.
55. Ueda S, Matsuoka K, Yamashita T, et al. Perirenal hematomas caused by SWL with EDAP LT-01 lithotripter. J Endourol 1993;7(1):11–5.
56. Fuselier HA, Prats L, Fontenot C, et al. Comparison of mobile lithotripters at one institution: healthtronics lithotron, Dornier MFL-5000, and Dornier Doli. J Endourol 1999;13(8):539–42.
57. Graber SF, Danuser H, Hochreiter WW, et al. A prospective randomized trial comparing 2 lithotriptors for stone disintegration and induced renal trauma. J Urol 2003;169(1):54–7.
58. Gerber R, Studer UE, Danuser H. Is newer always better? A comparative study of 3 lithotriptor generations. J Urol 2005;173(6):2013–6.
59. Evan AP, Mcateer JA, Connors BA, et al. Independent assessment of a wide-focus, low-pressure electromagnetic lithotripter: absence of renal bioeffects in the pig. BJU Int 2008;101(3):382–8.
60. Mcateer JA, Pishchalnikov YA, Vonderhaar JN, et al. Independent evaluation of the LithoGold LG-380 lithotripter: invitro acoustic characteristics and assessment of renal injury in the pig model. J Urol 2009; 181(Suppl 4):665–6.
61. Xi X, Zhong P. Improvement of stone fragmentation during shock-wave lithotripsy using a combined EH/PEAA shock-wave generator-in vitro experiments. Ultrasound Med Biol 2000;26(3):457–67.
62. Zhou Y, Cocks FH, Preminger GM, et al. Innovations in shock wave lithotripsy technology: updates in experimental studies. J Urol 2004;172(5 Pt 1):1892–8.
63. Weizer AZ, Zhong P, Preminger GM. New concepts in shock wave lithotripsy. Urol Clin North Am 2007; 34(3):375–82.

64. Fernandez F, Fernandez G, Loske AM. Treatment time reduction using tandem shockwaves for lithotripsy: an in vivo study. J Endourol 2009;23(8): 1247–53.
65. Sokolov DL, Bailey MR, Crum LA. Use of a dual-pulse lithotripter to generate a localized and intensified cavitation field. J Acoust Soc Am 2001;110(3 Pt 1):1685–95.
66. Sokolov DL, Bailey MR, Crum LA. Dual-pulse lithotripter accelerates stone fragmentation and reduces cell lysis in vitro. Ultrasound Med Biol 2003;29(7): 1045–52.
67. Handa RK, Mcateer JA, Evan AP, et al. Assessment of renal injury with a clinical dual head lithotriptor delivering 240 shock waves per minute. J Urol 2009;181(2):884–9.
68. Sheir KZ, Elhalwagy SM, Abo-Elghar ME, et al. Evaluation of a synchronous twin-pulse technique for shock wave lithotripsy: a prospective randomized study of effectiveness and safety in comparison to standard single-pulse technique. BJU Int 2008; 101(11):1420–6.
69. Owen NR, Bailey MR, Crum LA, et al. The use of resonant scattering to identify stone fracture in shock wave lithotripsy. J Acoust Soc Am 2007; 121(1):EL41–7.
70. Orkisz M, Farchtchian T, Saighi D, et al. Image based renal stone tracking to improve efficacy in extracorporeal lithotripsy. J Urol 1998;160(4):1237–40.
71. Chang CC, Liang SM, Pu YR, et al. In vitro study of ultrasound based real-time tracking of renal stones for shock wave lithotripsy: Part 1. J Urol 2001; 166(1):28–32.
72. Bohris C, Bayer T, Lechner C. Hit/Miss monitoring of ESWL by spectral Doppler ultrasound. Ultrasound Med Biol 2003;29(5):705–12.
73. Chiong E, Hwee ST, Kay LM, et al. Randomized controlled study of mechanical percussion, diuresis, and inversion therapy to assist passage of lower pole renal calculi after shock wave lithotripsy. Urology 2005;65(6):1070–4.
74. Kekre NS, Kumar S. Optimizing the fragmentation and clearance after shock wave lithotripsy. Curr Opin Urol 2008;18(2):205–9.
75. Pace KT, Tariq N, Dyer SJ, et al. Mechanical percussion, inversion and diuresis for residual lower pole fragments after shock wave lithotripsy: a prospective, single blind, randomized controlled trial. J Urol 2001;166(6):2065–71.
76. Shah A, Harper JD, Cunitz BW, et al. Focused ultrasound to expel calculi from the kidney. J Urol 2012; 187(2):739–43.

Advances in Ureteroscopy

Michael S. Borofsky, MD[a], Ojas Shah, MD[b,*]

KEYWORDS

• Ureteroscopy • Endourology • Laser • Lithotripsy • Stone • Basket • Technology • Advances

KEY POINTS

- Several digital ureteroscopes have been introduced over the past few years.
  - Benefits of digital ureteroscopes include larger, clearer images with a decreased need for accessory equipment.
  - Disadvantages include a larger tip diameter and increased baseline cost.
- Holmium laser lithotripsy remains the most common method of stone fragmentation during ureteroscopy, and there are increasing efforts in adapting technology to prevent laser damage to the scope.
- Hybrid guidewires are the most popular guidewires, yet several types are available with different indications for use depending on the scenario.
- Nitinol stone baskets have replaced stainless steel ones and they are now available at very small sizes as thin as 1.3F.
- Numerous antiretropulsion devices are now available, each with novel methods of preventing proximal stone migration during ureteroscopy and lithotripsy.

INTRODUCTION

Over the past 3 decades, endourology has undergone a remarkable evolution with the advent and incorporation of new technologies. The development of smaller, more flexible ureteroscopes, higher-definition cameras, and a wide variety of novel instruments have changed the role of the field from one of diagnostics to one of treatment. In this review, the authors highlight the latest technologic achievements in ureteroscopy.

FLEXIBLE URETEROSCOPES

Advancements in flexible ureteroscopes have had perhaps the greatest impact in changing endourology. Smaller sizes and increased capabilities in terms of optics, deflection, and instrumentation have now made it possible to access the entirety of the urinary tract. The rate of technologic improvement in this field has been staggering, with new ureteroscopes introduced each year (**Table 1**). Representations of the deflection characteristics and tip appearances of some of the newer flexible ureteroscopes can be seen in **Figs. 1** and **2**.

One of the most significant changes has been a change from fiberoptic to digital imaging. This change has been made possible through the advancement and miniaturization of the charge couple device and complementary metal oxide semiconductor image sensors. These chips are now small enough to be directly incorporated at the tip of the ureteroscope creating the so-called *chip on the stick* scope. Such technology eliminates the need for internal optics within the shaft of the scope potentially allowing for more durable

Funding: None.
Disclosures: Ojas Shah, MD, Consultant for Boston Scientific and Cook Inc.
[a] Department of Urology, NYU Langone Medical Center, New York University School of Medicine, 150 East 32nd Street, 2nd Floor, New York, NY 10016, USA; [b] Division of Endourology and Stone Disease, Department of Urology, NYU Langone Medical Center, New York University School of Medicine, 150 East 32nd Street, 2nd Floor, New York, NY 10016, USA
* Corresponding author.
E-mail address: Ojas.Shah@nyumc.org

Urol Clin N Am 40 (2013) 67–78
http://dx.doi.org/10.1016/j.ucl.2012.09.009

Table 1
Currently available flexible ureteroscope models

Manufacturer	Model	Digital	Tip Diameter (F)	Proximal Diameter (F)	Channel Size (F)	Deflection (Up/Down) (Degrees)	Length (cm)
Karl Storz (Tuttlingen, Germany)	Flex- X^2	No	7.5	8.5	3.6	270/270	67.5
Karl Storz	Flex-Xc	Yes	8.5	8.5	3.6	270/270	70
Olympus (Tokyo, Japan)	URF-P5	No	5.4	8.4	3.6	180/275	70
Olympus	URF-V	Yes	8.5	9.9	3.6	180/275	67
Olympus Gyrus ACMI (Southborough, Massachusetts)	DUR-8E	No	6.75	10.81	3.6	170/180	64
Olympus Gyrus ACMI	DUR-D	Yes	87.0	9.3	3.6	250/250	65
Stryker (Stryker Inc, Portage, MI)	Flexvision U-500	No	6.9	—	3.6	275/275	64
Wolf (Richard Wolf, Knittlington, Germany)	Viper	No	6.0	8.8	3.6	270/270	68
Wolf	Cobra	—	6.0	9.9	3.3	270/270	68

deflection mechanisms and equipment overall.[1] An additional advantage is eliminating the need for several pieces of equipment, including a separate camera; camera cord; light source or light cord; and several cumbersome steps, such as focusing and white balancing.[2] Furthermore, without the need for fiberoptic bundles within the shaft, larger working channels can be used.[3] Although

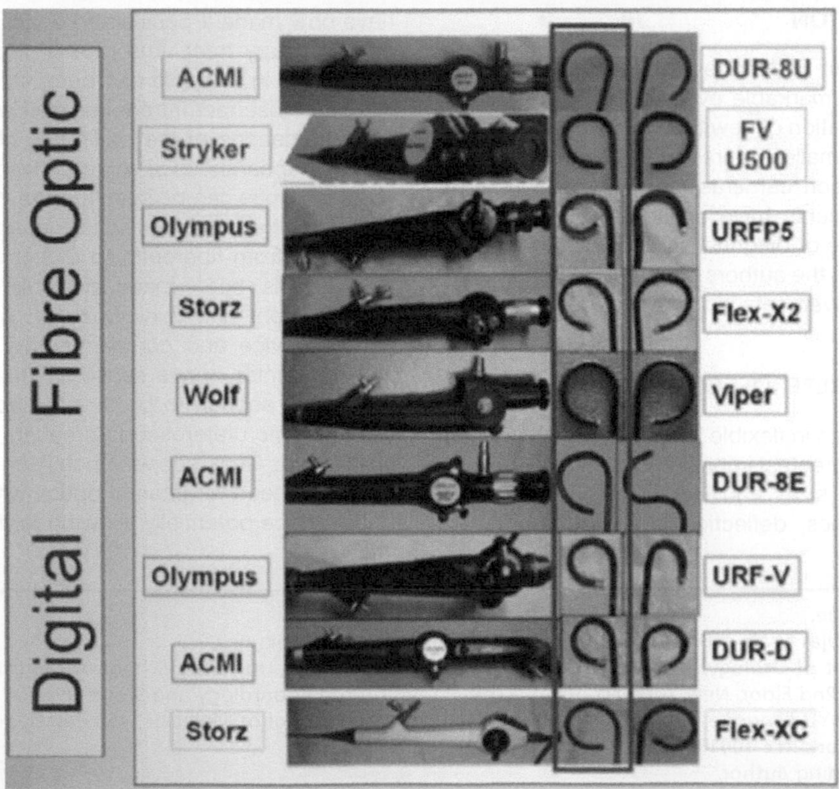

Fig. 1. Deflection characteristics of currently available flexible ureteroscopes. (*From* Traxer O. Digital and video flexible ureterorenoscopes: the future is now. AUA News 2012;17(7):1–9; with permission.)

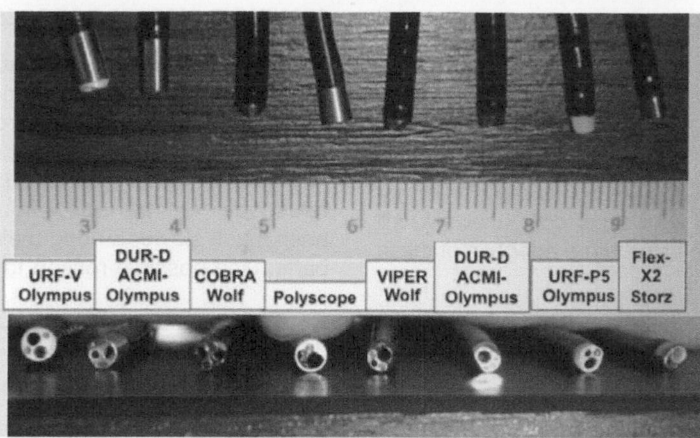

Fig. 2. Distal tips of currently available flexible ureteroscopes. (*From* Traxer O. Digital and video flexible ureterorenoscopes: the future is now. AUA News 2012;17(7):1–9; with permission.)

promising, the improvements do come at the expense of a larger-tip diameter, generally 8F or greater, making passage into narrow areas slightly more challenging. Additionally, the use of these scopes occasionally requires prestenting the ureter, ureteral balloon dilation, or the concomitant use of a ureteral access sheath to obtain access.

The image obtained with a digital scope is generally larger and clearer than that obtained with traditional fiberoptic scopes. Additionally, there is no honeycomb/pixelation pattern (Moiré effect) on the screen (**Fig. 3**). The first flexible digital ureteroscope was introduced in 2007. This scope, the DUR-D (Gyrus ACMI, Southborough, Massachusetts) has been estimated to have an increased image size up to 150% larger than its fiberoptic counterparts.[4] When compared with the Storz Flex X[2] (Karl Storz, Tuttlingen, Germany) fiberoptic flexible ureteroscope, it was associated with a faster stone fragmentation rate and corresponding decrease in total operative time.[5] The next digital scope to be introduced was the Olympus URF-V (Olympus Corporation, Tokyo, Japan) flexible digital ureteroscope in 2008. When compared with its fiberoptic counterpart, the Olympus URF-P5, it was found to have a higher resolution at a variety of distances and created an image size 5.3 times as large.[6] Multescu and colleagues[7] also compared this scope with the Storz Flex X flexible fiberoptic ureteroscope, and they found that the digital scope had more difficulty accessing narrow infundibula 4 mm or less in width. They did, however, find the digital scope to be superior in terms of visibility, maneuverability, and loss of deflection after repeated use. The most recent of the flexible digital ureteroscopes is the Storz Flex-Xc, which is the smallest digital ureteroscope on the market at 8.5F but has not yet been compared with a fiberoptic counterpart. It is not available in the United States at the time of this article; however, it is being used in several European countries.[8]

Although these newer digital scopes are more expensive than their fiberoptic predecessors, proposed improvements in durability may ultimately

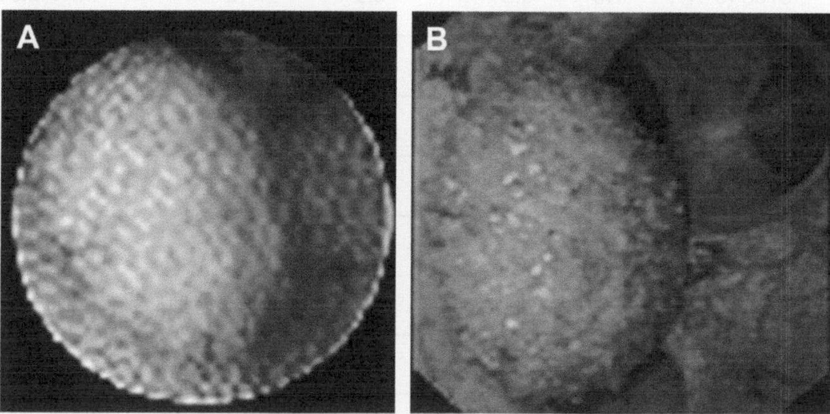

Fig. 3. Comparison of conventional fiberoptic ureteroscopic image[59] (*A*) versus digital ureteroscopic image using URF-V (*B*). (Olympus Corporation, Tokyo, Japan.)

offset differences in price. Knudsen and colleagues[9] analyzed scope durability among 4 of the most recent fiberoptic flexible ureteroscopes and found a mean range of 5.3 to 18.0 cases until the need for repair. With typical repair costs estimated between $3000 and $6000, the need for improved durability cannot be overemphasized.[10] Further comparative studies as well as cost analyses will likely play a large role in the future adoption of these scopes.

SEMIRIGID URETEROSCOPES

Semirigid ureteroscopes (**Table 2**) have had a slower evolution in terms of technologic improvement relative to flexible ureteroscopes but remain the most commonly used type of scope for access to the upper urinary tract.[11] Unlike in flexible ureteroscopy, the transition to digital scopes has been much slower among their semirigid counterparts. One possible reason to explain this slower

Table 2
Currently available semirigid ureteroscope models

Manufacturer	Model	Digital	Tip Diameter (F)	Proximal Diameter (F)	Number of Channels	Channel Size (F)	Length (cm)
Karl Storz	27001 K/L	No	7.0	13.5	1	5.0	34, 43
Karl Storz	27002 K/L	No	8.0	13.5	1	5.0	34, 43
Karl Storz	27003 K/L	No	9.0	15.0	1	5.0	34, 43
Karl Storz	27010 K/L	No	7.0	9.9	1	3.4	34, 43
Karl Storz	27011 K/L	No	7.0	13.5	1	5.0	34, 43
Karl Storz	27012 K/L	No	8.0	13.5	1	6.0	34, 43
Karl Storz	27014 K/L	No	9.0	15.0	1	5.0	34, 43
Olympus	OES Pro Single	No	6.4	7.8	1	4.2	33, 43
Olympus	OES 4000 Double	No	7.5	7.5	2	3.4 + 2.4	33, 43
Olympus	Pro Video	Yes	8.5	9.9	1	4.2	43
Olympus Gyrus ACMI	MR-6A Bagley	Yes	6.9	10.2	2	3.4 + 2.3	33, 41
Olympus Gyrus ACMI	MRO-733A	No	7.7	10.8	1	5.4	33
Olympus Gyrus ACMI	MRO-742-A	No	7.0	11.2	1	5.4	42
Stryker	SRU-6X	No	6.9	10.0	2	3.4 + 2.5	33, 43
Wolf	8702 (0.517, 0.518)	No	6.0	7.5	1	4.0	33, 43
Wolf	8703 (0.517, 0.518)	No	8.0	9.8	1	5.0	33, 43
Wolf	8708 (0.517, 0.518)	No	6.5	8.5	2	4.2 + 2.55	33, 43
Wolf	8702 (0.523, 0.524)	No	6.0	7.5	1	4.0	31.5, 43.0
Wolf	8703 (0.523, 0.524)	No	8.0	9.8	1	5.0	31.5, 43.0
Wolf	8704 (0.523, 0.524)	No	8.5	11.5	1	6.0	31.5, 43.0
Wolf	8701 (0.533, 0.534)	No	4.5	6.5	1	3.0	31.5, 43.0
Wolf	8702 (0.533, 0.544)	No	6.0	7.5	1	4.0	31.5, 43.0
Wolf	8703 (0.533, 0.534)	No	8.0	9.8	1	5.0	31.5, 43.0
Wolf	8708 (0.533, 0.534)	No	6.5	8.5	2	4.2 + 2.55	31.5, 43.0

adoption is the fact that the rigid shaft design allows for an increased density of fiberoptic bundles, which in turn allows for decreased image degradation[12] Currently there is only one major manufacturer of ureteroscopes that sells a digital semirigid instrument, the Olympus Pro Video scope (also known as the EndoEye ureteroscope). Image properties obtained with a digital scope are favorable. One previous study found that the image size was approximately 2.5 times greater with a digital semirigid scope. One downside, however, is that the current tip diameter is relatively large (8.5F/9.9F) compared with the fiberoptic versions.[2,13] Multescu and colleagues[14] examined the performance of the Olympus EndoEYE compared with a traditional fiberoptic semirigid ureteroscope and graded visibility and maneuverablity on a 5-point scale after each case that it was used. Overall, the digital scope had improved visibility (4.5 vs 3.5) but poorer maneuverability (3.93 vs 4.57) when the patient was not prestented. Furthermore, there was a lower success rate without prestenting among the cases where the digital scope was used (84% vs 98%). Decreasing the diameter of the scope is, thus, the logical next step in the evolution of this equipment and will likely be the rate-limiting step before widespread adoption of this technology is seen.

ADVANCED IMAGE SETTINGS

The introduction of high-definition cameras and video has brought visualization capabilities in ureteroscopy to an all-time high; however, there are several other advanced imaging technologies on the horizon. One is the use of narrow band imaging (NBI). NBI, developed by Olympus, is proposed to facilitate the detection of urothelial tumors. This technology works by enhancing the color contrast of increased vascular patterns caused by angiogenesis in tumor formation. In NBI, two wavelengths of light, 415 nm (blue) and 540 nm (green), are used to illuminate tissue. These wavelengths of light are strongly absorbed by hemoglobin, making tissue with increased vascularity (tumors) appear dark relative to surrounding normal mucosa (**Fig. 4**).[15] Currently, the only ureteroscope to offer such capabilities is the Olympus URF-V. To date, only one published study has investigated the clinical utility of using NBI in the diagnosis of upper tract urothelial carcinoma, though results were promising with an improved tumor detection relative to white light imaging by approximately 23%.[16]

Another advancement to expect in the next several years is the application of 3-dimensional technology. The use of 3-dimensional vision has been shown to enhance surgeon performance in laparoscopic and robotic settings,[17] and the application to endoscopy would be a logical next step.

Virtual endoscopy is yet another technology that is currently being developed. The idea for this is that the combination of ureteroscopy and computer-engineered software might help construct a reliable, 3-dimensional image of the ureteral anatomy. This technology might help identify tumors and could play a useful role in the surveillance of upper tract urothelial carcinomas; however, this technology is currently in its early infancy.[18,19]

Finally, in 2011, a pilot study was performed demonstrating the use and efficacy of robotic flexible ureteroscopy. This platform was converted from a robotic console designed for intracardiac applications but modified for use in ureteroscopy (**Fig. 5**). Eighteen patients were successfully treated with this method. Benefits mentioned by

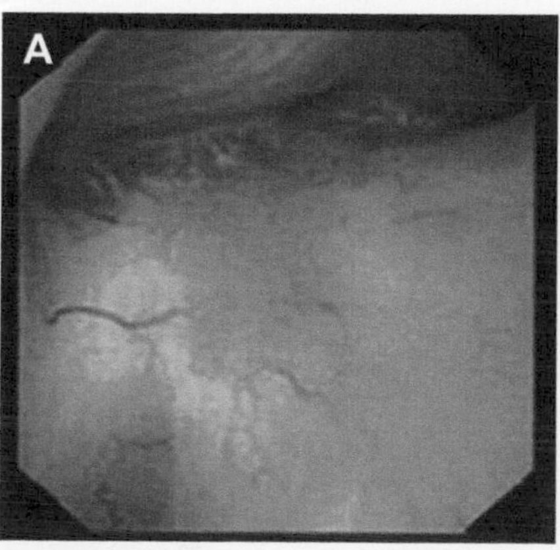

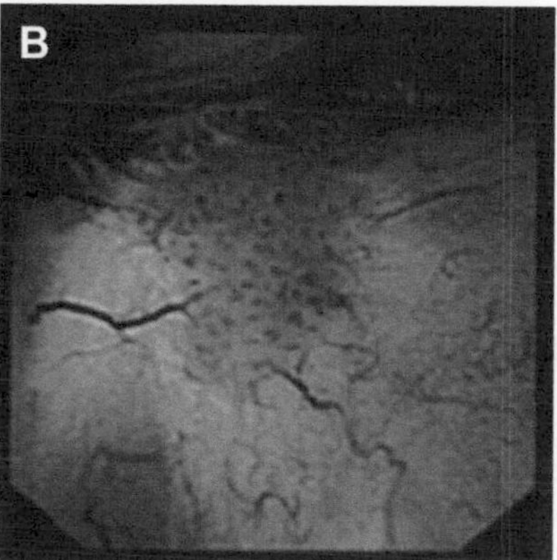

Fig. 4. Appearance of upper tract urothelial tumor during digital ureteroscopy using conventional white light (*A*) and Narrow-Band Imaging (*B*). (*From* Traxer O, Geavlete B, de Medina SG, et al. Narrowband imaging digital flexible ureteroscopy in detection of upper urinary tract transitional-cell carcinoma: initial experience. J Endourol 2011;25(1):19–23; with permission.)

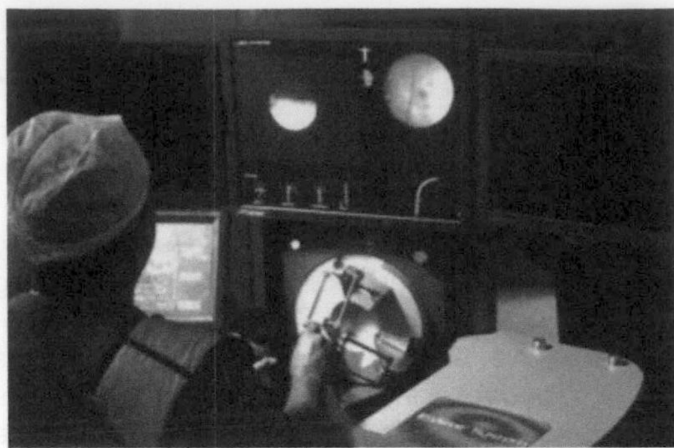

Fig. 5. Robotic flexible ureteroscopy.[20]

the investigators included the ergonomic advantage of being seated and using the robotic console as well as the ability to scale and fine tune motion to a very small degree based on stone fragment size. Disadvantages included the large size of the robotic sheath (14F), which required prestenting in all cases, and the procedure being quite cumbersome in its infancy.[20] Time will tell whether there is a role and benefit to this technique.

LITHOTRIPSY DEVICES

Numerous lithotriptors have been previously used for the purpose of stone fragmentation, including electrohydraulic (EHL), pneumatic, and ultrasonic. Lasers, however, are by far and away the most commonly used intracorporeal lithotripsy devices. Their use for this purpose was initially described in 1987[21]; and in the time since, they have revolutionized endourology. Currently, the holmium:yttrium-aluminum-garnet (Ho:YAG) laser is the most commonly used laser for lithotripsy[22] because of its superior complication and stone-free rates compared with pneumatic[23] and EHL[24] lithotriptors. The Ho:YAG laser works via the creation of laser pulse energy, which is absorbed by the targeted structure causing destruction.[25] The advantages of the Ho:YAG laser over other lasers are its ability to fragment stones of essentially all compositions[26] with minimal retropulsion[27] and surrounding tissue damage. It has been estimated that the absorption depth of this laser is as low as 0.4 mm.[22] Additionally, it has been shown to achieve smaller stone fragments than other lasers or lithotripsy devices, maximizing the likelihood of stone passage.[28]

It is likely that in the coming years there will be new lasers available on the market. The most likely candidates are the erbium:YAG (Er:YAG) fiber and the thulium laser fiber.[29] The potential benefit of the Er:YAG laser is a higher high-temperature water absorption coefficient, which has been shown to correspond with a 2 to 3 times increased stone fragmentation efficiency in vitro.[30] However, this laser requires a less flexible, more expensive midinfrared fiber that has limited its clinical applicability compared with the silica fibers used with the Ho:YAG laser.[29] Another laser that has been investigated for use in lithotripsy is the thulium laser, which also has a higher high-temperature water absorption coefficient and has been found to achieve stone vaporization rates 5 to 10 times higher than the Ho:YAG laser.[31] Additional clinical trials using these novel lasers for the purpose of lithotripsy will be necessary before determining their clinical utility. For the time being, they are not available in the United States.

One of the few challenges when using a Ho:YAG laser is that the size of the laser can decrease the scope flexion. The 365-μm laser fibers have been estimated to lead to a loss of 24° to 45°, whereas the 200-μm laser fiber has been estimated to lead to a loss of 9° to 19°.[32,33] Several companies manufacture a 150-μm laser fiber, which has been shown to be the most flexible of the currently available laser fibers[34]; and it is possible that even smaller laser fibers will be created. The authors recommend using a 365-μm–type fiber when using a rigid ureteroscope and a 200-μm–type or smaller fiber when using a flexible ureteroscope. The 200-μm fiber allows better deflection, thereby allowing better access to the upper urinary tract. It also likely leads to better durability of the scope by decreasing stress on the deflection mechanisms. However, the 200-μm fiber can have more burn back (or degradation) of the fiber, especially when treating a harder and/or larger stone burden. The larger fibers work well in the rigid ureteroscopes because the working channels are also more capacious, which allows better irrigation flow.

Another potential limitation in using lasers is the potential for scope damage with the introduction of the laser fiber or accidental activation of the fiber when it is still within the scope. Durak and colleagues[35] evaluated the utility of a protective laser sheath called the Flexguard (Lisa Laser Products, Katlenburg-Lindau, Germany), which they found was able to decrease the amount of force necessary to insert the fiber through the working channel. However, it was unable to protect the scope from laser damage and additionally led to a loss in deflection capability and irrigant flow rate. One subsequent study, however, demonstrated that this device reduced mechanical damage to the flexible ureteroscope after approximately 40 to 50 uses.[36]

Another device meant to address the potential for laser damage to the ureteroscope is the endoscope protection system (EPS) (Gyrus ACMI,

Southborough, Massachusetts) available with the DUR-D flexible ureteroscope. The EPS works by immediately terminating holmium laser energy when it is drawn back into the ureteroscope. In vitro, it was shown to successfully shut down the laser 120 out of 120 times with retraction.[37] In 20 cases whereby the EPS was used in vivo, the system shut down the laser in 50% of the cases when the laser was still safely outside the scope, likely from stone fragments or dust interfering with detection capability. However, the EPS was successful in shutting down the laser in all 80 attempts made at different speeds to retract the active laser into the scope.[38]

Another method of protecting the inner channel of the flexible ureteroscope and laser fiber tip is by only advancing the laser through the tip of the scope when the scope is not deflected (at the zero degree position). Acknowledging the potential for scope damage when a laser is inserted through a deflected scope tip, Boston Scientific (Natick, Massachusetts) has recently released the TracTip fiber, which is a 200-μm fiber with a ball tip that allows the fiber to be advanced while the scope is deflected because the ball tip can likely protect damage to the inner channel.

Finally, although lasers have recently dominated the market, pneumatic lithotripters may be making a return. The LMA StoneBreaker (Cook Inc, Bloomington, Indiana) is a high-powered single-pulse pneumatic lithotripter that causes stone fragmentation via direct contact. It is powered by carbon dioxide gas cartridges. Nerli and colleagues[39] used it to treat ureteral stones in 110 cases and found a mean number of only 8 shocks necessary to fully fragment the stone into sizes suitable for clearance. There were no complications or subjective ureteral trauma in any case. Benefits of this device are the fact that it is reusable and relatively inexpensive, with an estimated cost of less than $5 per carbon dioxide cartridge. It was recently compared with the Ho:YAG laser for use with rigid ureteroscopy for distal ureteral stones in a randomized controlled study, with no differences seen for operative time, complication rate, or stone-free rate.[40]

ACCESSORY INSTRUMENTS

Guidewires

A wide variety of accessory instruments have been introduced over the past several years with the intent of improving the ease and ability to treat stones. Guidewires remain critical in gaining access to the upper tracts. Although several different guidewires exist commercially, each has its unique advantages. Clayman and colleagues[41] found that the Glidewire (Boston Scientific) is the safest owing to increased flexibility and a tendency to bend when a point of obstruction is encountered. They also demonstrated that the Amplatz super stiff wires (Boston Scientific, Applied Medical [Rancho Santa Margarita, California]) were the most resistant to bending and were the best choice for passing instruments.

The current trend in guidewires has been the introduction and widespread adoption of the hybrid guidewire. These wires offer the advantage of hydrophilic distal tips ideal for bypassing obstructing stones as well as a stiff body optimized to maintain rigidity and to allow for the passage of instruments.[3] A recent comparison of 2 commonly used hybrid wires, the U-Nite (Bard Medical, Covington, Georgia) and Sensor (Boston Scientific), found that the Sensor wire had a greater friction force, potentially indicating it as a better choice for use as a safety wire because of its decreased likelihood of accidentally being pulled out. The Sensor wire was also found to have a more flexible tip, potentially indicating that it would be a better choice to maneuver around obstructing stones. The U-Nite, on the other hand, was found to have a rounder tip under electron microscopy, potentially meaning it is less likely to cause urothelial injury, such as submucosal tunneling.[42]

URETERAL ACCESS SHEATHS

The last several years have also brought about several conceptual changes in terms of access sheaths. Although conventional wisdom used to be that the larger the access sheath, the greater the flow, a recent study by Ng and colleagues[43] found minimal differences between a variety of different-sized access sheaths (10F to 16F) when the working channel was occupied. The same group introduced 2 novel configurations that did improve flow dynamics. In one configuration, they used a 4F ureteral access catheter solely for irrigation inflow adjacent to a 10F access sheath; in the other, they used a 5F ureteral access catheter within a 16F sheath. They found that these two configurations created the highest flow rates. Meanwhile, the potential for ureteral injury when an access sheath is used may be higher than previously thought. Traxer and colleagues[44] recently evaluated 136 patients who had ureteral access sheaths used during retrograde intrarenal stenting. They found some degree of ureteral wall injury estimated in approximately 50% of all cases, though these numbers were significantly lower among patients who were prestented, raising consideration that a routine ureteral access sheath may not be ideal.

STONE RETRIEVAL DEVICES

In terms of stone retrieval devices, nitinol baskets have essentially replaced stainless steel baskets completely owing to improved memory and increased flexibility with less resulting loss of scope deflection.[45] Today there are a wide variety of commercially available nitinol stone baskets (**Table 3**). The most recent generations of baskets are available in small sizes, often less than 1.5F, with the goal of preserving maximum irrigation during procedures. Korman and colleagues compared 3 of the smaller baskets on the market, including the Boston Scientific Optiflex (1.3F), Cook N-Circle (Cook Inc, Bloomington, IN) (1.5F), and Sacred Heart Medical Halo (1.5F) (Sacred Heart Medical Inc, Minnetonka, Minnesota) in a series of studies. Of the 3, they found the Sacred Heart basket to have the greatest radial dilating force and led to the fastest stone extraction times when tested in a ureteral model.[46,47] The Optiflex was associated with significantly slower extraction times. Magheli and colleagues[48] later compared the same 3 baskets; in this case, they found that the 1.3F Optiflex led to a significantly decreased loss of deflection and increased flow rate relative to the two other 1.5F devices.

Aside from smaller sizes, there have been several other unique basket designs recently introduced. The Escape basket (Boston Scientific) allows for simultaneous laser lithotripsy with a 200-μm holmium laser fiber via an inner channel within the basket wiring while the stone is held in the basket. Although this basket has been demonstrated to be both safe and effective in vivo,[49] there are currently no published studies comparing its use with other available stone baskets. Another is the N-Gage basket (Cook Inc, Bloomington, IN) whose design combines the entrapment capabilities of traditional baskets with the superior release capabilities of pronged graspers. The improved ability to easily release the stone helps optimize the surgeon's ability to reposition the stones into the upper pole where lasering is potentially more efficacious. Simultaneously, this basket's improved catch-and-release properties decrease the likelihood of stones becoming trapped in the device, thereby potentially preventing ureteral injury.

One of the remaining problems with retrieval baskets in general is that the number of times they need to be used in a single case to achieve true stone-free status can be cumbersome. To address this, Tan and colleagues[50] recently investigated a method of magnetizing calcium stone particles using paramagnetic microparticles with the intention of attracting smaller fragments to a magnetic instrument. They then invented an 8F magnetic tool able to be back loaded through a standard flexible ureteroscope to the collecting system. Although there was no significant difference compared with using a nitinol stone basket, they did retrieve more small stones (1.5–2.0 mm in size) using the magnetic device.

ANTIRETROPULSION DEVICES

Antiretropulsion devices are another novel type of accessory instrument gaining popularity in the world of ureteroscopy. Proximal stone migration remains a bothersome occurrence in many lithotripsy cases; therefore, a variety of ureteral occlusion and antiretropulsion devices have been created (**Fig. 6**). Three of the studied devices include the Stone Cone (Boston Scientific), Accordion (Percutaneous Systems Inc, Palo Alto, California), and NTrap (Cook Inc, Bloomington, IN). The Stone Cone was the first to become commercially available. It consists of a nitinol wire coiled in the shape of a cone that is covered in a 3F polytetrafluoroethylene cover that can be inserted distal to the area of a stone and prevent proximal migration. It has previously been demonstrated to be both safe and effective. Eisner and Dretler[51] studied its use in 133 cases of ureteroscopy for ureteral stones and found evidence of only 2 retropulsed fragments greater than 2 mm in size. It has also been estimated to have a 20% increase in the stone-free rate compared with controls. The NTrap was the second antiretropulsion device made commercially available. It is a deployable wire mesh net created of tightly wound nitinol wires. A recent meta-analysis found that cases in which the NTrap device was used had threefold higher stone-free rates as well as a decreased need for auxiliary shockwave lithotripsy procedures than controls.[52] More recently, the Accordion device has been introduced. This device is comprised of a flexible polyurethane film that, when deployed, conforms to the ureter to prevent stone retropulsion. In vitro studies have demonstrated an excellent ability to prevent retropulsion as well as associated improvement in terms of fragmentation rate with its use.[53] Additionally, there is a suggestion that it may be a more durable device owing to the improved ability to withstand laser damage.[54] A recent in vivo study demonstrated improved fragmentation efficiency and stone clearance with a significant reduction in retrograde migration during fragmentation.[55] All 3 of these devices have the issue that the scope needs to be placed beside the device; therefore, they could be difficult to use in cases with a baseline narrow distal ureter.

Table 3
List and features of current nitinol stone retrieval baskets

Manufacturer	Model	Available Sizes (F)	Available Basket Sizes (mm)	Available Lengths (cm)	Features
Bard	Dimension	2.4, 3.0	10, 13, 16	115	Articulating basket, 4-wire design, zero tip
Bard	Expand212	3.0	11	90, 115	Articulating basket, 2-1-2-1 wire design, filiform tip
Boston Scientific	Escape	1.9	11, 15	90, 120	4-wire cage, 2-port adapter allows simultaneous use of 200-μm laser fiber
Boston Scientific	Optiflex	1.3	6, 7, 9, 11	90, 120	Able to articulate and rotate 360°, small size preserves irrigation and deflection
Boston Scientific	Zerotip	1.9, 2.4, 3.0	12, 16	90, 120	Zero tip allows atraumatic use adjacent to parenchyma
Cook	NCircle	2.4	10, 20	115	Triangular shape allows very large wire mass, tipless design
Cook	NForce	2.2, 3.2	—	115	3-wire basket with maximal radial dilating ability suited for ureteral opening
Cook	NGage	1.7, 2.2	8, 11	115	Suited for optimal engage and release to allow repositioning
Sacred Heart (Minnetonka, Minnesota)	Halo	1.5	12	90, 120	Tipless, small size maximizes deflection and flow
Sacred Heart	Vantage	2.4, 3.0	16	90, 120	
Sacred Heart	Paragon	2.4, 3.0	10	90, 120	2 single and 2 paired wire design optimizes radial force, ideal for ureteral stone capture
Sacred Heart	Apex	2.4	15	90, 120	Zero tip for atraumatic use

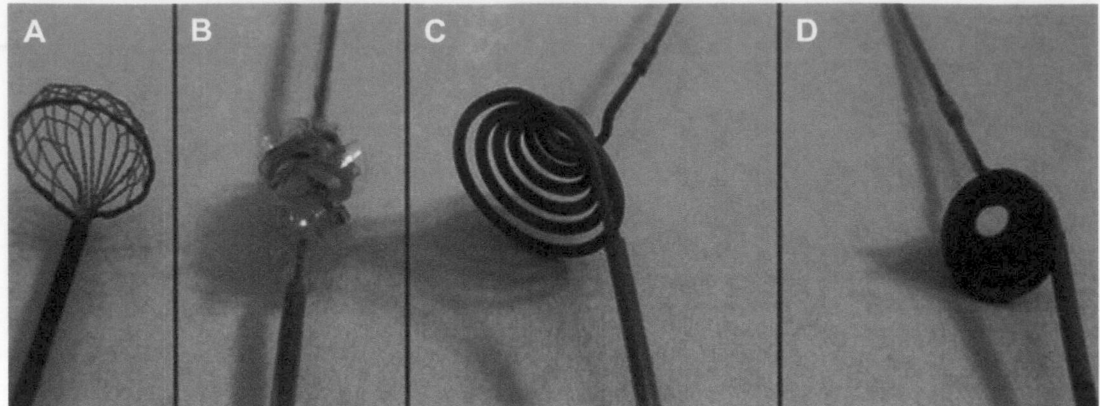

Fig. 6. Currently available antiretropulsion devices. (*A*) N-trap (Cook Inc, Bloomington, IN), (*B*) Accordion (Percutaneous Systems Inc. Palo Alto, CA), (*C & D*) Stone Cone 10 mm and 7 mm (Boston Scientific, Natick, MA).[57]

There are only a few studies available that have compared these devices with each other. Both the NTrap and Stone Cone were shown to have excellent ability of blocking proximal migration of fragments as small as 1.5 mm in a porcine model, although the NTrap was found to be capable of blocking even smaller fragments.[56] Ahmed and colleagues[57] compared the different physical characteristics of each device. Most importantly, the 3 devices seemed to be comparable and equally effective in terms of preventing stone migration. However, they did find that the Stone Cone required the most attempts and force to deploy, whereas the Accordion took the most time. The NTrap was found to have the greatest tip stiffness, potentially increasing the likelihood of ureteral injury; however, this difference was not statistically significant.

Two new devices have recently been introduced with unique features distinguishing them from the other available antiretropulsion devices currently on the market. The XenX (Xenolith Medical LTD, Kiryat-Gal, Israel) serves the dual purpose of both an occlusion device as well as a guidewire through which the surgeon is be able to place a stent at the end of the procedure. Although this device is not yet commercially available, early results have been promising. Sarkissian and colleagues[54] tested this device in a porcine model and found it to be comparable in terms of ease of passage to the NTrap and Stone Cone. They also found that the XenX was superior in terms of preventing stone migration in vitro. The other new device currently being marketed is Backstop (Boston Scientific). Backstop is a reverse thermosensitive water-soluble polymer that allows temporary occlusion of the desired segment of ureter. The polymer is applied using a small ureteral access catheter and can then be flushed away with irrigation of cold saline. The proposed benefit of Backstop is the fact that it does not require leaving a mechanical element in the ureter while operating that can potentially interfere with the procedure. To date, there has been only one published study analyzing outcomes of its use. Rane and colleagues[58] prospectively randomized 68 patients with solitary ureteral stones to either ureteroscopy or lithotripsy with or without Backstop. They found a statistically significant decrease rate of retropulsion in the Backstop group (8.8% vs 52.9%), with no adverse events in this group.

SUMMARY

Ureteroscopic technology continues to improve at a rapid pace. Recent advancements in both imaging equipment and instrumentation have not only improved the operator's ability to treat stone disease but have also led to improved outcomes. It is likely that the continued evolution of such technologies will continue to push the conventional limits of a retrograde treatment approach to the upper urinary tract.

REFERENCES

1. Afane JS, Olweny EO, Bercowsky E, et al. Flexible ureteroscopes: a single center evaluation of the durability and function of the new endoscopes smaller than 9Fr. J Urol 2000;164(4):1164–8.
2. Beiko DT, Denstedt JD. Advances in ureterorenoscopy. Urol Clin North Am 2007;34(3):397–408.
3. Khanna R, Monga M. Instrumentation in endourology. Ther Adv Urol 2011;3(3):119–26.
4. Andonian S, Okeke Z, Smith AD. Digital ureteroscopy: the next step. J Endourol 2008;22(4):603–6.
5. Binbay M, Yuruk E, Akman T, et al. Is there a difference in outcomes between digital and fiberoptic

flexible ureterorenoscopy procedures? J Endourol 2010;24(12):1929–34.
6. Zilberman DE, Lipkin ME, Ferrandino MN, et al. The digital flexible ureteroscope: in vitro assessment of optical characteristics. J Endourol 2011;25(3): 519–22.
7. Multescu R, Geavlete B, Georgescu D, et al. Conventional fiberoptic flexible ureteroscope versus fourth generation digital flexible ureteroscope: a critical comparison. J Endourol 2010;24(1):17–21.
8. Kruck S, Anastasiadis AG, Gakis G, et al. Flow matters: irrigation flow differs in flexible ureteroscopes of the newest generation. Urol Res 2011; 39(6):483–6.
9. Knudsen B, Miyaoka R, Shah K, et al. Durability of the next-generation flexible fiberoptic ureteroscopes: a randomized prospective multi-institutional clinical trial. Urology 2010;75(3):534–8.
10. Landman J, Lee DI, Lee C, et al. Evaluation of overall costs of currently available small flexible ureteroscopes. Urology 2003;62(2):218–22.
11. Krambeck AE, Murat FJ, Gettman MT, et al. The evolution of ureteroscopy: a modern single-institution series. Mayo Clin Proc 2006;81(4):468–73.
12. Smith AD. Smith's textbook of endourology. 3rd edition. Chichester (West Sussex): Wiley; 2012.
13. Springhart WP, Maloney M, Sur RL, et al. Digital video ureteroscope: a new paradigm in ureteroscopy. J Urol 2005;173(Suppl 4):428.
14. Multescu DR, Mirciulescu V, Gevlete B, et al. Digital semirigid ureteroscopy: a new standard in endoscopic imaging. Eur Urol 2009;(Suppl 8):686.
15. Jichlinski P, Lovisa B. High magnification cystoscopy in the primary diagnosis of bladder tumors. Curr Opin Urol 2011;21(5):398–402.
16. Traxer O, Geavlete B, de Medina SG, et al. Narrow-band imaging digital flexible ureteroscopy in detection of upper urinary tract transitional-cell carcinoma: initial experience. J Endourol 2011;25(1):19–23.
17. Wagner OJ, Hagen M, Kurmann A, et al. Three-dimensional vision enhances task performance independently of the surgical method. Surg Endosc 2012;26(10):2961–8.
18. Battista G, Sassi C, Schiavina R, et al. Computerized tomography virtual endoscopy in evaluation of upper urinary tract tumors: initial experience. Abdom Imaging 2009;34(1):107–12.
19. Natalin RA, Landman J. Where next for the endoscope? Nat Rev Urol 2009;6(11):622–8.
20. Desai MM, Grover R, Aron M, et al. Robotic flexible ureteroscopy for renal calculi: initial clinical experience. J Urol 2011;186(2):563–8.
21. Dretler SP, Watson G, Parrish JA, et al. Pulsed dye laser fragmentation of ureteral calculi: initial clinical experience. J Urol 1987;137(3):386–9.
22. Lee J, Gianduzzo TR. Advances in laser technology in urology. Urol Clin North Am 2009;36(2):189–98, viii.
23. Jeon SS, Hyun JH, Lee KS. A comparison of holmium: YAG laser with lithoclast lithotripsy in ureteral calculi fragmentation. Int J Urol 2005;12(6):544–7.
24. Teichman JM, Rao RD, Rogenes VJ, et al. Ureteroscopic management of ureteral calculi: electrohydraulic versus holmium: YAG lithotripsy. J Urol 1997;158(4):1357–61.
25. Bader MJ, Eisner B, Porpiglia F, et al. Contemporary management of ureteral stones. Eur Urol 2012;61(4): 764–72.
26. Leveillee RJ, Lobik L. Intracorporeal lithotripsy: which modality is best? Curr Opin Urol 2003;13(3): 249–53.
27. Cinman NM, Andonian S, Smith AD. Lasers in percutaneous renal procedures. World J Urol 2010;28(2): 135–42.
28. Teichman JM, Vassar GJ, Bishoff JT, et al. Holmium: YAG lithotripsy yields smaller fragments than lithoclast, pulsed dye laser or electrohydraulic lithotripsy. J Urol 1998;159(1):17–23.
29. Matlaga BR, Lingeman JE. Surgical management of stones: new technology. Adv Chronic Kidney Dis 2009;16(1):60–4.
30. Lee H, Kang HW, Teichman JM, et al. Urinary calculus fragmentation during Ho: YAG and Er: YAG lithotripsy. Lasers Surg Med 2006;38(1):39–51.
31. Blackmon RL, Irby PB, Fried NM. Holmium: YAG (lambda = 2,120 nm) versus thulium fiber (lambda = 1,908 nm) laser lithotripsy. Lasers Surg Med 2010; 42(3):232–6.
32. Kuo RL, Aslan P, Zhong P, et al. Impact of holmium laser settings and fiber diameter on stone fragmentation and endoscope deflection. J Endourol 1998; 12(6):523–7.
33. Poon M, Beaghler M, Baldwin D. Flexible endoscope deflectability: changes using a variety of working instruments and laser fibers. J Endourol 1997;11(4):247–9.
34. Mues AC, Teichman JM, Knudsen BE. Evaluation of 24 holmium: YAG laser optical fibers for flexible ureteroscopy. J Urol 2009;182(1):348–54.
35. Durak E, Hruby G, Mitchell R, et al. Evaluation of a protective laser sheath for application in flexible ureteroscopy. J Endourol 2008;22(1):57–60.
36. Herrmann TR, Bach T, Imkamp F, et al. Insertion sheaths prevent breakage of flexible ureteroscopes due to laser fiber passage: a video endoluminal study of the working channel. J Endourol 2010; 24(11):1747–51.
37. Sung C, Singh H, Schwartz M, et al. Evaluation of efficacy of novel optically activated digital endoscope protection system against laser energy damage. Urology 2008;72(1):57–60.
38. Xavier K, Hruby GW, Kelly CR, et al. Clinical evaluation of efficacy of novel optically activated digital endoscope protection system against laser energy damage. Urology 2009;73(1):37–40.

39. Nerli RB, Koura AC, Prabha V, et al. Use of LMA Stonebreaker as an intracorporeal lithotrite in the management of ureteral calculi. J Endourol 2008; 22(4):641–4.
40. Salvado JA, Mandujano R, Saez I, et al. Ureteroscopic lithotripsy for distal ureteral calculi: comparative evaluation of three different lithotriptors. J Endourol 2012;26(4):343–6.
41. Clayman M, Uribe CA, Eichel L, et al. Comparison of guide wires in urology. Which, when and why? J Urol 2004;171(6 Pt 1):2146–50.
42. Sarkissian C, Korman E, Hendlin K, et al. Systematic evaluation of hybrid guidewires: shaft stiffness, lubricity, and tip configuration. Urology 2012;79(3): 513–7.
43. Ng YH, Somani BK, Dennison A, et al. Irrigant flow and intrarenal pressure during flexible ureteroscopy: the effect of different access sheaths, working channel instruments, and hydrostatic pressure. J Endourol 2010;24(12):1915–20.
44. Traxer O, Thomas A, Alqahtani S, et al. Ureteral wall injuries induced by ureteral access sheath during retrograde intra-renal surgery (prospective evaluation). Eur Urol 2011;10(2):I–XIV.
45. Netsch C, Herrera G, Gross AJ, et al. In vitro evaluation of nitinol stone retrieval baskets for flexible ureteroscopy. J Endourol 2011;25(7):1217–20.
46. Korman E, Hendlin K, Monga M. Small-diameter nitinol stone baskets: radial dilation force and dynamics of opening. J Endourol 2011;25(9):1537–40.
47. Korman E, Hendlin K, Chotikawanich E, et al. Comparison of small diameter stone baskets in an in vitro caliceal and ureteral model. J Endourol 2011;25(1):123–7.
48. Magheli A, Semins MJ, Allaf ME, et al. Critical analysis of the miniaturized stone basket: effect on deflection and flow rate. J Endourol 2012;26(3): 275–7.
49. Kesler SS, Pierre SA, Brison DI, et al. Use of the Escape nitinol stone retrieval basket facilitates fragmentation and extraction of ureteral and renal calculi: a pilot study. J Endourol 2008;22(6):1213–7.
50. Tan YK, McLeroy SL, Faddegon S, et al. In vitro comparison of prototype magnetic tool with conventional nitinol basket for ureteroscopic retrieval of stone fragments rendered paramagnetic with iron oxide microparticles. J Urol 2012;188(2):648–52.
51. Eisner BH, Dretler SP. Use of the stone cone for prevention of calculus retropulsion during holmium: YAG laser lithotripsy: case series and review of the literature. Urol Int 2009;82(3):356–60.
52. Ding H, Wang Z, Du W, et al. NTrap in prevention of stone migration during ureteroscopic lithotripsy for proximal ureteral stones: a meta-analysis. J Endourol 2012;26(2):130–4.
53. Eisner BH, Pengune W, Stoller ML. Use of an antiretropulsion device to prevent stone retropulsion significantly increases the efficiency of pneumatic lithotripsy: an in vitro study. BJU Int 2009;104(6): 858–61.
54. Sarkissian C, Paz A, Zigman O, et al. Safety and efficacy of a novel ureteral occlusion device. Urology 2012;80(1):32–7.
55. Pagnani CJ, El Akkad M, Bagley DH. Prevention of stone migration with the Accordion during endoscopic ureteral lithotripsy. J Endourol 2012;26(5): 484–8.
56. Holley PG, Sharma SK, Perry KT, et al. Assessment of novel ureteral occlusion device and comparison with stone cone in prevention of stone fragment migration during lithotripsy. J Endourol 2005;19(2):200–3.
57. Ahmed M, Pedro RN, Kieley S, et al. Systematic evaluation of ureteral occlusion devices: insertion, deployment, stone migration, and extraction. Urology 2009;73(5):976–80.
58. Rane A, Bradoo A, Rao P, et al. The use of a novel reverse thermosensitive polymer to prevent ureteral stone retropulsion during intracorporeal lithotripsy: a randomized, controlled trial. J Urol 2010;183(4): 1417–21.
59. Al-Qahtani SM, Geavlette BP, de Medina SG, et al. The new Olympus digital flexible ureteroscope (URF-V): initial experience. Urol Ann 2011;3(3): 133–7.

Management of Stones in Abnormal Situations

Yung K. Tan, MBBS, MRCS, Doh Yoon Cha, MD, Mantu Gupta, MD*

KEYWORDS

• Nephrolithiasis • Pregnancy • Horseshoe kidney • Urinary diversions • Calyceal diverticulum • Pelvic kidneys • Transplant kidneys • Autosomal dominant polycystic kidney disease

KEY POINTS

- The management of urinary calculi in abnormal situations continues to pose challenges to urologists. Abnormal situations include pregnancy, aberrant anatomy, kidney transplants, calyceal diverticuli, urinary diversions and autosomal dominant polycystic kidney disease.
- A combination of aberrant anatomy, urinary tract infections, and metabolic changes predispose these patients to an increased incidence of stone formation.
- Metabolic evaluation and medical therapy are arguably more important in these patients, as metabolic abnormalities can be rather common.

INTRODUCTION

The management of urinary calculi in abnormal situations continues to pose challenges to urologists. Abnormal situations include pregnancy, aberrant anatomy, kidney transplants, calyceal diverticuli, urinary diversions, and autosomal dominant polycystic kidney disease (ADPKD). A combination of aberrant anatomy, urinary tract infections, and metabolic changes predispose these patients to an increased incidence of stone formation. The aims of treatment are similar to normal situations. That is an attempt at complete clearance of all stone fragments with the least invasive means possible while trying to minimize secondary procedures and complications. Unfortunately, the aberrant anatomy makes access and clearance of these calculi more difficult to accomplish.

Metabolic evaluation and medical therapy are arguably more important in these patients, as metabolic abnormalities can be rather common, as will be discussed later. These changes often lead to progression of remnant stones requiring secondary treatments and increasing morbidity to the patient.

The options for treatment include open procedures, extracorporeal shockwave lithotripsy (ESWL), percutaneous nephrolithotomy (PCNL), laparoscopy, and ureteroscopy. The choice of procedure must take into account difficulties with access and the anatomic configuration of the kidney and stone. In general, our experience is that most if not all urinary calculi can be managed by minimally invasive procedures, obviating the need of open procedures, although we do acknowledge that in the situations of a lack of access to equipment or inexperience, open procedures may be the safer option with better stone-free rates.

HORSESHOE KIDNEYS

Horseshoe kidneys are the most common renal malformation with an incidence of 1 in 400 births. There is also a preponderance toward males with a 2:1 ratio.[1] As the renal units ascend during fetal development there is abnormal fusion of the mesonephric blastemas. This leads to incomplete ascension and also malrotation of the kidneys. The final product is a fused kidney in the shape of

Department of Urology, Columbia University Medical Center, 630 West 168th Street, New York, NY 10032, USA
* Corresponding author.
E-mail address: drmantugupta@gmail.com

Urol Clin N Am 40 (2013) 79–97
http://dx.doi.org/10.1016/j.ucl.2012.10.001

a horseshoe that is limited by the inferior mesenteric artery and lies more caudally (**Fig. 1**). The kidney calyces tend to be posterior and medial and the upper pole calyces lie more cranial and lateral (**Fig. 2**).[2] The ureters have a high insertion and deviate more anteriorly, as they have to cross the renal isthmus (**Fig. 3**). This high insertion and crossing of the renal isthmus may lead to increased incidence of urinary stasis.

Horseshoe kidneys are associated with up to 100% incidence of urinary metabolic abnormalities, 40% recurrent urinary tract infections, and 35% incidence of suboptimal urinary outflow.[3] There is a 20% median incidence of stones in horseshoe kidneys[1] with most in the posterior lower pole calyx and the renal pelvis. Most of these stones are calcium oxalate.

As the innervation of the horseshoe kidney is the same as that of the normal kidney, symptoms of renal colic are similar; however, atypical presentations of vague abdominal pain or emesis may occur owing to the different lie of the kidneys.

The decision of treatment option will have to take into consideration aberrations in anatomy that may include aberrant vasculature, distortions of the renal collecting system, and interposing bowel between skin and kidney. The presence of ureteropelvic junction (UPJ) obstruction should also be determined before treatment, as it will affect outcomes of certain procedures. The options for treatment include ESWL, ureteroscopy, PCNL, laparoscopy, and open surgery.

ESWL

ESWL is the least invasive modality of treatment for horseshoe kidney stones. There are a number of factors that may make shockwave therapy less efficacious. The horseshoe kidney sits lower

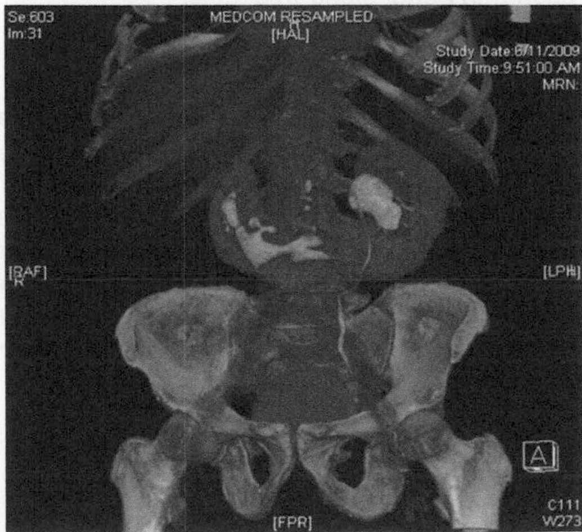

Fig. 1. Horseshoe kidney.

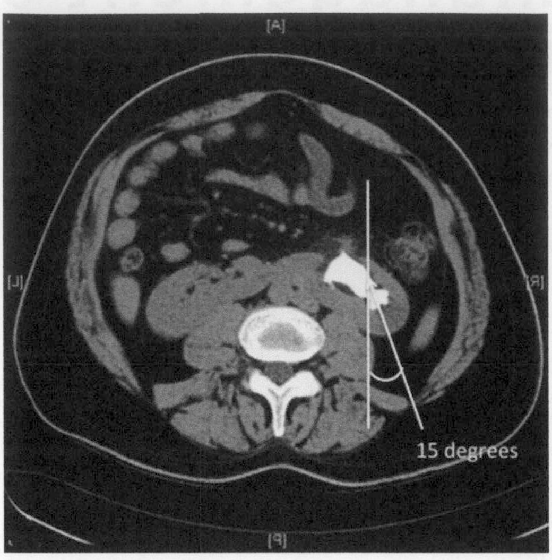

Fig. 2. Horseshoe kidney with stone. Note the access angle is 15° as opposed to the 30° for normal kidneys.

in the abdominal cavity and tends to be more medial. The end result of these changes is that vertebral bodies, transverse processes, bony pelvis, and bowel gas shadows may obscure targeting of the stone. Furthermore, if the stone lies below the pelvic brim, a prone ESWL will have to be attempted and this has a higher chance of traumatizing the overlying bowel.

The second problem is the high insertion and kinking of the ureter as it crosses the renal isthmus. Contrast studies and excretory studies may also need to be done to exclude UPJ obstruction in these kidneys. The net effect is that even if the stones are fragmented, there is poor passage of fragments.

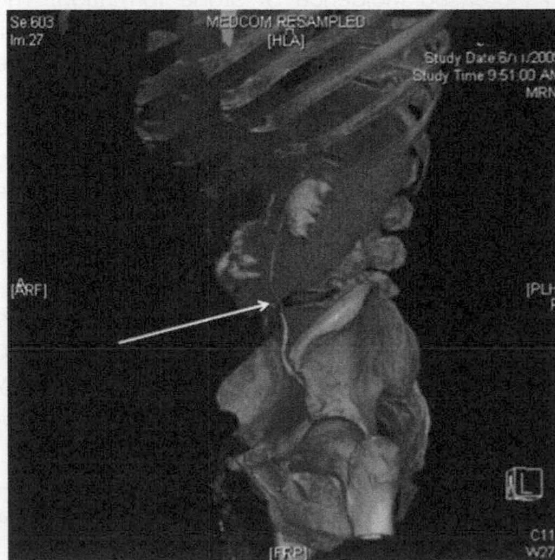

Fig. 3. Anterior deviating ureter with kink over the isthmus.

There have been a number of studies looking at the efficacy of shockwaves for stones in horseshoe kidneys and the success rates range from 28% to 80%.[4–6] Many of these stones required multiple sessions of shockwave and even the definitions of success are debatable, as remnant stone fragments smaller than 4 mm were considered as successful treatments in some of these articles.

Size of stones treated influences the success of ESWL in these patients. Sheir and colleagues[7] documented a success rate of 79% for stones smaller than 15 mm, which dropped to 53% once stones were larger than 15 mm. **Table 1** shows the results of studies attempting to clear stones in horseshoe kidneys with ESWL. Clayman[8] suggested that percutaneous treatment maybe more appropriate for stones larger than 10 to 15 mm.

In one of the largest studies to date, Ray and colleagues[9] treated 41 horseshoe kidneys with stones with ESWL. They managed single treatment success of 25% and stone free rate of 9.1%. Overall success was 63.6% with stone-free rate of 39.1%; 73.0% of the patients needed auxiliary treatments that included repeat ESWL, percutaneous nephrolithotomy, or ureterorenoscopy.

The consensus is that ESWL should be reserved for stones smaller than 20 mm, in nondependent locations of the renal pelvis with minimal renal collecting system dilation. UPJ obstruction should also be excluded before proceeding. If the patient is not stone free after ESWL, ureteroscopy or percutaneous clearance of stones should be considered.

Ureteroscopy

The aberrant anatomy of horseshoe kidneys with anterior, tortuous, and high insertions of the ureters make semirigid ureteroscopic treatment of the upper ureteric or renal calculi challenging in the best of circumstances. With the advent of flexible ureteroscopes and lasers there have been a number of small series that have explored the use of ureteroscopy for the management of renal calculi in horseshoe kidneys. Andreoni and colleagues[10] in a case report described the use of an access sheath and flexible ureteroscope to clear 3 stones, the largest being 12 mm, leaving no fragments larger than 2 mm. In a later series, Weizer and colleagues[11] treated 4 patients with stones in a horseshoe kidney with a flexible ureteroscope. The average size was 1.4 cm, with a mean operative time of 126 minutes and a success rate of 75%. The largest series by Molimard and colleagues[12] consisted of 17 patients; 70% of the patients were treated with flexible ureteroscopy after failure with either PCNL or ESWL. Average stone burden was 16 mm and average operative time was 106 minutes; 41% required staged procedures. They were able to achieve a stone-free rate of 88.2% as defined by no remnant stones larger than 3 mm. Ureteroscopic management continues to be challenging. Its indication is limited to stones smaller than 2 cm. Access sheaths and ureteric dilators are often required and patients who choose this modality must be prepared for staged procedures.

PCNL

Ever since the publications by Wickham and Kellett[13] and Clayman and colleagues,[14] percutaneous nephrolithotomy has become the standard of care for stones larger than 2 cm or for cases that have failed ESWL.[15] An understanding of anatomy is critical for the urologist who desires to attempt PCNL. The horseshoe kidney lies lower and is malrotated such that the posterior calyx lies in an anterior-posterior plane with the renal pelvis lying anteriorly. The upper pole calyx lies

Table 1
Results of SWL patients with horseshoe kidneys

Investigator, Y	Mean Stone Diameter, mm	No. of Patients	Fragmentation Rate, %	Stone-Free Rate, %	Retreatment Rate, %
Esuvaranathan,[122] 1991	12	7	Not Reported	59	50
Kirkali et al,[5] 1996	24	18	78	28	57
Smith,[123] 1989	Not Reported	14	Not Reported	79	29
Bhatia and Biyani,[2] 1994	28	27	Not Reported	70	48
Sheir et al,[7] 2003	13.5	49	Not Reported	71	71
Tunc et al,[6] 2004	22	46	Not Reported	66	Not Reported
Ray et al,[9] 2011	9.5	41	Not Reported	39.1	71

posterior-lateral and sits lower than in the normal kidney. Other associated abnormalities include a higher incidence of UPJ obstruction (15%–33%)[16] and aberrant vasculature as the vessels enter the isthmus dorsally, precluding percutaneous access there.[17] Another consideration is the possibility of a retrorenal colon, which would affect access (**Fig. 4**). A computed tomography (CT) scan with contrast and possibly functional nuclear medicine studies are important to look for these abnormalities.

Access is best achieved via the upper pole posterior calyx. This access gives direct access toward the renal pelvis and is associated with a low risk of pneumothorax, as the upper pole lies well below the costophrenic angles of the lung.[18] As the horseshoe kidney lies more anteriorly, the access tract tends to be longer. This is especially so for obese patients. The horseshoe kidney, by virtue of its position, is more fixed and excessive torque on the kidney can lead to bleeding.[19] A full complement of baskets and flexible nephroscopes should be available for the successful clearance of stones.

The aim of PCNL should be complete stone-free status. This is especially so as the high ureteric insertion leads to stasis and even small residual fragments may have difficulty passing and may in time act as a nidus for stone formation. Success rates in PCNL range from 65.5% to 75.0%.[1,20] These numbers are contentious, as in many of the articles there is no consistent definition of stone-free status.

Complications are similar to PCNL in a normal kidney. These include urinary tract infection (UTI), hematuria, renal hematomas, urine leak, and

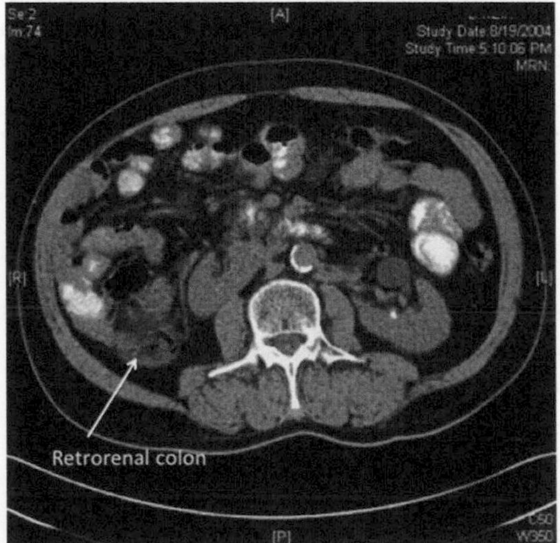

Fig. 4. Retrorenal colon.

obstruction, although, as previously mentioned, risks of pneumothorax and hydrothorax with an upper pole access is much lower because the kidney is low lying.[18]

Laparoscopy

This is a rarely used modality of treatment for stones in horseshoe kidneys. The anterior location of the kidney and its renal pelvis suggests that access to the stones via a laparoscopic pyelolithotomy should be easier. Another added advantage of a laparoscopic approach would be the ability to treat a UPJ obstruction with a laparoscopic pyeloplasty. Nambirajan and colleagues[21] described a successful bilateral laparoscopic pyelolithotomy and more recently Symons and colleagues[22] described the laparoscopic management of a large staghorn stone. Surgical time was 3 hours and the patient was discharged without complications.

In conclusion, for stones smaller than 2 cm in nondependent locations, ESWL is a viable option for treatment. PCNL should be reserved for stones larger than 2 cm or after ESWL failure. Ureteroscopy and laparoscopy are alternatives that show promise, although the experience in the literature is limited. In the setting of UPJ obstruction secondary to a crossing vessel, laparoscopy would be the treatment of choice, as it allows concomitant treatment of the obstruction.

PELVIC KIDNEY

The pelvic kidney occurs owing to a failure of ascent of the kidney during development. Its incidence is estimated at 1:2200 to 1:3000. Pelvic kidneys have a significant portion of the kidney below the pelvic brim (**Fig. 5**). They are malrotated and have high insertion of the ureter, which may predispose them to urinary stasis and calculi formation.[23] There is also an increased incidence of UPJ obstruction. This low position in the pelvis, associated with other abnormalities, provides unique challenges to management of urolithiasis in these kidneys.

Like the horseshoe kidney, innervation of the kidney follows that of the normally positioned kidney and symptoms are typical as for a kidney in the normal position.

ESWL

As part of the workup for ESWL for calculi in the pelvic kidney, it is important to exclude UPJ obstruction, as this would have consequences on stone fragment passage after ESWL. Because of the low-riding position of the pelvic kidney, the

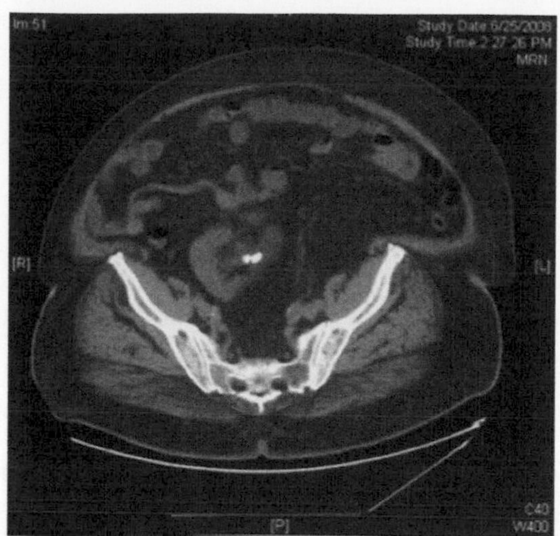

Fig. 5. Right pelvic kidney with stones: note it lies below the pelvic brim.

patient often has to have treatment in the prone position, as the bony pelvis would get in the way of the ESWL shockwaves. Loops of bowel anterior to the pelvic kidney can also reduce the efficacy of the shockwaves.

Data for ESWL treatment of stones in pelvic kidneys is limited to small case series. Stone-free outcomes range from 25% to 92%.[24–26] The numbers are contentious, as there are different definitions of stone-free status. For example, Talic[27] treated 14 patients with a mean stone size of 2.35 cm^2 with an absolute stone-free status of 57.2%, and 35.7% of patients had remnant stones smaller than 4 mm. The more successful studies tried to exclude obstruction at the UPJ and oftentimes the patients underwent multiple procedures for stone clearance. Overall, there is relatively good stone clearance if there is no concomitant obstruction.

Ureteroscopy

There are a few reports of ureteroscopic management of pelvic kidney stones. Weizer and colleagues[11] treated 4 patients with pelvic kidney urolithiasis with flexible ureteroscopy. The mean stone size was 14 mm with a stone-free rate of 75%. Mean operative time was 126 minutes. This is comparable to success rates with ESWL without the need for secondary procedures. These investigators encouraged the use of access sheaths to help straighten the ureter. The access sheaths also allowed for rapid access to the upper ureter but its use must be cautioned, as these tortuous, anterior ureters have a risk of trauma from passage of the access sheaths. An effort should be made to achieve stone-free status, as the ureters usually have a high insertion and remnant stones have poor potential to pass spontaneously.

PCNL

Unlike horseshoe kidneys, the location of the kidney within the pelvis makes PCNL challenging. The PCNL will need to be performed in the supine position and requires a transperitoneal approach. As can be imagined, this approach has the potential for significant injury to intra-abdominal contents, in particular the bowel. There is also the problem of urine leak, which if it occurs is not limited to the retroperitoneum, as is in the case with a retroperitoneal PCNL.

Desai and Jasani[28] reported on the use of ultrasound-guided supine transperitoneal PCNL. In brief, the ultrasound is used for both calyceal localization and also as a tool to push away bowel to reduce the risk of bowel injury during the access. They achieved a 100% stone-free status in 16 patients with 1 case of bowel injury that was managed conservatively.

Watterson and colleagues[29] reported a posterior approach via the sciatic foramen; unfortunately, this approach was associated with postoperative femoral neuropathy.

Others have tried a laparoscopic-assisted transabdominal percutaneous approach to the kidney. Eshghi and colleagues[30] reported the first such procedure in 1985. The patient is positioned in a Trendelenburg position and 3 to 4 ports are inserted. A ureteral catheter is placed so that percutaneous access can be directed both visually and fluoroscopically. Once puncture of the kidney is successful, it is dilated as per usual PCNL. It should be noted that the distances that need to be traversed are longer and long instruments may be needed.

There have been variations on this combined laparoscopic/percutaneous nephrolithotomy technique. Zafar and Lingeman[31] described the laparoscopic suturing of the nephrotomy so that percutaneous drainage is not required. A total extraperitoneal approach was described by Holman and Toth.[32] A space maker balloon was inserted into the extraperitoneal space and the percutaneous access was directed both visually and fluoroscopically. An advantage of this last variation is that if there is a leak, it is into the extraperitoneal space.

Laparoscopy

In pure laparoscopic pyelolithotomy, ports are placed transperitoneally in a patient who is in the Trendelenburg position.[33] Bowel is displaced and a pyelotomy is made sharply. Stones are then extracted laparoscopically with graspers under direct vision. Flexible nephroscopes can then be passed into the collecting system and stones can then be extracted by basket. A double J stent is usually recommended, as leakage into the peritoneal cavity can have serious consequences. Ramakumar and Segura[34] achieved 90% and 80% stone free rates at 3 months and 12 months respectively in 19 patients using this approach.

Laparoscopy also allows simultaneous management of a UPJ obstruction. The pyelotomy can be extended distally as a fengerplasty or a formal dismembered pyeloplasty can be performed.

There have been a series of cases in which retroperitonoscopy was performed. The space was created by a balloon but it was noted in some instances that there was difficulty creating the space.[35] When the renal pelvis was accessed successfully the success rate was 83%.

In the age of robotic surgery, a number of cases of robot-assisted laparoscopic pyelolithotomy have been performed. The advantages of the robot relate to improved optics and also easier closure of the pyelotomy. This is especially advantageous in the patient who undergoes concomitant pyeloplasty. The stone-free rates approach 80% to 100%.[36,37]

Our opinion is that ESWL or ureteroscopy is a possible first treatment option for stones smaller than 2 cm if UPJ obstruction has been excluded. In the presence of stones larger than 2 cm or if UPJ obstruction is present, laparoscopy or PCNL may be a better option as first-line therapy.

CALYCEAL DIVERTICULAR STONES

Calyceal diverticula are nonsecretory, transitional cell epithelium-lined cystic cavities within the renal parenchyma with an incidence of less than 1% (**Fig. 6**).[38] They may have narrow infundibuli that may predispose them to recurrent infections, pain, and stone formation. The incidence of stone formation is between 10% and 50%.[39,40]

Most stones are calcium oxalate or mixed stones; in a urine metabolic evaluation of patients with diverticular calculi by Auge and colleagues,[41] it was found that all patients with diverticular calculi had metabolic abnormalities.

Indications for treatment include, pain, recurrent infections, hematuria, and progressive stone growth.[42]

ESWL

When ESWL is chosen as the primary treatment modality, stone-free rates are low, ranging from 20% to 58%.[43–45] Streem and Yost,[43] who had one of the higher success rates when treating calyceal diverticular stones, suggest that patient selection plays an important role in treatment success. In their study, 21 renal units were treated with ESWL. Inclusion criteria for treatment was stones smaller than 1.5 cm in calyceal diverticuli with a wide and short infundibulum. They achieved a 58% stone-free rate with 1 treatment.

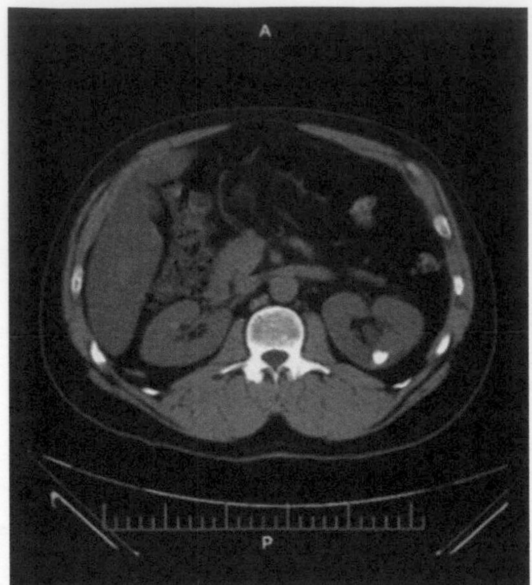

Fig. 6. Left calyceal diverticulum stone.

Surprisingly, even with dismal stone-free rates, pain-free rates after ESWL are much higher, ranging from 65% to 75%.[44,45] There are a number of theories to this. First, pain in the flank may not necessarily be caused by the calyceal diverticuli stone, and relief of pain may be related to improvements in musculoskeletal back pain. Another theory is that the fragmented stones maybe less symptomatic than the actual stones.

Ureteroscopy

Outcomes from ureteroscopy have been equivocal with stone-free rates of 19% to 58% and symptom-free rates of 38% to 68%.[46,47] There are a number of technical challenges associated with ureteroscopy for the treatment of diverticular stones. An infundulotomy will often need to be performed. This has the dual purpose of allowing access to the stone and also to externalize the calyceal diverticulum into the pyelocalyceal cavities.[48] Lower pole diverticuli are difficult to treat, as there are limits to the deflection of the flexible ureteroscopes. The complications associated with retrograde management of diverticula include bleeding, cautery-induced tissue injury, ureteral perforation, and infection.

PCNL

PCNL is the favored treatment option for calyceal diverticular calculi. Stone-free rates are in the range of 70% to 100% and recurrence rates of 0% to 30%.[40,49,50] Apart from rendering the diverticuli stone-free, PCNL allows for the fulguration/ablation of the diverticuli and either an infundibuloplasty or the ablation of the infundibulum.[48]

Percutaneous access can be achieved directly into the diverticulum or indirectly via a neighboring calyx following the wall of the diverticulum that is perforated or the diverticulum is accessed via a retrograde fashion.[51] The direct approach is usually favored, as it provides better stone-free rates[52] and as such the indirect approach is usually reserved for small diverticuli or upper pole diverticuli. In situations in which the infundibulum is sternotic, a variation of the direct access involves the creation of a neoinfundibulotomy. In this instance, the diverticuli is accessed and the access needle is further advanced into the main collecting system. Both the access tract and a neoinfundibulum are dilated. The stone is then cleared and a nephrostomy tube is advanced beyond the neoinfundibulum into the renal pelvis and kept in place for a week to allow for epithelialization of the neoinfundibulum.[53]

PCNL can be challenging, as the diverticuli are usually small and the infundibulum can be difficult to locate if there is a plan to do an infundibulotomy. Percutaneous access to anterior diverticuli can also predispose to increased bleeding from the longer distance that the tract has to traverse through renal parenchyma.

Laparoscopy

There have been a few case series of laparoscopic extraction of diverticular stones. Most of these studies have small numbers. Miller and colleagues,[54] in a study of 5 patients, managed to achieve 100% stone clearance and fulguration of the diverticular cavity and infundibulum. This technique has more relevance for calyceal stones with thin overlying parenchyma. Laparoscopy, however, is far more morbid then the other options and should be reserved only for anterior calyceal stones with thin overlying parenchyma.

In conclusion, for stones smaller than 1 cm with a short and wide infundibulum in patients who would prefer the least-invasive means of stone clearance, ESWL would be a treatment option. Ureteroscopy would be an alternative to ESWL in these same circumstances and would likely achieve a higher stone clearance rate in the appropriately selected patient. For larger stones or stones with narrow infundibuli, PCNL would give the best stone clearance rates with the additional ability to fulgurate and ablate the diverticular cavity. Laparoscopy should be reserved for larger stones in anterior calyces with thin overlying parenchyma and in which laparoscopic experience is available.

TRANSPLANT KIDNEYS

The incidence of calculi in transplant kidneys ranges from 0.4% to 1%.[55,56] These calculi can occur de novo or could have been present in the preoperative donor kidney. There are a number of factors that may predispose the donated kidney to stone formation. Patients with chronic kidney disease often have secondary or tertiary hyperparathyroidism. This predisposes the patient to have hypercalcemia and consequent hypercalciuria. Nonabsorbable sutures can also act as a potential nidus for stone formation if mistakenly used during the transplantation. Additionally, the immunocompromised state of the patient may predispose to recurrent UTI and subsequent infection of stones.[57]

The most common stone type is calcium oxalate. Cyclosporine A used as an immunosuppressant can predispose toward hyperuricosuria. The urate in urine can act as nidus for calcium oxalate stone formation. Uric acid stones are relatively uncommon probably owing to the concentrated alkali production often seen in transplant kidneys.[55]

The transplant kidney is in essence a solitary kidney and it is paramount that calculi be aggressively managed in these patients to prevent obstruction and its sequelae. These patients are especially susceptible to the loss of the renal unit, as they are more prone to infections.[58]

Calculi in transplant kidneys often present late. The transplant kidney is not innervated, so pain is not a typical symptom of obstruction, although the patient may complain of vague discomfort around the graft site from the stretching of the pseudocapsule during hydronephrosis. Presentations may include fever without localizing signs, hematuria, decreased urine output, and rising serum creatinine levels.[57] It is important to have a high index of suspicion in such instances.

Imaging can also be difficult. Because of its pelvic location, KUB x-rays may not be able to visualize the stone because of the overlap with the pelvic bones. Ultrasounds of the graft may not yield good images because of the possibility of overlapping gas shadows.[56] CT scans are the most useful imaging modality to determine the presence of calculi.

Observation

Observation of renal calculi in transplant kidneys should be reserved only in a select group of patients. Klingler and colleagues[59] successfully observed patients with nonobstructing stones smaller than 4 mm. As the kidney is denervated, pain is often not an early sign of obstruction. These patients will have to be followed closely with serum creatinine levels. The role of serial imaging is not well defined in this population but ultrasound imaging may offer the best compromise, as there is no risk of ionizing radiation and new dilatation of the renal pelvis would be a definitive sign of obstruction. The threshold for intervention in this group should be very low.

ESWL

The transplant kidney, owing to its location, offers unique challenges to ESWL as a treatment modality. The graft kidney overlies the pelvic bones and the treatment will have to be performed in the prone position. Unlike the horseshoe kidney, the graft kidney usually lies anterior to bowel, although there maybe instances in which there may be interposed bowel. This would limit the efficacy of the shockwaves and possibly lead to trauma to the overlying bowel. Challacombe and colleagues,[55] in a small series, treated 13 patients with ESWL; 8 required adjuvant treatments, such as stents and percutaneous nephrostomy tubes or repeat shockwaves, to achieve stone free status. Klinger and colleagues[59] in a separate study treated 7 patients successfully with ESWL, although 3 required percutaneous nephrostomy tubes. Both studies indicate that ESWL can be efficacious for stones smaller than 1.5 to 2.0 cm. The threshold to the use of stents and nephrostomy tubes should be low, as steinstrasse would be a serious complication in the solitary transplant kidney.

Ureteroscopy

Anatomy of the transplant kidney plays an important part in the success of ureteroscopy for stones in transplant kidneys. First, localizing and access of the transplant ureteric orifice can be a challenge. This may be found in the dome or anterior surface of the bladder. The orifice and ureter maybe tortuous, especially if the transplant ureter is long and redundant. Special catheters like the cobra (**Fig. 7**) and kumpe catheter (**Fig. 8**) may be required to gain access to the renal pelvis. A curved tip hydrophilic wire with good torque control can greatly help with access to the system. Newer flexible ureteroscopes with good secondary deflection will help especially with access to the lower pole calyces. Del Pizzo and colleagues[57] successfully treated 6 of 7 patients and more recently, Basiri and colleagues[60] reported a 67% success rate.

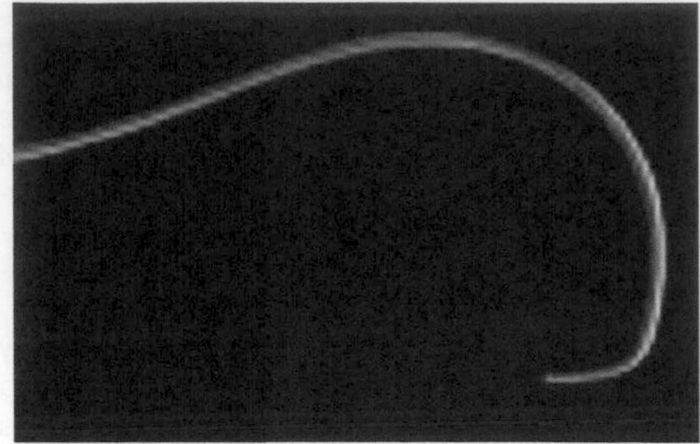

Fig. 7. A 6F cobra catheter.

Hyams and colleagues[61] also described a nondilating antegrade approach to the ureteroscopic management of the transplant lithiasis. Briefly, percutaneous access was obtained before ureteroscopy. A wire was then passed down the nephrostomy tube and passed down into the bladder with the aid of an angiographic catheter. A safety wire was then placed with the aid of a coaxial catheter and the nephroscope could then be advanced into the collecting system antegradely via one of the wires. An access sheath was used based on the surgeon's discretion.

PCNL

The approach to PCNL is similar to a pelvic kidney but in a more anterior location.[62] The patient is placed supine and access is best achieved with an ultrasound-guided or CT-guided puncture, as there is risk of overlying bowel.[58,63] Another important aspect to PCNL of a transplant kidney is the tough fibrous capsule that forms around transplant kidneys. Coaxial metal dilators may be more efficacious at breaching this tough fibrous capsule.[63,64] For transplant ureteral stones, these can be quite often treated without requiring tract dilation in an antegrade manner with a flexible ureteroscope.[61]

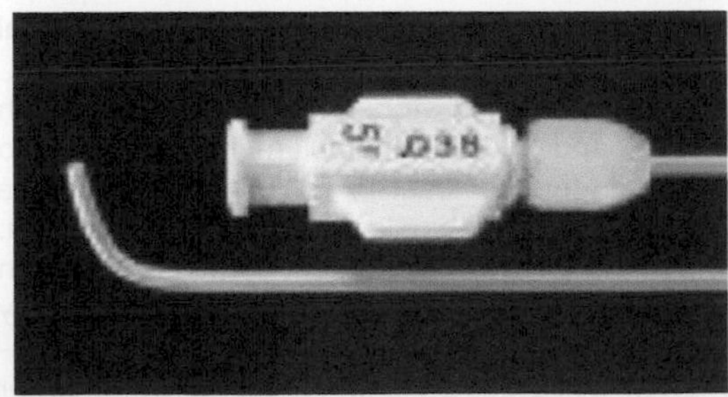

Fig. 8. A 5F kumpe catheter.

The kidney is fixed in its capsule and excessive torque could lead to massive hemorrhage. Flexible nephroscopes and ureteroscopes along with baskets should be used liberally to clear the stones.[55] Rifiaoglu and colleagues[65] reported on 15 anterior PCNL cases performed for transplant kidneys. They achieved 100% success rates with the liberal use of flexible scopes and baskets.

Potential complications include bleeding, urosepsis (as the patients are immunocompromised), and delayed wound healing (secondary to concomitant steroid therapy), which can lead to prolonged urine leaks.

In summary, conservative management of stones in the kidney should be taken with caution. This should be reserved for stones smaller than 4 mm, and close follow-up is required; there should be a low index of suspicion for intervention. ESWL or ureteroscopy is possible as a first-line treatment for stones smaller than 1.5 cm in diameter. There should be a low threshold to stenting, as steinstrasse could have catastrophic consequences for these patients. PCNL should be considered in stones larger than 1.5 to 2.0 cm.

CROSS-FUSED RENAL ECTOPIA

The incidence of ectopic kidney is 1:2000. There are 6 different kinds of ectopia, most (90%) being fused, with the orthotopic kidney cephalad (**Fig. 9**). There is usually some degree of malrotation that places the parenchyma posterior and the pelvis anterior, not unlike a horseshoe kidney. This can lead to hydronephrosis purely from malrotation; however, other causes can be associated with UPJ obstruction or vesicoureteric reflux.

Owing to the variety of ectopias, most of the literature is based on case reports and an emphasis is made on the individualization of treatment based on anatomy. A CT scan is an important prerequisite, as it helps delineate rotation and other aberrant anatomy and is thus the most appropriate imaging modality for treatment. For example, in a patient with an anterior pelvis, distension of the pelvis may bring it up to the anterior abdominal wall, allowing an anterior supine PCNL with the aid of fluoroscopy. To achieve a successful and safe access, the C arm would have to be placed in full lateral so that the distance

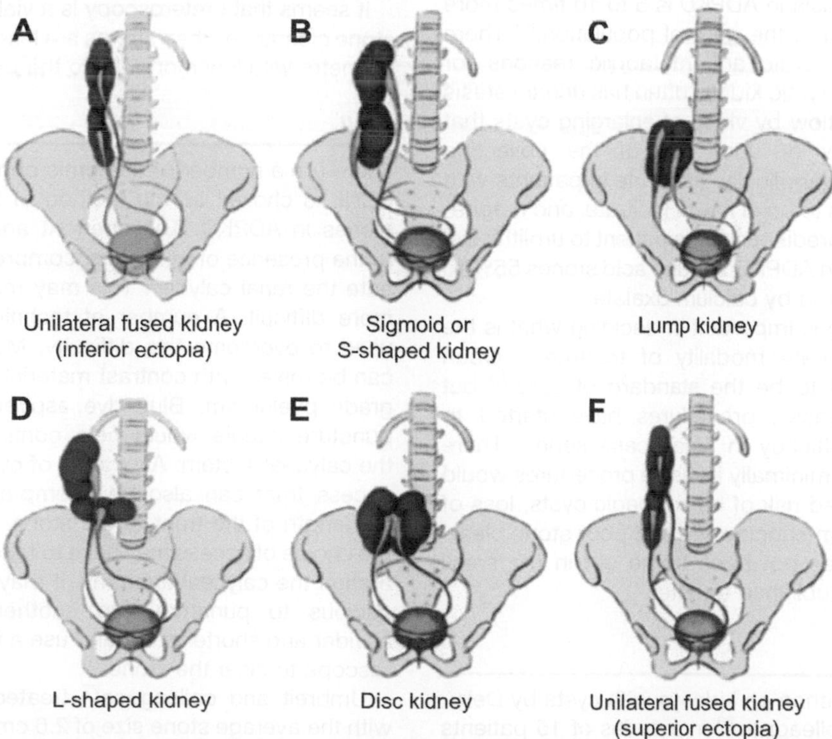

Fig. 9. Cross-fused ectopia. (*A*) Unilateral fused kidney (inferior ectopia). (*B*) Sigmoid or S-shaped kidney. (*C*) Lump kidney. (*D*) L-shaped kidney. (*E*) Disc kidney. (*F*) Unilateral fused kidney (Superior Ectopia). (*Reprinted from* Shapiro E, Bauer SB, Chow JS. Anomalies of the Upper Urinary Tract. In: Wein AJ, Kavoussi LR, Novick AC, et al, editors. Campbell-Walsh Urology. 10th Edition. Elsevier; 2012. Figure 117-13A-F; with permission.)

between the dilated pelvis and the anterior abdominal wall can be appreciated to avoid bowel injury.

Other approaches have involved laparoscopy, ureteroscopy, and ESWL. Tokgoz and colleagues[66] reported on 2 patients with L-shaped kidneys treated with ESWL. They achieved success in 1 patient with a renal pelvis stone after 3 ESWL sessions. The other patient failed treatment and required ureteroscopy.

Laparoscopy has also been attempted. Modi and colleagues[67] performed a transperitoneal laparoscopic pyeloplasty and pyelolithotomy on a pediatric patient with stone-free status up to the 6-month follow-up.

AUTOSOMAL DOMINANT POLYCYSTIC KIDNEY DISEASE

ADPKD is one of the most common inheritable diseases affecting 1:500 to 1:1000 live births.[68] It is a proliferation of tubular epithelial cells leading to blockage of the tubules and subsequent cyst formation. There are 2 variants: the polycystin-1 (PKD-1) mutation is associated with onset of cysts at an earlier age and end-stage renal failure by the fifth or sixth decade of life.

Nephrolithiasis in ADPKD is 5 to 10 times more common than in the general population.[69] There are both anatomic and metabolic reasons for this. The polycystic kidney often has urinary stasis and poor outflow by virtue of enlarging cysts that obstruct flow of urine out of the collecting system.[70] Metabolically, the urine in patients with ADPKD tends to be of low pH, citrate, and magnesium.[71] This predisposes the patient to urolithiasis. Most stones in ADPKD are uric acid stones 55% to 71%,[72] followed by calcium oxalate.

CT imaging is important in deciding what is the most appropriate modality of treatment. Open surgery used to be the standard of care,[70] but minimally invasive procedures have started to show their efficacy in small case series. There was fear that minimally invasive procedures would have increased risk of hemorrhagic cysts, loss of nephrons from shockwave, and poor stone clearance. This has not been borne out in the small case series published to date.

ESWL

Earlier experience on kidneys with cysts by Deliveliotis and colleagues[73] in a series of 15 patients treated with ESWL achieved an overall stone free rate of 60%. In the subgroup with polycystic kidneys, the success was 25.0% and rose to 83.3% in the subgroup with solitary cysts. This discrepancy points to the issues of attenuation of shockwaves as they travels through the cystic medium. Also, cysts may obstruct the pelvicalyceal outflow making stone passage more difficult. Delakas and colleagues,[74] on the other hand, achieved stone-free status in 85% of 13 patients with 16 treated renal units. Most stones were smaller than 2 cm and a stent was used in 57% of the patients. There was no incidence of hemorrhagic cysts. We conclude that ESWL can be an efficacious treatment modality for stones less than 2 cm and stenting may help with overcoming the likely obstruction from the aberrant anatomy.

Ureteroscopy

There are few reports on the use of ureteroscopy for ADPKD. Liu and colleagues[75] attempted flexible ureteroscopy in 13 patients. All stones were smaller than 2 cm with a mean stone size of 5.6 mm. Most of the stones were located in the renal pelvis and on average each renal unit had 3.2 stones. There was extensive use of ureteral access sheaths and post-procedural stenting. He was able to achieve stone-free rates of 84.5% and 92.3% with a second procedure. There were 3 complications:1 low grade fever, 1 flank pain and 1 stent-associated pain.

It seems that ureteroscopy is a viable option for stone clearance when stones are less than 2 cm in diameter with low morbidity to the patient.

PCNL

There are a number of anatomic considerations if PCNL is chosen as the method of treatment for stones in ADPKD. The aberrant anatomy owing to the presence of cysts may compress and elongate the renal calyces. This may make puncture more difficult. A number of techniques can be used to overcome this difficulty. Methylene blue can be mixed with contrast material for the retrograde pyelogram. Blue dye aspirated from the puncture needle would help confirm entry into the calyceal system. Aspiration of cysts along the access tract can also be attempted to shorten the length of the tract to the stone. Alternatively, the choice of access may have to take into consideration the calyceal anatomy. It maybe more efficacious to puncture into another calyx with a wider and shorter calyx and use a flexible nephroscope to clear the stone.[76]

Umbreit and colleagues[77] treated 11 kidneys with the average stone size of 2.6 cm. The investigators required 2 access tracts in 5 of the kidneys and achieved an 82% stone-free rate. There were no significant complications and no blood transfusions were required. Al-Kandari and colleagues,[76] in one of the largest studies to date, performed PCNL on 20 kidneys. Six cases had access achieved by the radiologist in the earlier part of the series. The other 13 had access achieved by the urologist. There were unable to achieve access for 1 case that eventually required an open nephrolithotomy. Three cases required second look PCNL. Most stones were larger than 2 cm. They achieved an 89.4% stone-free rate. They had 3 complications, 1 fever, 1 bleeding via the nephrostomy tract that was managed conservatively, and 1 mild postoperative hematuria.

In ADPKD, stones smaller than 2 cm are best treated by ureteroscopy or ESWL. When stones are larger than 2 cm, PCNL may be a better option. The theoretical risks of hemorrhage into cysts have not been reported in recent studies.

PREGNANCY AND STONE DISEASE

Symptomatic urolithiasis occurs in approximately 1:1500 pregnancies[78] and is comparable to the incidence in women in age-matched groups.[78,79] Most cases occur in the second or third trimester.[78,80]

There are a number of physiologic and anatomic changes related to increased stone formation. These include dilatation of the renal collecting system and ureters owing to the effects of compression of the gravid uterus and also smooth muscle dilatory effects of progesterone on the ureter.[81] Interestingly, the predominant stone type is calcium phosphate (65.6%), as opposed to age-matched women in whom calcium phosphate comprised 34.6% of the stones.[78] This may be related to gestational hypercalciuria, hyperuricemia, and an elevated urinary pH.[78]

Rosenberg and colleagues,[82] in a retrospective review of more than 219,000 pregnancies, found 195 pregnancies complicated by urolithiasis over a 20-year span. They found that nephrolithiasis during pregnancy could be associated with recurrent abortions, mild preeclampsia, caesarian deliveries, gestational diabetes mellitus, and chronic hypertension. There was also association with urinary tract infections, hydronephrosis, and hydroureter, but surprisingly no association with preterm labor or adverse perinatal complications. This is opposed to findings from most other article, which seem to indicate increased risk of preterm labor.[80,83] Andreoiu and MacMahon[80] found that there was a 4.3% to 14.3% incidence of premature labor in pregnant patients with symptomatic nephrolithiasis depending if intervention was performed.

One of the issues of urolithiasis in pregnancy is related to the problems of diagnosis. As mentioned earlier, dilation of the ureter and renal pelvis may be related to the physiologic changes of pregnancy and not to the presence of obstructing calculi.[80] The use of x-rays and ionizing radiation to the unborn fetus is a concern. Currently, ultrasound is the mainstay for diagnosis. Unfortunately ultrasonography is operator dependent with an accuracy to detect stones of 56.2% and rising to 71.9% when resistive indices and presence of ureteric jets (**Fig. 10**) are incorporated into the study.[80] MR urography may be useful but its major disadvantage is that the stone cannot be directly visualized and secondary signs such as a filling defect on T2-weighted imaging, transition point of hydroureteronephrosis or double-kink signs are noted. Gadolinium is not recommended to be used in pregnancy, as there is a theoretical risk of fetal loss and long-term neurotoxicity and retardation of growth. This has been seen in animal studies,[84] but in the limited literature in humans, has not been borne out at this time.[85,86]

There has been increasing interest in the use of low-dose CT (less than 10mSV) for the detection of stones. The issue with low-dose CT is the increase in noise, although to a certain extent this can be mitigated by newer algorithms. The best study looking at stone detection between standard and low-dose CT was a cadaveric study by Jin and colleagues[87] that showed that the sensitivity for stones smaller than 2 mm was 29% versus approximately 47% to 59% sensitivity in conventional-dose CT. For stones larger than 4 mm, most studies indicate that low-dose CT (regardless of the protocols) do provide adequate sensitivities for the pickup of calculi.[88,89] It should be noted that none of these studies was performed in pregnancy. White and colleagues[90] looked at the issue of low-dose CT in pregnancy. In a cohort of 20 patients they picked up 13 patients with stones.

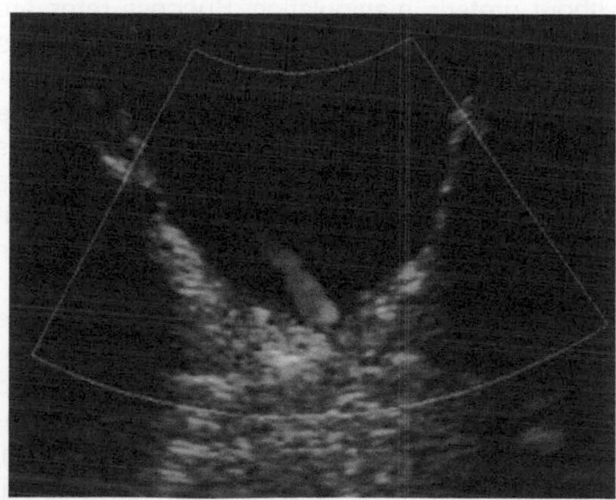

Fig. 10. Normal left ureteric jet.

Unfortunately, the sensitivity cannot be assessed, as there was no gold standard assessment of stones for obvious reasons. The American Congress of Obstetrics and Gynecology in a position paper[91] states that the concern over ionizing radiation should not preclude the use of x-rays from being used if medically indicated, although nonionizing imaging modalities should be considered first. The pregnant patient should be informed of the risks and consent should be obtained before the procedure.

Conservative Management

Conservative management involves bed rest, hydration, and analgesia.[92] Success rates range from 66.6% to 81.0%.[78,93] Age-matched nonpregnant women on the other hand have a spontaneous passage rate of 46%.[78] Interestingly, Burgess and colleagues[94] looked at spontaneous passage rates in pregnancy and found a rate of only 48%. They defined colic as attributable to stone only if the stone was seen on imaging, observed on passage, seen during intervention, or seen in postpartum imaging. They found that up to 25% of diagnoses of renal colic did not have stones, based on their definitions. Thus, the inappropriate diagnosis of renal colic from stone could lead to the belief that stones in pregnancy have a higher spontaneous passage rate.

Percutaneous Drainage and Stenting

Ureteral stenting and percutaneous nephrostomies can be used as temporizing measures to manage symptomatic stones during pregnancy. Percutaneous nephrostomies can act as a bridge to ureteric stenting or more definitive stone management with ureteroscopy or deferring treatment until after delivery. Their advantages include effective decompression of obstruction and can be performed with local anesthesia in patients with sepsis without ureteric manipulation. Success rates are from 90% to 100%.[95,96] Possible complications for percutaneous nephrostomies include urosepsis, hematuria, and renal hemorrhage. Also, the patient has to deal with the social consequences of having an externalized appliance. These tubes can also be dislodged and should be changed at 4-week to 6-week intervals to prevent the problem of early encrustation in pregnancy.

Ureteral stenting is another temporizing measure that can be used to relieve obstruction and symptoms of colic such that stones can then be treated after delivery. Stenting can be performed retrograde (typically with general or regional anesthesia) or antegrade, occasionally with local anesthesia. Positioning can be checked with ultrasonography[97] or limited fluoroscopy if there are difficulties with insertion. The main disadvantages of stenting include irritative stent symptoms, injury to the ureters during stent manipulation, urinary tract infections, hematuria, and stent encrustation and blockage owing to absorptive hypercalciuria and hyperuricosuria.[98] Stents should be exchanged every 4 to 6 weeks to avoid the problem of encrustation. Recurrent stent changes stand to cause more morbidity in pregnancy; thus, it is often recommended that for early pregnancy, a nephrostomy tube might be a more appropriate approach to urinary diversion and a stent for third-trimester pregnancies.

ESWL

ESWL is contraindicated in pregnancy, as the shockwaves are transmitted through the body and the fetus with the potential for fetal death.[99] There have, however, been case reports of patients having undergone ESWL without realizing pregnancy who went on to have a normal delivery and healthy baby.[100]

Ureteroscopy and Lithotripsy

Advances in ureteroscopes and lasers have improved the outcomes of ureteroscopic management of symptomatic stones in pregnancy. Ureteroscopic management has been shown to have a 70% to 100% efficacy of stone clearance.[97,101–103] Complications rates are similar to that of nonpregnant patients. In a meta-analysis by Semins and colleagues,[104] there was an 8.6% complication rate, most being Clavien grade 1 and 2. When obstetric complications were looked at specifically, there was a 4% complication rate with no fetal loss.[105] A number of modifications should be made to reduce the risks to mother and child. This includes increased use of spinal anesthesia or even sedation. Avoid using ionizing radiation by using ultrasound and direct visualization and only using fluoroscopy sparingly when there are access issues.[106,107] The use of Holmium laser for stone fragmentation is recommended, as there is little dissipation of heat beyond the ureter and depth of energy penetration is less than 0.5 mm.[101] Sound intensities generated are also less than that from electrohydraulic probes. Electrohydraulic probes are discouraged because of high peak pressures that could potentially harm the fetus.[108]

PCNL

There are 2 case reports of PCNL in early pregnancy, both with good outcomes.[109,110] PCNL is not recommended, however, as it typically requires prone positioning, fluoroscopy, and general anesthesia.

In summary, nephrolithiasis can be difficult to diagnose and challenging to treat in pregnant patients. Up to 25% of patients with renal colic may be misdiagnosed with nephrolithiasis. Older treatment algorithms involving stenting and percutaneous nephrostomy tubes are fraught with problems of encrustation and require frequent changes. Newer data seem to point to the safety and efficacy of ureteroscopy as a means of treatment of stones in pregnancy.

URINARY DIVERSION

Urolithiasis in urinary diversions poses a unique challenge to the urologist. There is a predisposition to stone formation in urinary diversions with an incidence of 3% to 43%.[111] Different types of diversions have different propensities toward stone formation. For example, Terai and colleagues[112] found that the incidence was 12.9% in patients with Indiana pouch versus 43% in patients with Koch pouch.

The risk factors can be divided into metabolic and anatomic factors. The anatomic factors include urinary stasis, obstruction from strictures, reflux of mucous, and foreign bodies that act as a nidus for stone formation. Metabolically, diversions involving ileum are associated with a hyperchloremic metabolic acidosis. Long segments of ileum also predispose to enteric hyperoxaluria. The dual problems of bacteriuria and reflux lead to urease-splitting organisms in the upper tracts and increased urinary ammonium, phosphate, and bicarbonate. Thus, the most common stone type is struvite stone; nevertheless, there are also calcium oxalate, uric acid, and calcium phosphate stones reported.[112]

In view of the difficult and varied anatomy, the imaging of choice is the CT scan with and without intravenous contrast with delayed images to help define collecting system anatomy. The choice of treatment is highly dependent on the location of the stone, its size, and the type of diversion that the patient has undergone.

ESWL

ESWL is probably best used for stones smaller than 2 cm or as an adjunct to other procedures.[113] The success rates range from 25.0% to 81.5%. This large disparity can be explained by patient selection. Cass and colleagues[114] attributed the low success rate to dilatation of the upper tracts and immobility of obese myelomeningocoele patients. On the other extreme Deliveliotis and colleagues[115] managed a 63.7% stone-free rate after 1 ESWL session, which rose to 81.8% after a follow-up session. This was a small study in which most patients were fit and had a cystectomy and ileal conduit for bladder cancer. Most of the patients did not have dilatation of the collecting system and, when it was present, it was attributed to obstruction from the stones.

If ESWL is attempted, it should be noted that there is a good chance that the patients may require some other form of antegrade or retrograde procedure. El-Assmy and colleagues[113] reported a success rate of 65.6% with a single ESWL treatment; 7.4% required secondary procedures for stone treatment and another 7.4% developed complications from obstruction caused by stone fragments, requiring antegrade ureteroscopy or percutaneous intervention. In the Deliveliotis and colleagues' study,[115] 18% of the patients required a secondary procedure. This consisted of percutaneous nephrolithotomy and an open ureterolithotomy.

Ureteroscopy

There are few studies describing the use of ureteroscopy for the management of urinary diversion stones. This can be attributed to the inherent difficulties of locating the implanted ureteric orifices. This is exacerbated if the bowel segment is convoluted. Furthermore, it can be difficult to traverse the uretero-enteric anastomosis especially if a stricture is present. Care must be taken in access to the left ureter, as it is usually slung under the sigmoid colon mesentery.

Hyams and colleagues[116] published a series of retrograde ureteroscopy for urinary diversion stones. They achieved successful access in 75% of renal units. The highest was in orthotopic neobladders (90%) and lowest in Indiana pouches (33%). The deflection capabilities of the flexible scopes can also be impaired if the reservoirs and ureters are capacious, as buckling at a proximal part of the scope can lead to a loss of deflection of the distal tip of the scope.[111]

Another approach would be a dual antegrade/retrograde approach. Delvecchio and colleagues[117] described a technique of percutaneous puncture, passage of a wire down the ureter into the diversion, which would allow antegrade access via an access sheath.

PCNL

Percutaneous access can be challenging in patients with urinary diversion. Cannulation of the ureters for retrograde contrast can be difficult. A number of techniques can be used to overcome this problem. In neobladders, the chimney can be accessed via a flexible cystoscope and indigo carmine given intravenously to aid in localization of the ureteral orifices. In ileal conduits, a loopogram can be performed and contrast can be allowed to reflux up into the collecting system to aid with access. Alternatively, a spinal needle (typically of small bore, such as a 22-gauge needle rather than an 18-gauge needle) can be punctured directly into the renal pelvis and contrast injected in. This would then allow the actual puncture to be performed fluoroscopically. Last, access can be performed via ultrasound guidance.

Stone-free rates following the use of PCNL with or without adjunct ESWL range from 75.0% to 87.5%.[114,118,119] In a meta-analysis, El-Nahas and Shokeir[120] found that the adjunct use of ESWL to clear remnant stone fragments improved stone-free status from 62.5% to 87.5%. Historical complication rates in these patients was up to 38%, but a recent article had lower complication rates of 8.3%.[118] These comprised 1 urine leak and 1 case of septicemia postprocedure.

Stones in Reservoirs

The risk factors for the formation of stones in urinary reservoirs include high residual urine volumes, bacterial colonization, and large amounts of mucous exacerbated by insufficient flushing of the reservoir and foreign body material.

The most common approach is that of a transurethral access for neobladders and for the cutaneous diversion via the cutaneous stoma or additional percutaneous tract. A problem with continent cutaneous diversions is that the act of transcutaneous access via the stoma may disrupt the continence mechanism.[111]

Another approach is a percutaneous approach to the conduit or reservoir. An ultrasound-guided or CT-guided puncture is preferred in this setting, as it is important to establish that there is no intervening bowel. The puncture can then be dilated with serial dilators or balloon dilation and laparoscopic ports or an Amplatz sheath can be inserted allowing access with a standard rigid or flexible nephroscope. There have also been descriptions of use of an endocatch bag to remove stones for more efficacious stone clearance (**Fig. 11**).[121] An added advantage is that crushing the stones within the bag protects the mucosa of the neobladder or conduit. **Fig. 12** gives an algorithm to the management of these pouch stones.

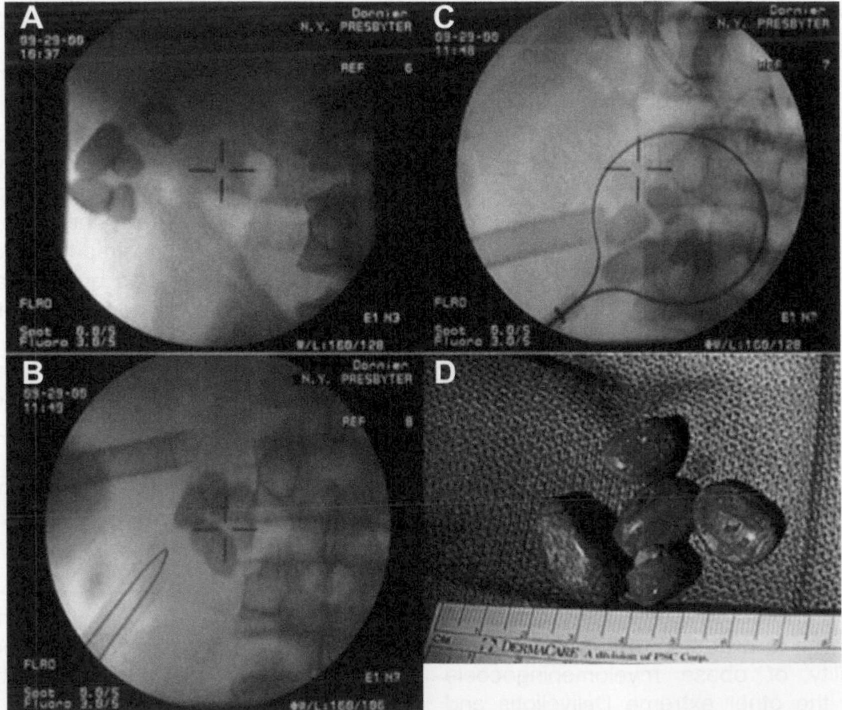

Fig. 11. (*A*) Stones in a continent cutaneous urinary diversion. (*B*) Dual access via catheterizable stoma and second percutaneous access. (*C*) Stones collected in entrapment bag. (*D*) Extracted stones.

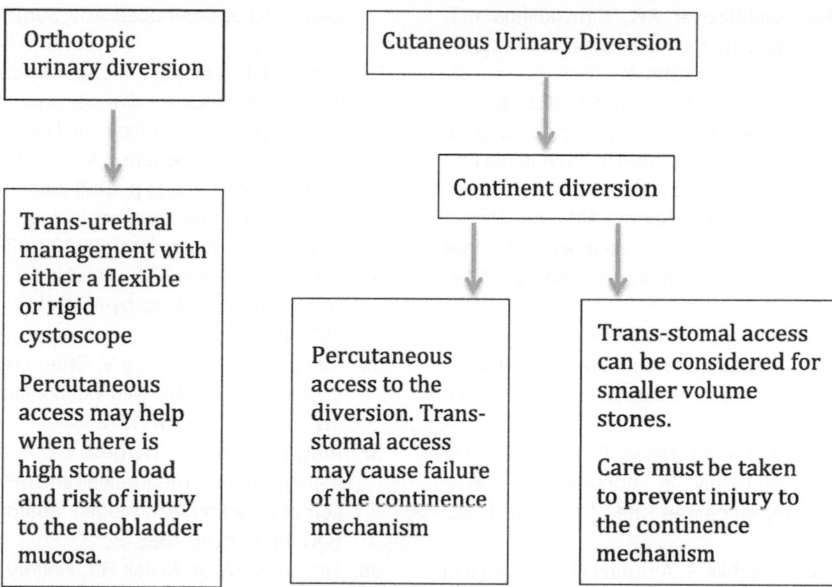

Fig. 12. Management of stones in continent urinary diversions.

SUMMARY

The management of stones in abnormal situations can be a nebulous topic; however, the principles remain the same: complete clearance of stone fragments by the least-invasive means. Treatment decisions should be individualized based on stone location, anatomic considerations, and function and location of the renal unit. Metabolic evaluation and management is especially important in this population of stone formers, as there is a high associated incidence of metabolic abnormalities.

REFERENCES

1. Raj GV, Auge BK, Weizer AZ, et al. Percutaneous management of calculi within horseshoe kidneys. J Urol 2003;170:48–51.
2. Bhatia V, Biyani CS. Urolithiasis with congenital upper tract anomalies: a 4-year experience with extracorporeal shock wave lithotripsy. J Endourol 1994;8:5–8.
3. Collado Serra A, Parada Moreno R, Rousaud Baron F, et al. Current management of calculi in horseshoe kidneys. Scand J Urol Nephrol 2000; 34:114–8.
4. Vandeursen H, Baert L. Electromagnetic extracorporeal shock wave lithotripsy for calculi in horseshoe kidneys. J Urol 1992;148:1120–2.
5. Kirkali Z, Esen AA, Mungan MU. Effectiveness of extracorporeal shockwave lithotripsy in the management of stone-bearing horseshoe kidneys. J Endourol 1996;10:13–5.
6. Tunc L, Tokgoz H, Tan MO, et al. Stones in anomalous kidneys: results of treatment by shock wave lithotripsy in 150 patients. Int J Urol 2004;11:831–6.
7. Sheir KZ, Madbouly K, Elsobky E, et al. Extracorporeal shock wave lithotripsy in anomalous kidneys: 11-year experience with two second-generation lithotripters. Urology 2003;62:10–5 [discussion: 5–6].
8. Clayman RV. Effectiveness of extracorporeal shockwave lithotripsy in the management of stone-bearing horseshoe kidneys. J Urol 1998; 160:1949.
9. Ray AA, Ghiculete D, D'A Honey RJ, et al. Shockwave lithotripsy in patients with horseshoe kidney: determinants of success. J Endourol 2011;25:487–93.
10. Andreoni C, Portis AJ, Clayman RV. Retrograde renal pelvic access sheath to facilitate flexible ureteroscopic lithotripsy for the treatment of urolithiasis in a horseshoe kidney. J Urol 2000;164: 1290–1.
11. Weizer AZ, Springhart WP, Ekeruo WO, et al. Ureteroscopic management of renal calculi in anomalous kidneys. Urology 2005;65:265–9.
12. Molimard B, Al-Qahtani S, Lakmichi A, et al. Flexible ureterorenoscopy with holmium laser in horseshoe kidneys. Urology 2010;76:1334–7.
13. Wickham JE, Kellett MJ. Percutaneous nephrolithotomy. Br J Urol 1981;53:297–9.
14. Clayman RV, Surya V, Miller RP, et al. Percutaneous nephrolithotomy. An approach to branched and staghorn renal calculi. JAMA 1983;250:73–5.
15. Yohannes P, Smith AD. The endourological management of complications associated with horseshoe kidney. J Urol 2002;168:5–8.

16. Jabbour ME, Goldfischer ER, Stravodimos KG, et al. Endopyelotomy for horseshoe and ectopic kidneys. J Urol 1998;160:694–7.
17. Glodny B, Petersen J, Hofmann KJ, et al. Kidney fusion anomalies revisited: clinical and radiological analysis of 209 cases of crossed fused ectopia and horseshoe kidney. BJU Int 2009;103:224–35.
18. Shokeir AA, El-Nahas AR, Shoma AM, et al. Percutaneous nephrolithotomy in treatment of large stones within horseshoe kidneys. Urology 2004; 64:426–9.
19. Skoog SJ, Reed MD, Gaudier FA Jr, et al. The posterolateral and the retrorenal colon: implication in percutaneous stone extraction. J Urol 1985; 134:110–2.
20. Skolarikos A, Binbay M, Bisas A, et al. Percutaneous nephrolithotomy in horseshoe kidneys: factors affecting stone-free rate. J Urol 2011;186: 1894–8.
21. Nambirajan T, Jeschke S, Albqami N, et al. Role of laparoscopy in management of renal stones: single-center experience and review of literature. J Endourol 2005;19:353–9.
22. Symons SJ, Ramachandran A, Kurien A, et al. Urolithiasis in the horseshoe kidney: a single-centre experience. BJU Int 2008;102:1676–80.
23. Gleason PE, Kelalis PP, Husmann DA, et al. Hydronephrosis in renal ectopia: incidence, etiology and significance. J Urol 1994;151:1660–1.
24. Gallucci M, Vincenzoni A, Schettini M, et al. Extracorporeal shock wave lithotripsy in ureteral and kidney malformations. Urol Int 2001;66:61–5.
25. Theiss M, Wirth MP, Frohmuller HG. Extracorporeal shock wave lithotripsy in patients with renal malformations. Br J Urol 1993;72:534–8.
26. Semerci B, Verit A, Nazli O, et al. The role of ESWL in the treatment of calculi with anomalous kidneys. Eur Urol 1997;31:302–4.
27. Talic RF. Extracorporeal shock-wave lithotripsy monotherapy in renal pelvic ectopia. Urology 1996; 48:857–61.
28. Desai MR, Jasani A. Percutaneous nephrolithotripsy in ectopic kidneys. J Endourol 2000;14:289–92.
29. Watterson JD, Cook A, Sahajpal R, et al. Percutaneous nephrolithotomy of a pelvic kidney: a posterior approach through the greater sciatic foramen. J Urol 2001;166:209–10.
30. Eshghi AM, Roth JS, Smith AD. Percutaneous transperitoneal approach to a pelvic kidney for endourological removal of staghorn calculus. J Urol 1985;134:525–7.
31. Zafar FS, Lingeman JE. Value of laparoscopy in the management of calculi complicating renal malformations. J Endourol 1996;10:379–83.
32. Holman E, Toth C. Laparoscopically assisted percutaneous transperitoneal nephrolithotomy in pelvic dystopic kidneys: experience in 15 successful cases. J Laparoendosc Adv Surg Tech A 1998;8: 431–5.
33. Kamat N, Khandelwal P. Laparoscopic pyelolithotomy—a technique for the management of stones in the ectopic pelvic kidney. Int J Urol 2004;11:581–4.
34. Ramakumar S, Segura JW. Laparoscopic surgery for renal urolithiasis: pyelolithotomy, caliceal diverticulectomy, and treatment of stones in a pelvic kidney. J Endourol 2000;14:829–32.
35. Gaur DD, Agarwal DK, Purohit KC, et al. Retroperitoneal laparoscopic pyelolithotomy. J Urol 1994; 151:927–9.
36. Ramakumar S, Lancini V, Chan DY, et al. Laparoscopic pyeloplasty with concomitant pyelolithotomy. J Urol 2002;167:1378–80.
37. Atug F, Castle EP, Burgess SV, et al. Concomitant management of renal calculi and pelvi-ureteric junction obstruction with robotic laparoscopic surgery. BJU Int 2005;96:1365–8.
38. Timmons JW Jr, Malek RS, Hattery RR, et al. Caliceal diverticulum. J Urol 1975;114:6–9.
39. Middleton AW Jr, Pfister RC. Stone-containing pyelocaliceal diverticulum: embryogenic, anatomic, radiologic and clinical characteristics. J Urol 1974;111:2–6.
40. Jones JA, Lingeman JE, Steidle CP. The roles of extracorporeal shock wave lithotripsy and percutaneous nephrostolithotomy in the management of pyelocaliceal diverticula. J Urol 1991;146:724–7.
41. Auge BK, Maloney ME, Mathias BJ, et al. Metabolic abnormalities associated with calyceal diverticular stones. BJU Int 2006;97:1053–6.
42. Kriegmair M, Schuller J, Schmeller N, et al. Diverticular calculi of the kidney calices—extracorporeal shockwave lithotripsy, percutaneous extraction or open surgery. Urologe A 1990;29:204–8 [in German].
43. Streem SB, Yost A. Treatment of caliceal diverticular calculi with extracorporeal shock wave lithotripsy: patient selection and extended followup. J Urol 1992;148:1043–6.
44. Ritchie AW, Parr NJ, Moussa SA, et al. Lithotripsy for calculi in caliceal diverticula? Br J Urol 1990; 66:6–8.
45. Turna B, Raza A, Moussa S, et al. Management of calyceal diverticular stones with extracorporeal shock wave lithotripsy and percutaneous nephrolithotomy: long-term outcome. BJU Int 2007;100: 151–6.
46. Auge BK, Munver R, Kourambas J, et al. Endoscopic management of symptomatic caliceal diverticula: a retrospective comparison of percutaneous nephrolithotripsy and ureteroscopy. J Endourol 2002;16: 557–63.
47. Batter SJ, Dretler SP. Ureterorenoscopic approach to the symptomatic caliceal diverticulum. J Urol 1997;158:709–13.

48. Gross AJ, Herrmann TR. Management of stones in calyceal diverticulum. Curr Opin Urol 2007;17:136–40.
49. Hulbert JC, Reddy PK, Hunter DW, et al. Percutaneous techniques for the management of caliceal diverticula containing calculi. J Urol 1986;135:225–7.
50. Monga M, Smith R, Ferral H, et al. Percutaneous ablation of caliceal diverticulum: long-term follow-up. J Urol 2000;163:28–32.
51. Hedelin H, Geterud K, Grenabo L, et al. Percutaneous surgery for stones in pyelocaliceal diverticula. Br J Urol 1988;62:206–8.
52. Krambeck AE, Lingeman JE. Percutaneous management of caliceal diverticuli. J Endourol 2009;23:1723–9.
53. Auge BK, Munver R, Kourambas J, et al. Neoinfundibulotomy for the management of symptomatic caliceal diverticula. J Urol 2002;167:1616–20.
54. Miller SD, Ng CS, Streem SB, et al. Laparoscopic management of caliceal diverticular calculi. J Urol 2002;167:1248–52.
55. Challacombe B, Dasgupta P, Tiptaft R, et al. Multimodal management of urolithiasis in renal transplantation. BJU Int 2005;96:385–9.
56. Rhee BK, Bretan PN Jr, Stoller ML. Urolithiasis in renal and combined pancreas/renal transplant recipients. J Urol 1999;161:1458–62.
57. Del Pizzo JJ, Jacobs SC, Sklar GN. Ureteroscopic evaluation in renal transplant recipients. J Endourol 1998;12:135–8.
58. Crook TJ, Keoghane SR. Renal transplant lithiasis: rare but time-consuming. BJU Int 2005;95:931–3.
59. Klingler HC, Kramer G, Lodde M, et al. Urolithiasis in allograft kidneys. Urology 2002;59:344–8.
60. Basiri A, Nikoobakht MR, Simforoosh N, et al. Ureteroscopic management of urological complications after renal transplantation. Scand J Urol Nephrol 2006;40:53–6.
61. Hyams E, Marien T, Bruhn A, et al. Ureteroscopy for transplant lithiasis. J Endourol 2012;26:819–22.
62. Benoit G, Blanchet P, Eschwege P, et al. Occurrence and treatment of kidney graft lithiasis in a series of 1500 patients. Clin Transplant 1996;10:176–80.
63. Francesca F, Felipetto R, Mosca F, et al. Percutaneous nephrolithotomy of transplanted kidney. J Endourol 2002;16:225–7.
64. Harper JM, Samuell CT, Hallson PC, et al. Risk factors for calculus formation in patients with renal transplants. Br J Urol 1994;74:147–50.
65. Rifaioglu MM, Berger AD, Pengune W, et al. Percutaneous management of stones in transplanted kidneys. Urology 2008;72(3):508–12.
66. Tokgoz H, Sen I, Tan MO, et al. Extracorporeal shock wave lithotripsy in L-shaped kidneys: report of two cases. Int Urol Nephrol 2005;37:685–9.
67. Modi P, Goel R, Dodia S. Case report: laparoscopic pyeloplasty with pyelolithotomy in crossed fused ectopia. J Endourol 2006;20:191–3.
68. Mufti UB, Nalagatla SK. Nephrolithiasis in autosomal dominant polycystic kidney disease. J Endourol 2010;24:1557–61.
69. Delaney VB, Adler S, Bruns FJ, et al. Autosomal dominant polycystic kidney disease: presentation, complications, and prognosis. Am J Kidney Dis 1985;5:104–11.
70. Grampsas SA, Chandhoke PS, Fan J, et al. Anatomic and metabolic risk factors for nephrolithiasis in patients with autosomal dominant polycystic kidney disease. Am J Kidney Dis 2000;36:53–7.
71. Torres VE, Wilson DM, Hattery RR, et al. Renal stone disease in autosomal dominant polycystic kidney disease. Am J Kidney Dis 1993;22:513–9.
72. Pak CY. Citrate and renal calculi: an update. Miner Electrolyte Metab 1994;20:371–7.
73. Deliveliotis C, Argiropoulos V, Varkarakis J, et al. Extracorporeal shock wave lithotripsy produces a lower stone-free rate in patients with stones and renal cysts. Int J Urol 2002;9:11–4.
74. Delakas D, Daskalopoulos G, Cranidis A. Extracorporeal shockwave lithotripsy for urinary calculi in autosomal dominant polycystic kidney disease. J Endourol 1997;11:167–70.
75. Yili L, Yongzhi L, Ning L, et al. Flexible ureteroscopy and holmium laser lithotripsy for treatment of upper urinary tract calculi in patients with autosomal dominant polycystic kidney disease. Urol Res 2012;40:87–91.
76. Al-Kandari AM, Shoma AM, Eraky I, et al. Percutaneous nephrolithotomy for management of upper urinary tract calculi in patients with autosomal dominant polycystic kidney disease. Urology 2009;74:273–7.
77. Umbreit EC, Childs MA, Patterson DE, et al. Percutaneous nephrolithotomy for large or multiple upper tract calculi and autosomal dominant polycystic kidney disease. J Urol 2010;183:183–7.
78. Meria P, Hadjadj H, Jungers P, et al. Stone formation and pregnancy: pathophysiological insights gained from morphoconstitutional stone analysis. J Urol 2010;183:1412–6.
79. Coe FL, Parks JH, Lindheimer MD. Nephrolithiasis during pregnancy. N Engl J Med 1978;298:324–6.
80. Andreoiu M, MacMahon R. Renal colic in pregnancy: lithiasis or physiological hydronephrosis? Urology 2009;74:757–61.
81. McAleer SJ, Loughlin KR. Nephrolithiasis and pregnancy. Curr Opin Urol 2004;14:123–7.
82. Rosenberg E, Sergienko R, Abu-Ghanem S, et al. Nephrolithiasis during pregnancy: characteristics, complications, and pregnancy outcome. World J Urol 2011;29:743–7.

83. Swartz MA, Lydon-Rochelle MT, Simon D, et al. Admission for nephrolithiasis in pregnancy and risk of adverse birth outcomes. Obstet Gynecol 2007;109:1099–104.
84. Colletti PM, Sylvestre PB. Magnetic resonance imaging in pregnancy. Magn Reson Imaging Clin N Am 1994;2:291–307.
85. Marcos HB, Semelka RC, Worawattanakul S. Normal placenta: gadolinium-enhanced dynamic MR imaging. Radiology 1997;205:493–6.
86. De Santis M, Straface G, Cavaliere AF, et al. Gadolinium periconceptional exposure: pregnancy and neonatal outcome. Acta Obstet Gynecol Scand 2007;86:99–101.
87. Jin DH, Lamberton GR, Broome DR, et al. Effect of reduced radiation CT protocols on the detection of renal calculi. Radiology 2010;255:100–7.
88. Ciaschini MW, Remer EM, Baker ME, et al. Urinary calculi: radiation dose reduction of 50% and 75% at CT—effect on sensitivity. Radiology 2009;251: 105–11.
89. Karmazyn B, Frush DP, Applegate KE, et al. CT with a computer-simulated dose reduction technique for detection of pediatric nephroureterolithiasis: comparison of standard and reduced radiation doses. AJR Am J Roentgenol 2009;192:143–9.
90. White WM, Zite NB, Gash J, et al. Low-dose computed tomography for the evaluation of flank pain in the pregnant population. J Endourol 2007; 21:1255–60.
91. ACOG Committee on Obstetric Practice. ACOG Committee Opinion. Number 299, September 2004 (replaces No. 158, September 1995). Guidelines for diagnostic imaging during pregnancy. Obstet Gynecol 2004;104:647–51.
92. Semins MJ, Matlaga BR. Management of stone disease in pregnancy. Curr Opin Urol 2010;20: 174–7.
93. Isen K, Hatipoglu NK, Dedeoglu S, et al. Experience with the diagnosis and management of symptomatic ureteric stones during pregnancy. Urology 2012;79:508–12.
94. Burgess KL, Gettman MT, Rangel LJ, et al. Diagnosis of urolithiasis and rate of spontaneous passage during pregnancy. J Urol 2011;186: 2280–4.
95. Khoo L, Anson K, Patel U. Success and short-term complication rates of percutaneous nephrostomy during pregnancy. J Vasc Interv Radiol 2004;15: 1469–73.
96. Dyer RB, Regan JD, Kavanagh PV, et al. Percutaneous nephrostomy with extensions of the technique: step by step. Radiographics 2002;22:503–25.
97. Jarrard DJ, Gerber GS, Lyon ES. Management of acute ureteral obstruction in pregnancy utilizing ultrasound-guided placement of ureteral stents. Urology 1993;42:263–7 [discussion: 7–8].
98. Cormier CM, Canzoneri BJ, Lewis DF, et al. Urolithiasis in pregnancy: current diagnosis, treatment, and pregnancy complications. Obstet Gynecol Surv 2006;61:733–41.
99. Streem SB. Contemporary clinical practice of shock wave lithotripsy: a reevaluation of contraindications. J Urol 1997;157:1197–203.
100. Deliveliotis CH, Argyropoulos B, Chrisofos M, et al. Shockwave lithotripsy in unrecognized pregnancy: interruption or continuation? J Endourol 2001;15: 787–8.
101. Watterson JD, Girvan AR, Beiko DT, et al. Ureteroscopy and holmium:YAG laser lithotripsy: an emerging definitive management strategy for symptomatic ureteral calculi in pregnancy. Urology 2002;60:383–7.
102. Lifshitz DA, Lingeman JE. Ureteroscopy as a first-line intervention for ureteral calculi in pregnancy. J Endourol 2002;16:19–22.
103. Polat F, Yesil S, Kirac M, et al. Treatment outcomes of semirigid ureterorenoscopy and intracorporeal lithotripsy in pregnant women with obstructive ureteral calculi. Urol Res 2011;39:487–90.
104. Semins MJ, Trock BJ, Matlaga BR. The safety of ureteroscopy during pregnancy: a systematic review and meta-analysis. J Urol 2009;181: 139–43.
105. Johnson EB, Krambeck AE, White WM, et al. Obstetric complications of ureteroscopy during pregnancy. J Urol 2012;188:151–4.
106. Ulvik NM, Bakke A, Hoisaeter PA. Ureteroscopy in pregnancy. J Urol 1995;154:1660–3.
107. Scarpa RM, De Lisa A, Usai E. Diagnosis and treatment of ureteral calculi during pregnancy with rigid ureteroscopes. J Urol 1996;155:875–7.
108. Evans HJ, Wollin TA. The management of urinary calculi in pregnancy. Curr Opin Urol 2001;11: 379–84.
109. Shah A, Chandak P, Tiptaft R, et al. Percutaneous nephrolithotomy in early pregnancy. Int J Clin Pract 2004;58:809–10.
110. Toth C, Toth G, Varga A, et al. Percutaneous nephrolithotomy in early pregnancy. Int Urol Nephrol 2005;37:1–3.
111. Okhunov Z, Duty B, Smith AD, et al. Management of urolithiasis in patients after urinary diversions. BJU Int 2011;108:330–6.
112. Terai A, Ueda T, Kakehi Y, et al. Urinary calculi as a late complication of the Indiana continent urinary diversion: comparison with the Kock pouch procedure. J Urol 1996;155:66–8.
113. El-Assmy A, El-Nahas AR, Mohsen T, et al. Extracorporeal shock wave lithotripsy of upper urinary tract calculi in patients with cystectomy and urinary diversion. Urology 2005;66:510–3.
114. Cass AS, Lee JY, Aliabadi H. Extracorporeal shock wave lithotripsy and endoscopic management of

renal calculi with urinary diversions. J Urol 1992; 148:1123–5.

115. Deliveliotis C, Varkarakis J, Argiropoulos V, et al. Shockwave lithotripsy for urinary stones in patients with urinary diversion after radical cystectomy. J Endourol 2002;16:717–20.
116. Hyams ES, Winer AG, Shah O. Retrograde ureteral and renal access in patients with urinary diversion. Urology 2009;74:47–50.
117. Delvecchio FC, Kuo RL, Iselin CE, et al. Combined antegrade and retrograde endoscopic approach for the management of urinary diversion-associated pathology. J Endourol 2000;14:251–6.
118. el-Nahas AR, Eraky I, el-Assmy AM, et al. Percutaneous treatment of large upper tract stones after urinary diversion. Urology 2006;68:500–4.
119. Wolf JS Jr, Stoller ML. Management of upper tract calculi in patients with tubularized urinary diversions. J Urol 1991;145:266–9.
120. El-Nahas AR, Shokeir AA. Endourological treatment of nonmalignant upper urinary tract complications after urinary diversion. Urology 2010;76:1302–8.
121. Miller DC, Park JM. Percutaneous cystolithotomy using a laparoscopic entrapment sac. Urology 2003;62:333–6 [discussion: 6].
122. Esuvaranathan K, Tan EC, Tung KH, et al. Stones in horseshoe kidneys: results of treatment by extracorporeal shock wave lithotripsy and endourology. J Urol 1991;146(5):1213–5.
123. Smith JE, Van Arsdalen KN, Hanno PM, et al. Extracorporeal shock wave lithotripsy treatment of calculi in horseshoe kidneys. J Urol 1989;142(3):683–6.

Advances in Percutaneous Nephrolithotomy

Jodi A. Antonelli, MD[a], Margaret S. Pearle, MD, PhD[a,b,*]

KEYWORDS

• Kidney • Kidney calculi • Percutaneous nephrolithotomy • Percutaneous nephrostomy
• Post-operative imaging • Intracorporeal lithotripsy

KEY POINTS

- Percutaneous nephrolithotomy (PCNL) is increasingly applied to moderate stone burdens, particularly for stones in the lower pole calyces.
- CT can be used to obtain percutaneous access when intraoperative fluoroscopic access is considered unsafe.
- Supine PCNL is associated with reduced operative times but has not demonstrated an advantage over traditional prone PCNL.
- Liberal use of flexible nephroscopy and prone retrograde ureteroscopy can reduce the need for multiple percutaneous accesses.
- New lithotrites, including a combination ultrasonic-pneumatic device, dual ultrasonic lithotripter, and pneumatic stone breaker have the potential to enhance the efficiency of stone fragmentation and add to the armamentarium of instrumentation for PCNL.
- A trend toward the use of smaller or no nephrostomy tube post-PCNL offers the advantage of shorter hospital stay, less analgesic requirements, and reduced urine leakage without an increased risk of hemorrhage.
- New imaging modalities offer the possibility of detecting residual fragments intraoperatively and obviating secondary procedures to retrieve residual stones.

INTRODUCTION

Percutaneous nephrolithotomy (PCNL) was first described in 1976,[1] just a few years before the introduction of shockwave lithotripsy (SWL). The strong initial interest in PCNL, however, was subsequently quelled by the explosion of SWL as the first noninvasive treatment of kidney and ureteral stones. Although early on SWL was used almost indiscriminately for the management of upper tract calculi, the limitations of the technique for large and complex stones became evident over time, and PCNL became firmly established in the therapeutic armamentarium of nephrolithiasis. In recent years, however, as the indications for ureteroscopic management of upper tract stones have expanded, ureteroscopy (URS) has, in some cases, supplanted SWL and PCNL for the treatment of some stones. Nonetheless, there have been efforts underway to reduce the morbidity and increase the efficiency and effectiveness of PCNL, making it more competitive with SWL and URS for the first-line management of upper tract stones. The contemporary advances in surgical technique, instrumentation, and perioperative care that continue to refine PCNL are reviewed here.

[a] Department of Urology, University of Texas Southwestern Medical Center, 5323 Harry Hines Boulevard, J8.106, Dallas, TX 75390-9110, USA; [b] Jane and Charles Pak Center for Mineral Metabolism, University of Texas Southwestern Medical Center, 5323 Harry Hines Boulevard, J8.106, Dallas, TX 75390-9110, USA
* Corresponding author. Department of Urology, University of Texas Southwestern Medical Center, 5323 Harry Hines Boulevard, J8.106, Dallas, TX 75390-9110.
E-mail address: margaret.pearle@utsouthwestern.edu

Urol Clin N Am 40 (2013) 99–113
http://dx.doi.org/10.1016/j.ucl.2012.09.012
0094-0143/13/$ – see front matter

INDICATIONS

One of the most important factors in selecting the optimal surgical modality for the patient with nephrolithiasis is stone size because size has been shown to strongly influence stone-free rate, need for secondary procedures, and complication rate for some treatment modalities. Historically, PCNL has been the treatment of choice for the management of large and/or complex stones. Indeed, the American Urologic Association (AUA) Guidelines for the Management of Staghorn Calculi states that "percutaneous nephrolithotomy should be the first treatment used for most patients" with stones. According to their meta-analysis of published clinical trials evaluating outcomes for surgical management of staghorn calculi, the stone-free rate for PCNL was 78% versus 71% for open surgery, 66% for combined PCNL and SWL, and 54% for SWL monotherapy. When comparing the total number of procedures required to successfully treat the stone and to manage complications, PCNL required 1.9, combination therapy 3.3, SWL 3.6, and open surgery 1.4 procedures.[2] Likewise, the European Association of Urology Guideline on Urolithiasis (updated Feb 2012) recommends PCNL for the treatment of all stones greater than or equal to 2 cm and lower pole stones greater than or equal to 1.5 cm.[3]

With improvements in the safety and efficacy of PCNL as a result of advances in instrumentation and a growing experience with the technique, some investigators have argued that the indications for PCNL should be broadened to include smaller stones throughout the kidney and specifically to those in the lower pole calyces. Deem and colleagues[4] randomized 32 subjects with moderate sized (1–2 cm, median 1.2 cm) upper or middle calyceal or renal pelvis stones to PCNL or SWL and evaluated them at 3 months with non-enhanced CT. PCNL stone-free rate was superior to SWL (85% vs 33%, respectively) and none of the PCNL patients required a secondary procedure, whereas 77% of the SWL subjects required at least one other procedure and 17% required more than one. Quality of life, as assessed by the short form (SF)-8 quality of life survey, also favored PCNL for both mental and physical domains.

Stone location is also an important determinant of stone-free rate for some treatment modalities. Lower pole location has been shown to be associated with poor stone-free rates for SWL, likely because of limited clearance of fragments from the dependent lower pole calyces.[5,6] On the other hand, PCNL stone-free rate is independent of stone burden.[5–8] The Lower Pole I Study Group conducted a prospective, multicenter randomized clinical trial (RCT) comparing SWL and PCNL for symptomatic, greater than 1.0 cm, lower pole stones and found that stone-free rates overall were threefold higher for PCNL compared with SWL (95% vs 37%, respectively, $P<.001$).[9] When stone-free rates were stratified by stone size (less than 1 cm, 1–2 cm, and greater than 2 cm), PCNL stone-free rates were relatively uniform at 100%, 93%, and 86%, respectively, whereas SWL stone-free rates were inversely related to stone size (63%, 23% and 14%, respectively).

PCNL has increasingly been used as an alternative to URS and SWL for large, proximal ureteral stones as well. Sun and colleagues[10] randomized subjects with greater than 1 cm proximal ureteral stones to PCNL or URS and found that PCNL with antegrade URS achieved a higher stone-free rate than retrograde ureterolithotripsy according to imaging obtained at discharge (95% vs 79.5%, $P = .027$) and 1 month postprocedure (100% vs 86%, $P = .026$). Several other series have corroborated these results.[11–14]

In addition to stone size and location, other factors, including stone composition, patient factors, and renal anatomy, can influence the success of specific treatment modalities.[15] SWL success is influenced by stone composition, with harder stones, such as cystine, calcium oxalate monohydrate, and brushite, being relatively shockwave-resistant; therefore, patients with these stone compositions are best treated endoscopically. Although one study suggested poorer outcomes for PCNL in subjects with increasing calcium phosphate content of their stones,[16] this finding was subsequently disputed by another group[17] and, in general, PCNL outcomes have not been definitively shown to be influenced by stone composition. Although predicting stone composition based on preoperative imaging has met with limited success, investigators have correlated CT attenuation coefficient (Hounsfield units [HU]) as a surrogate for stone composition with SWL success and found an inverse relationship between the two.[18] Perks and colleagues,[19] and others,[20,21] have shown that harder stones, particularly those with HU greater than 900, are less likely to be successfully treated with SWL and may, therefore, be more amenable to PCNL or URS. Skin-to-stone-distance (SSD), another CT-derived parameter, has been shown to correlate with SWL success and can be used to identify patients in whom endoscopic management, PCNL or URS, is advisable.[22] Perks and colleagues[19] showed that an SSD greater than 9 cm is associated with diminished SWL success (79% for subjects with SSD <9 cm vs 57% for subjects with SSD >9 cm). On the other hand, PCNL is not affected by body mass index with respect to stone-free rate, complication rate, or cost.[23,24]

POSITIONING

PCNL has historically been performed with the patient in a prone position. Retrograde placement of a ureteral catheter before PCNL has traditionally been performed with the patient in the dorsal lithotomy position before repositioning the patient prone. The prone split-leg approach was introduced as a modification to prone positioning to increase efficiency and decrease the number of operative interventions required for patients with both upper and lower tract pathology.[25] This approach has become widely accepted for PCNL because it obviates patient repositioning, thereby decreasing operative time and need for operative staff for multiple patient transfers.

Another extension of the prone position is the prone-flexed position. Ray and colleagues[26] conducted an anatomic survey of subjects in the prone, prone-flexed (30°), and supine positions using triphasic CT. They found that the distance from the posterior iliac crest to the 12th and 11th ribs was increased by 2.9 cm and 3.0 cm, respectively ($P<.001$), with prone-flexed positioning compared with prone positioning. Consequently, in 5 of 11 subjects (45.5%) upper pole access above the 11th rib was converted to access above the 12th rib or access above the 12th rib was converted to infracostal access by using the prone-flexed position. This same group later reported on 318 subjects who underwent PCNL in the prone-flexed position and found that most (>85%) of single tract punctures of upper pole calyces could be accomplished below the 11th rib, thereby reducing morbidity.[27]

Although prone positioning in general has proven successful, it does have notable drawbacks. Obese patients and those with cardiopulmonary comorbidities often do not tolerate being in the prone position for long periods of time. In addition, repositioning the patient from lithotomy to prone, if a split-leg table is not used, is time consuming. In an effort to overcome these drawbacks and streamline the procedure, supine PCNL was introduced.

Valdivia and colleagues[28] first described PCNL in the supine position in 1987 and later published a series of 557 consecutive subjects undergoing supine PCNL with favorable outcomes, including a transfusion rate of 1%, no colonic injuries, and greater than 90% of subjects describing little or no pain.[29] Since that time several other series of supine PCNL have been published with similar results.[30–35]

A Cochrane-based systematic review and meta-analysis comparing supine and prone PCNL included two RCTs and two case-controlled studies that met inclusion criteria.[36] Operative time was shorter for supine PCNL, but complication, transfusion, and fever rates were similar for the two approaches. Only a single colonic injury was reported in the supine setting.[36] Another subsequent meta-analysis comparing the two approaches included the previous four studies in addition to 27 case series (8 supine and 19 prone).[37] This analysis also found a significant difference in operative time between the supine and prone groups (65 ± 15 minutes vs 90 ± minutes, respectively, $P = .0009$) but detected no significant differences between the two groups with respect to stone-free (82% vs 82%, respectively) and transfusion rates (9% vs 4%, respectively).[37]

Overall, the safety and efficacy of supine and prone PCNL seems to be equivalent and, at this time, there is no demonstrable advantage of one technique over the other. However, both the sample sizes and methodological quality of the studies included in the meta-analyses were limited and, therefore, a large, prospective, multicenter, RCT is needed to more reliably compare the two approaches.

In addition to the supine position, other modifications to the traditional prone position have been proposed over the years. Published series have reported on the supine oblique,[38] semisupine,[39] lateral decubitus,[40] split-leg modified lateral,[41] flank,[42] and flank prone position.[43] Many of these positions have demonstrated the advantage of allowing for simultaneous antegrade and retrograde access to the kidney, enabling access to stones remote from the nephrostomy tract without the need for additional percutaneous punctures.

ACCESS

The key to a successful percutaneous procedure is well-placed access into the kidney. The percutaneous puncture can be performed under fluoroscopic, ultrasound, MRI, or CT guidance, and it can be obtained from an antegrade or retrograde approach. In 2003, three-quarters of the practicing urologists in the North Central Section of the AUA who responded to a survey reported feeling comfortable performing PCNL, but only 11% of that group routinely obtained percutaneous access without the assistance of a radiologist.[44] Today, it remains true that most practicing urologists, including endourologists, in the United States do not obtain their own percutaneous renal access. Despite this, several studies have demonstrated that access obtained by a urologist is comparable or favorable to access obtained by an interventional radiologist.

Watterson and colleagues[45] retrospectively reviewed 103 PCNL procedures at a single institution in which access was obtained by a radiologist in 54 subjects and by a urologist in 49 subjects. They found fewer complications (5 vs 15, respectively) and higher stone-free rates (86% vs 61%, respectively) in the urologist-directed access group compared with the radiologist-directed access group. Similar retrospective reviews with larger numbers of subjects have corroborated these findings.[46,47] Tomaszewski and colleagues[48] also compared 195 subjects with urologist-directed access with 38 subjects with radiologist-directed access and found comparable complication rates between the two groups. However, the stone-free rate was higher with urologist-obtained access (99% vs 92%, respectively), and access obtained by a radiologist was considered unsuitable in 37% of subjects, necessitating access by a urologist at the time of surgery. Of note, however, access obtained by a radiologist was often done solely for the purpose of renal decompression, without the foresight or opportunity to communicate with the urologist about the suitability of the access for future surgical intervention. These data underscore the advantage of the urologist over the radiologist in obtaining appropriate access, which is that the urologist can apply his or her knowledge and expertise in renal anatomy and surgical technique to select a puncture site that minimizes the number of procedures and improves outcomes.

Intraoperative percutaneous access is most commonly performed using fluoroscopic guidance. Inherent to this modality is exposure to ionizing radiation for the surgeon, operating room staff, and patient. The dose of radiation in this setting is not inconsequential to the physicians or staff who perform these surgeries daily, or to the recurrent stone formers who often undergo repeated surgical interventions. Kumari and colleagues[49] sought to quantify the radiation exposure received by the urologist, operating room staff, and patient during PCNL using lithium fluoride thermo-luminescent dosimeter chips to monitor incident radiation exposure in 50 consecutive PCNL procedures. With a mean operating time of 75 minutes and mean fluoroscopy time of 6 minutes (1.8–12.16 minutes), the mean incident radiation exposure to the finger of the operating urologist and assisting resident were 0.28 mSv and 0.36 mSv, respectively, and to the subject was 0.56 mSv. Although the mean radiation dose at the level of the trunk of the operating urologist was 60 μSv, the radiation dose to the anesthesiologist and floor nurse was minimal. Of note, the National Commission on Radiation Protection states that the maximum permissible dose equivalent for occupational exposure in 1 year for the combined whole body is 50,000 mSv. Although the average radiation exposure during PCNL described by Kumari and others[49] is well under the permissible yearly amount, it is important to keep in mind that radiation dose can vary greatly depending on complexity and length of procedure and can accumulate quickly, particularly for those urologists and/or staff largely dedicated to endourology and for those patients afflicted with chronic stone-forming conditions.

An alternative to fluoroscopy is ultrasound-guided percutaneous access. The advantages of ultrasound-guidance include lack of ionizing radiation to the patient and physician, the ability to identify nearby organs such as bowel, spleen or liver, widespread availability, and low cost. However, ultrasound-guidance is quite operator dependent and has limited ability to delineate fine detail of renal anatomy, particularly in obese patients or those with nondilated collecting systems.[50] Despite these limitations, ultrasound-guided percutaneous puncture of the collecting system is ideal for pregnant[51–53] and pediatric patients and for those in whom retrograde placement of a ureteral catheter is difficult or impossible (eg, those with urinary diversions or renal transplants[54,55]).

Several groups of investigators have examined the safety and efficacy of ultrasound-guided percutaneous renal access, all of which concluded that ultrasound-guided access has satisfactory outcomes with few complications and less radiation exposure compared with conventional fluoroscopic-guided access.[56–59] Agarwal and colleagues[60] prospectively evaluated 224 subjects undergoing PCNL who were randomized to fluoroscopic or ultrasound-guided access. They found a shorter mean access time (1.8 minutes vs 3.2 minutes, $P<.01$) and fewer mean puncture attempts (1.5 vs 3.3, $P<.01$) to achieve access into the desired calyx in the ultrasound group compared with the fluoroscopy group. Furthermore, mean duration of radiation exposure was shorter for ultrasound compared with fluoroscopic guidance (14.4 seconds vs 28.6 seconds, respectively, $P<.01$) and all subjects in both groups were stone free at 1 month based on noncontrast CT.

MRI has recently been described as an alternative means of nonionizing radiation that can be used to guide percutaneous renal access.[61] Kariniemi and colleagues[62] prospectively evaluated eight subjects undergoing percutaneous access using an open-configuration, C-arm shaped MRI and reported success in seven of the eight attempts, with the only failed attempt occurring in a nondilated system. The investigators noted that a significant drawback of this technique, however, is difficulty visualizing the guidewire with MRI.

For patients with unusual anatomy, such as spinal cord deformity in spina bifida or scoliosis, percutaneous access under fluoroscopic guidance can predispose to a higher likelihood of adjacent organ injury. In these instances, CT-guided percutaneous renal access obtained at a setting separate from PCNL provides an advantage over the traditional fluoroscopic approach. Matlaga and colleagues[63] reported that 3% of 154 percutaneous nephrolithotomies underwent CT-guided access because of spinal deformity, retrorenal colon, or transplant kidney, and subsequently underwent successful PCNL.

Because percutaneous renal access is not a skill set that is routinely included in the curriculum of urologic residency, some practitioners have favored using the more familiar retrograde approach to the kidney. Lawson and colleagues,[64] and Hunter and colleagues,[65] described directing a steerable catheter in a retrograde fashion into the desired calyx, then advancing a puncture wire out through the catheter to the skin, creating through-and-through access. Since their first reports, contemporary modifications of the technique have been described, including the use of endoscopic assistance to visually direct the puncture wire out through the targeted calyx.[66]

Endoscopic assistance has also been used to facilitate antegrade access to the kidney when a percutaneous puncture cannot be successfully performed or when a wire cannot be navigated out of an obstructed calyx. The initial report in 1995 described the use of simultaneous retrograde URS and fluoroscopic percutaneous renal access.[67] Kidd and Conlin[68] reported three clinical scenarios, morbid obesity, renal ptosis, and a large staghorn calculus, in which endoscopic assistance was a valuable adjunct to traditional fluoroscopic or ultrasound-guided antegrade renal access. Other investigators have advocated for the routine use of ureteroscopic-guided percutaneous renal access because they argue that endoscopic-assisted access provides for safer, more precise placement of the working sheath, potentially translating into less bleeding, and that the use of a ureteroscopic access sheath facilitates drainage, passage of fragments, and easy access to calyces that are inaccessible via the nephroscope.[69] Although this technique adds to troubleshooting options available to assist with difficult access, routine use is arguably unnecessary, time-consuming, and cost-inefficient.

One of the advantages of PCNL in treating large or complex stones is the large caliber of the access tract, which allows for intact removal of large stones and the use of fragmentation devices that incorporate suction capability. However, morbidity of the procedure is often attributed to the large size of the nephrostomy tract (typically 30F). A review of data derived from the Clinical Research Office of the Endourology Society (CROES) global database of over 5000 PCNLs showed that the probability of bleeding was higher with larger caliber working sheaths (odds ratio 1.42, $P = .0001$).[70] In an effort to decrease the morbidity of PCNL, there has been interest in reducing the size of the working sheath and/or the size of the nephrostomy tube.

The technique of using a small caliber working sheath, known as the mini-perc, was originally an extension of a pediatric technique that used an 11-15 F peel-away vascular access sheath.[71] Jackman and colleagues[72] later substituted a 13 F ureteral access sheath for the flimsy vascular access sheath because of it offered superior stability. The technique involves conventional percutaneous access to the collecting system using an 18-gauge needle. After passage of two guide wires down the ureter, a 13 F sheath is passed directly over the working wire, without the need for sequential dilation. In a small series of nine mini-percs on stones with an average cross-sectional area of 1.5 cm^2, Jackman and colleagues[72] reported stone-free rates comparable to standard PCNL with no transfusions and modest pain medication requirements.

Three prospective trials compared the safety and efficacy of mini-perc with standard PCNL. Knoll and colleagues[73] randomized 50 subjects with solitary lower pole or renal pelvic calculi to mini-perc (25 subjects, 18 F outer sheath) or standard PCNL (24 subjects, 26 F outer sheath). Of note, mean stone size in the standard group was slightly larger than in the mini-perc group (22 mm vs 18 mm) and postoperative management differed between the two groups (subjects undergoing uncomplicated mini-percs were left tubeless, while all subjects undergoing standard PCNL were left with 22 F nephrostomy tubes). Operative times, stone-free rates, and complication rates were comparable between the two groups, but the mini-perc group reported slightly lower postoperative pain scores and had a significantly shorter hospital stay (3.8 vs 6.9 days) compared with the standard PCNL group. Cheng and colleagues[74] performed an RCT that compared 72 subjects undergoing mini-perc using a 16 F sheath with 115 subjects undergoing standard PCNL using a 24 F sheath. Although mini-perc was associated with a lower transfusion rate ($P<0.05$), the procedure was significantly longer than standard PCNL. Finally, Mishra and colleagues[75] prospectively compared mini-perc with standard PCNL in subjects with 1 to 2 cm renal stones and found longer operative times but significantly less blood loss, lower analgesic use, and reduced hospital stay for mini-perc compared with standard PCNL.

Mini-perc is the predecessor of the microperc, a technique that furthers the concept of downsizing renal access. Bader and colleagues[76] initially described using an "all-seeing needle," which allowed visualization of the punctured calyx and stone before proceeding with dilation to 30 F for standard PCNL. The group subsequently used this needle to obtain access and perform PCNL in a single-step. After obtaining percutaneous access with the 16-gauge all-seeing needle under optical guidance, the inner bevel of the needle is removed, leaving the 4.85 F outer sheath in place. A three-way connector is attached to the proximal end of the sheath to allow for irrigation and passage of a 200 μm laser fiber and a micro-optic (**Fig. 1**).[77] This technique may have an advantage compared with SWL for the treatment of intermediate-sized lower pole stones because it allows for direct visualization of the stone and active clearance of fragments using pressurized irrigation. Micro-perc is applicable to stones in calyceal diverticuli and in horseshoe and ectopic kidneys.[77] Further studies, ideally in a randomized, controlled setting, are needed to define the safety, efficacy, and applicability of this innovative technique.

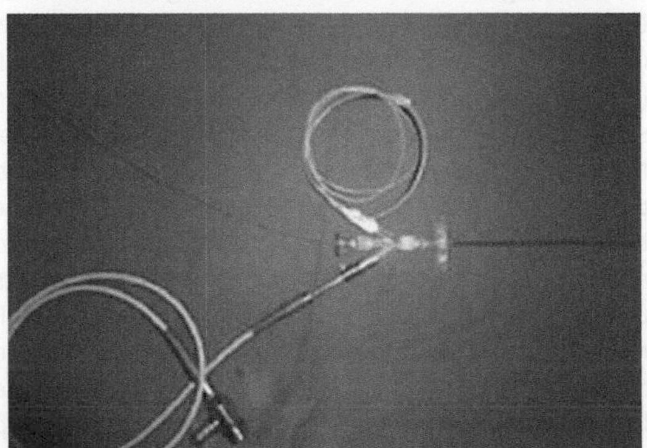

Fig. 1. Fully assembled microperc set-up, including. 4.85 F needle sheath fitted with a 3-way adapter accommodating irrigation tubing above, telescope cable below, and laser fiber passing through the center of the sheath. (*From* Desai MR, Sharma R, Mishra S, et al. Single-step percutaneous nephrolithotomy (microperc): the initial clinical report. J Urol 2011;186:140–1, Fig. 2D; with permission.)

For complex stones, multiple percutaneous accesses are often needed to removal stones from disparate locations. However, the use of multiple accesses carries a higher risk of bleeding and complications, including potentially a detrimental effect on renal function, compared with single access.[78,79] Accordingly, measures that reduce the need for multiple accesses are desirable. Wong and Leveillee[80] made liberal use of flexible nephroscopy and holmium:YAG laser lithotripsy in their series of 45 subjects with >5 cm partial or complete staghorn calculi in which a single upper percutaneous renal access was obtained. With a mean of 1.6 procedures per subject and a transfusion rate of 2.2%, they achieved a 95% stone-free rate. Other investigators have described the use of same-procedure URS to access and retrieve calyceal stones inaccessible from the percutaneous nephrostomy tract. Landman and colleagues[81] reported on nine subjects with partial or compete staghorn calculi in whom a ureteral access sheath was placed before lower pole percutaneous puncture. Inaccessible stones were retrieved ureteroscopically and placed in a position where they could be removed percutaneously. They achieved a stone-free rate of 78% with an estimated blood loss of only 290 cc. Likewise, Marguet and colleagues[82] performed initial URS and treated or displaced stones they anticipated would be remote from the planned percutaneous access tract before repositioning the subject prone and proceeding with standard PCNL using a single percutaneous access.

Finally, in another effort to reduce the number of percutaneous accesses, Miller and colleagues[83] described the use of a nondilated puncture to facilitate access to a stone that is remote from the nephrostomy tract for which the associated infundibulum is either not identifiable or is inaccessible. The technique involves percutaneous needle puncture directly into the stone-bearing calyx with subsequent injection of contrast-stained saline or air that can be identified endoscopically with a flexible nephroscope (**Fig. 2**). In some cases, the nephroscope can then be advanced into the stone-bearing calyx to fragment or retrieve the stone or, in some cases, the stone may be able to be irrigated out of the calyx via saline injection through the needle.

TRACT DILATION

Historically, a variety of methods have been used to dilate the nephrostomy tract, including metal telescoping Alken dilators, sequential Amplatz dilators, and balloon dilation.[84] In general, balloon dilation is thought to be quicker than fascial

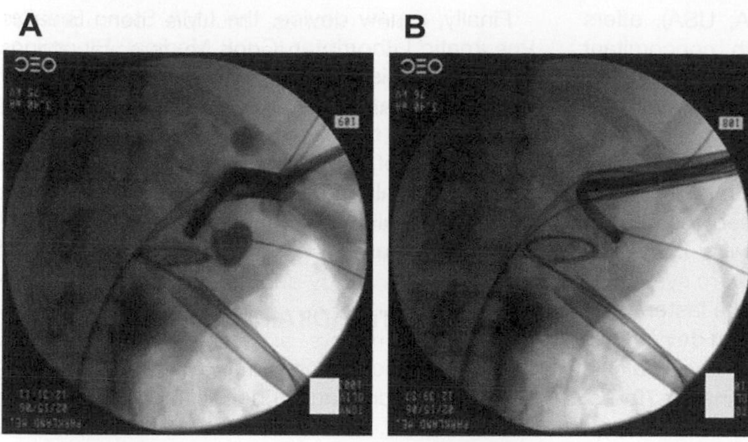

Fig. 2. Nondilated percutaneous access to facilitate identification of a stone-bearing calyx that could not be located endoscopically. (*A*) Percutaneous needle puncture into a stone-bearing calyx visualized fluoroscopically but not accessible with a flexible nephroscope via either of the two established nephrostomy tracts. (*B*) The flexible nephroscope has been advanced into the previously inaccessible calyx via an upper pole access tract after air or contrast had been injected through the needle, enabling endoscopic identification of the infundibulum.

dilation, which requires numerous passes of metal or plastic dilators. Additionally, the numerous passes that are required during dilation with sequential dilators increase the likelihood of wire dislodgement or perforation of the collecting system, which can increase the risk of hemorrhage.[85,86] On the other hand, balloon dilation is more costly and arguably less effective in the setting of a previously operated kidney.[87,88]

The introduction of the X-Force N30 dilating balloon (Bard Medical, Covington, GA, USA), with a burst pressure of 30 ATM (atmospheres) instead of the standard 17 ATM, offers the potential for greater efficacy in the setting of the patient undergoing reoperation. Hendlin and Monga[89] reported a 100% success rate in dilating 60 consecutive percutaneous tracts with a 30 ATM balloon compared with the historic 5% to10% failure rate with a 17 ATM balloon.[89]

Despite a general consensus in the literature regarding the superior safety and efficacy of balloon dilation over metal or plastic dilators, a recent analysis of the CROES database assessing PCNL operative times and bleeding complications in 5537 tract dilations (2277 balloon dilations and 3260 telescopic or serial dilations) demonstrated higher median operating time, bleeding, and transfusion rates in the balloon dilation group compared with the telescoping-serial dilation group.[70] Furthermore, on multivariate analysis, independent predictors of bleeding complications included sheath size, operating time, stone size, and caseload but did not include dilation method. Of note, this was not a randomized comparison, and it is possible that there are other unidentified confounding factors.

In an effort to streamline traditional two-step dilation (balloon dilation and passage of the working sheath over the balloon), a novel device called the Pathway Balloon Expandable PCNL Sheath (Onset Medical, Irvine, CA, USA) was developed that is comprised of a polyester balloon housed in an expandable Teflon access sheath. The device allows for simultaneous tract dilation and sheath placement in one step. Pathak and Bellman[90] compared the safety and efficacy of this dilation system (Pathway Access Sheath [PAS]) to standard balloon dilation in 21 randomly assigned subjects undergoing PCNL and found a shorter insertion time with the PAS system compared with standard balloon dilation (3 minutes vs 5.7 minutes, respectively) but no significant difference in blood loss or cost. The investigators admitted that potential drawbacks to the design include a less stiff body compared with the Amplatz sheath and a slightly oblong shape, which may hinder the removal of very round stones.

LITHOTRIPSY DEVICES

Successful and efficient PCNL relies heavily on the effectiveness of the lithotripsy device. Ultrasonic lithotripsy has historically constituted the mainstay of stone fragmentation because it effectively fragments most stones and incorporates an efficient suction device for aspiration of fragments. A disadvantage of ultrasonic lithotripsy is its relative inability to effectively fragment and, therefore clear, hard stones, including those with a significant proportion of cystine, calcium oxalate monohydrate, and brushite compositions.[91] Pneumatic lithotripsy is more efficient in fragmenting hard stones than ultrasonic lithotripsy, but pneumatic devices have no or limited suction capability.[92] A dual modality device that combines both of these lithotrites, the Swiss LithoClast Ultra (Boston

Scientific Corporation, Natick, MA, USA), offers efficient stone fragmentation with concomitant suction. The device consists of a 3.3 mm diameter ultrasonic probe and hand piece as well as a 1.1 mm diameter pneumatic probe and hand piece. The hand pieces interlock, with the pneumatic probe resting within the lumen of ultrasonic probe, and the two modalities can be used together or separately. The efficacy of the Swiss LithoClast Ultra was tested in a hands-free in vitro system by Kuo and colleagues[93] who reported a faster mean penetration time with the combination device than either an ultrasonic or pneumatic device alone, with the pneumatic portion accounting for 79% of the total time improvement. Of note, at 100% ultrasonic power the investigators did report "occasional overheating and device malfunction."

The CyberWand dual ultrasonic lithotriptor (Gyrus ACMI, Southborough, MA, USA) is another relatively new lithotripsy device that is comprised of an ultrasonic hand piece with dual high frequency-low frequency coaxial concentric probes (2.77 mm diameter inner probe and a 3.75 mm diameter outer probe). The probes act in synergy to more efficiently comminute stones than a single probe alone while retaining suction capabilities. In a direct comparison of the CyberWand to the Swiss LithoClast Ultra in an in vitro system, the CyberWand produced significantly shorter penetration times compared with the Swiss LithoClast Ultra (4.8 vs 8.1 seconds, $P<.0001$) with no adverse events or malfunctions reported in either group.[94]

In an RCT comparing the Swiss Lithoclast Ultra with a standard ultrasonic lithotripter (LUS-II, Olympus, Waltham, MA, USA) in 20 subjects undergoing PCNL, Pietrow and colleagues[95] demonstrated superiority of the Lithoclast Ultra with respect to mean time to stone clearance (21 vs 44 minutes, $P = .036$) and rate of clearance (40 mm^2/min vs 17 mm^2/min, $P = .028$). However, despite in vitro evidence of more efficient stone fragmentation with the CyberWand compared with the Lithoclast Ultra, a multicenter RCT of 57 subjects undergoing PCNL for greater than 2 cm renal calculi showed no advantage in the performance of the CyberWand compared with the Lithoclast Ultra with regard to time to stone clearance, stone-free rate, or complication rate.[96] The investigators did report eight device malfunctions in the CyberWand group and five in the LUS-II group that temporarily interrupted the procedures. An updated version of the CyberWand probe was released midstudy that was used for the second half of subjects in the CyberWand group. Although none of the new probes malfunctioned, subset analysis showed no improvement in stone clearance and stone-free rates with the new CyberWand.

Finally, a new device, the LMA Stone Breaker Pneumatic Lithotripter (Cook Medical, Bloomington, IN, USA) is comprised of a cordless reusable handpiece that uses CO_2 cartridges and disposable probes to generate high velocity at the probe-tip to effect stone fragmentation. Although no clinical trials have compared this device with the other available lithotrites, it is marketed for use on very hard stones.

POSTOPERATIVE DRAINAGE OPTIONS

The final surgical decision of PCNL is the need for and type of drainage tube. Historically, a large-bore catheter, such as a 24 F Councill catheter, a reentry Malecot catheter, or a nephroureteral stent, was placed at the end of the procedure and left indwelling for several days to provide drainage and tamponade the nephrostomy tract. The advantages of a large-bore catheter include reliable and efficient drainage, maintenance of the tract for a secondary percutaneous procedure, and prevention of bleeding from the tract. However, larger tubes are thought to be associated with increased patient discomfort and may in fact not limit postoperative blood loss as initially thought.

Several studies have compared the outcomes of percutaneous renal procedures using nephrostomy tubes of different sizes. Maheshwari and colleagues[97] prospectively studied 40 subjects undergoing PCNL who were left with either a 28 F nephrostomy tube or a 9 F pigtail catheter postoperatively and found a comparable incidence of hematuria in the two groups. However, the pigtail group required less analgesia and had less urinary leakage and a shorter hospital stay. Pietrow and colleagues[98] found similar results in a trial of 30 subjects randomized to postoperative drainage with either a 22 F Councill catheter or a 10 F pigtail catheter.

Wickham first described leaving no nephrostomy tube after PCNL in 1984.[99] However, the practice of omitting the nephrostomy tube fell out of favor after reported occurrences of postoperative hemorrhage.[100] Bellman and colleagues[101] introduced the term "tubeless" PCNL in 1997 with their report of 50 subjects undergoing percutaneous procedures in whom the first 30 subjects were managed with an indwelling ureteral stent and 22 F nephrostomy tube that was removed 2 to 3 hours later and the last 20 subjects who were left with only an indwelling ureteral stent. These tubeless subjects were compared with a historical control group of 50 subjects drained with a standard 22 F nephrostomy tube. The tubeless group had a shorter hospital stay, lower analgesic requirement, quicker return to normal activity, and no increased complication rate compared with the standard nephrostomy group.

The optimal choice of drainage tube after PCNL has been evaluated in randomized trials that have compared outcomes with different size or no nephrostomy tubes postprocedure. Desai and colleagues[102] randomized 30 subjects to large-bore (22 F nephrostomy tube), small-bore (9 F pigtail), and no nephrostomy tube (6 F double-J stent) and found similar blood loss among the groups but the highest analgesic requirement in the large-bore group and the shortest duration of urinary leakage and shortest hospital stay in the tubeless group. Marcovich and colleagues[103] also randomized 60 subjects to 24 F reentry catheter, 8 F pigtail catheter, or double-J stent and, likewise, found no difference in blood loss or transfusion rates among the three groups. However, they discerned no advantage with regard to analgesic use or hospital stay among any the three drainage routines.

The concept of tubeless PCNL has been further tested with the introduction of the "totally tubeless" PCNL, which involves no internal or external urinary drainage tubes.[104–106] Crook and colleagues[106] identified 100 PCNL procedures over a 10-year period during which the decision was made to leave no external or internal urinary drainage tube in the setting of no significant bleeding or residual stones appreciated by the surgeons. They concluded that, in the properly selected patient, a totally tubeless approach is associated with outcomes comparable to standard PCNL.

In an effort to compare the available data regarding drainage options after PCNL, several systematic reviews and meta-analyses have been performed. Zilberman and colleagues[107] identified 50 papers with appropriate data regarding drainage after PCNL and summarized the complications and outcomes of tubeless versus standard PCNL to create a set of recommendations regarding the indications for tubeless PCNL. They determined that major complications with tubeless PCNL were "anecdotal" and occurred in only one to two subjects per series, and they found comparable major and minor complications for tubeless and standard PCNL. However, outcomes such as cost, postoperative pain, hospital stay, and return to normal activities were all superior in the tubeless approach. The investigators concluded that nephrostomy tube placement after PCNL should be reserved for patients in whom more than two access tracts are required and/or there is significant collecting system perforation, intraoperative bleeding, likely need for second-look nephroscopy, or risk of pleural violation.

Yuan and colleagues[108] also performed a meta-analysis to evaluate the safety and efficacy of tubeless versus standard PCNL and identified 14 randomized, controlled trials with appropriately expressed data that were included in the analysis. Patients who underwent standard PCNL were subdivided into those managed with a small caliber nephrostomy tube (4–10 F) and those left with a large caliber tube (14–24 F). Overall, the investigators found that tubeless PCNL had the lowest analgesic requirement and shorter hospital stay compared with standard PCNL, regardless of tube size. Additionally, tubeless procedures were associated with significantly shorter operative times, reduced postoperative pain, and less urine leakage than were the small-tube group (**Fig. 3**). Although the small sample size of the small nephrostomy group may preclude meaningful comparisons, there seems to be an advantage to no nephrostomy tube compared with any size tube with regard to patient morbidity.

Finally, Wang and colleagues[109] also performed a meta-analysis of tubeless versus standard PCNL and identified seven randomized controlled trials from 2006 to 2010 that were included in their analysis. They found no difference in mean operative time or blood loss between the two groups but did find that tubeless PCNL was associated with lower analgesic requirements and shorter hospital stay compared with standard PCNL.

It is evident that there is an increasing trend toward performing tubeless PCNL in appropriately selected patients because of reduced patient morbidity. However, the disadvantage of losing access for second-look flexible nephroscopy in the event of residual fragments has not been fully explored. Proponents of tubeless PCNL argue

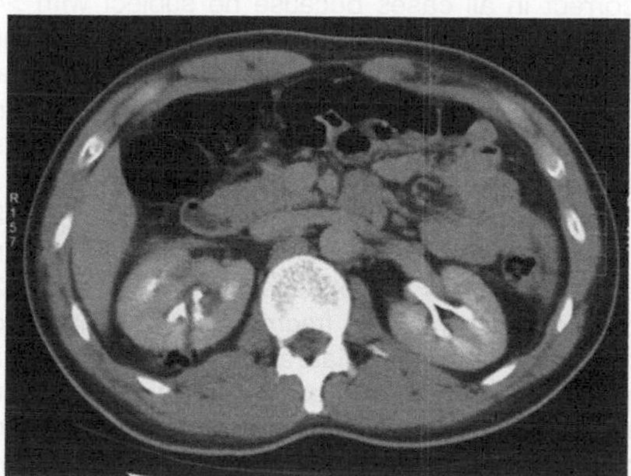

Fig. 3. Contrast-enhanced CT performed on postoperative day 1 after right tubeless PCNL demonstrates no renal hematoma or urinary extravasation. Note the nephrostomy tract and air around the right kidney.

that second-look flexible URS is as effective as second-look nephroscopy, but the likelihood that the patient actually undergoes a secondary procedure after being discharged from the hospital has not been investigated.

MANAGEMENT OF RESIDUAL FRAGMENTS

The goal of any surgical stone procedure is complete stone removal. Although the single procedure stone-free rate for PCNL is higher than for SWL or URS for comparable sized stones,[4,9] the likelihood of residual fragments after PCNL for large renal calculi is as high as 67%, using strict CT criteria.[110] As such, secondary percutaneous procedures to retrieve residual stones and achieve a stone-free state have been encouraged. Likewise, there has been interest in ways to enhance the identification of residual fragments at the time of initial PCNL so as to avoid the need for a secondary procedure. Portis and colleagues[111] described the use of high-resolution fluoroscopy at the time of initial PCNL to improve the likelihood of detecting and removing all fragments at the initial procedure. Among 36 subjects undergoing PCNL who were thought to be stone free, further high resolution fluoroscopy demonstrated residual fragments in 36%, resulting in an additional seven of nine subjects being rendered stone free on post-PCNL CT. However, despite these measures the stone-free rate was only 60% on postoperative CT. Portis and colleagues[112] further attempted to assess residual stone burden intraoperatively among 74 subjects undergoing PCNL and used their assessment of stone-free status to guide the need for nephrostomy tube placement. Based on the investigators assumption that ≤4 mm residual fragments can be safely left behind after PCNL, they considered their decision to place a tube correct in all cases because no subject with >4 mm residual fragments were left tubeless, and all subjects left tubeless had no or ≤4 mm residual fragments. However, the investigators' assumption that less than or equal to 4 mm residual fragments are harmless is subject to debate.

The natural history of fragments after PCNL largely depends on their size and location. Raman and colleagues[113] retrospectively reviewed 42 subjects with residual fragments after PCNL and determined by multivariate analysis that a maximum residual stone size exceeding 2 mm and location in the renal pelvis or ureter independently predicted an adverse stone-related event at a median follow-up of 32 months. Raman and colleagues[114] further performed a cost-effectiveness analysis and found that at their institution routine second-look nephroscopy on all patients undergoing PCNL patients was not cost-effective and that an observational strategy for patients with less than 4 mm residual fragments was cost-effective, whereas second-look nephroscopy for patients with residual stones >4 mm in size was cost-advantageous.

POSTPROCEDURE IMAGING

Postoperative imaging after PCNL is aimed at identifying renal and extrarenal complications, such as pleural violation, colonic, splenic or hepatic injury, or urinary extravasation or hemorrhage, and at assessing stone-free status. One of the more common extrarenal complications is the occurrence of hydrothorax associated with pleural transgression during percutaneous access. Historically, many urologists have routinely obtained a chest radiograph in the postanesthesia care unit after PCNL, especially in patients who have undergone supracostal access.

Ogan and colleagues[115] prospectively compared intraoperative chest fluoroscopy with postoperative recovery room portable chest radiography, and postoperative day 1 CT scan that included imagines of the lung bases in 100 subjects undergoing PCNL. They found that intraoperative chest fluoroscopy was adequate to detect clinically meaningful hydrothoracies and that it could be used to guide the need for intraoperative tube thoracostomy, thereby avoiding a delay in diagnosis and additional cost incurred with the use of routine postoperative imaging.

In an effort to reduce radiation exposure to stone patients at risk of accumulating a significant amount of radiation over their lifetimes, Bjurlin and colleagues[116] reviewed 214 percutaneous procedures to determine whether routine postoperative chest radiography was necessary for all patients undergoing PCNL. Despite supracostal access in 21% of cases, they found an incidence of hydrothorax diagnosed by postoperative chest radiography of only 1% and both subjects were symptomatic. The investigators concluded that it is safe and cost-effective to perform selective postoperative chest radiography after PCNL, targeting those patients with supracostal access and/or those with symptomatic manifestations of potential pulmonary pathology.

Postprocedural imaging to detect residual stone burden typically includes kidney, ureter, bladder (KUB), plain nephrotomograms, CT, and/or antegrade nephrostogram. Denstedt and colleagues[117] showed that KUB and nephrotomograms missed residual stones found at the time of second-look flexible nephroscopy in 34% and 17% of cases, respectively. On the other hand, Pearle and colleagues[110] demonstrated that CT was 100%

sensitive and 62% specific in detecting residual stones postoperatively in a group of 31 subjects with 41 renal units evaluated prospectively with postoperative day 1 CT and flexible nephroscopy in all subjects regardless of CT findings. As such, CT constitutes the optimal post-PCNL imaging modality to detect residual fragments. Whether low-dose CT will prove to retain sufficient sensitivity to detect most residual stones remains to be seen, but it may represent a reasonable compromise that maintains high sensitivity but with reduced radiation exposure.

Cone beam CT is a novel imaging modality that uses an imaging head similar to that of a conventional C-arm but provides high-resolution axial CT-like images and may have potential future application in the setting of PCNL. Roy and colleagues[118] described the use of this imaging modality in conjunction with PCNL to detect residual fragments intraoperatively, thereby providing the opportunity to retrieve residual stones at the time of initial PCNL and obviating the need for secondary procedures. Although the utility of this imaging modality has yet to be definitively demonstrated, it holds promise in increasing the ability to detect residual fragments intraoperatively.

SUMMARY

PCNL was developed in an effort to reduce the morbidity and mortality associated with open renal surgery but still represents the most morbid of the minimally invasive surgical modalities for stone removal. However, in recent years, efforts to reduce the morbidity and increase the effectiveness and efficiency of the procedure have brought PCNL closer to SWL and URS as the optimal first-line treatment of a variety of renal and ureteral calculi.

REFERENCES

1. Fernstrom I, Johansson B. Percutaneous pyelolithotomy. A new extraction technique. Scand J Urol Nephrol 1976;10(3):257–9.
2. Preminger GM, Assimos DG, Lingeman JE, et al. Chapter 1: AUA guideline on management of staghorn calculi: diagnosis and treatment recommendations. J Urol 2005;173(6):1991–2000.
3. Tiselius HG, Ackermann D, Alken P, et al. Guidelines on urolithiasis. Eur Urol 2001;40(4):362–71.
4. Deem S, Defade B, Modak A, et al. Percutaneous nephrolithotomy versus extracorporeal shock wave lithotripsy for moderate sized kidney stones. Urology 2011;78(4):739–43.
5. Lingeman JE, Siegel YI, Steele B, et al. Management of lower pole nephrolithiasis: a critical analysis. J Urol 1994;151(3):663–7.
6. Unsal A, Resorlu B, Kara C, et al. The role of percutaneous nephrolithotomy in the management of medium-sized (1–2 cm) lower-pole renal calculi. Acta Chir Belg 2011;111(5):308–11.
7. Carr LK, DAH J, Jewett MA, et al. New stone formation: a comparison of extracorporeal shock wave lithotripsy and percutaneous nephrolithotomy. J Urol 1996;155(5):1565–7.
8. Chen RN, Streem SB. Extracorporeal shock wave lithotripsy for lower pole calculi: long-term radiographic and clinical outcome. J Urol 1996;156(5):1572–5.
9. Albala DM, Assimos DG, Clayman RV, et al. Lower pole I: a prospective randomized trial of extracorporeal shock wave lithotripsy and percutaneous nephrostolithotomy for lower pole nephrolithiasis-initial results. J Urol 2001;166(6):2072–80.
10. Sun X, Xia S, Lu J, et al. Treatment of large impacted proximal ureteral stones: randomized comparison of percutaneous antegrade ureterolithotripsy versus retrograde ureterolithotripsy. J Endourol 2008;22(5):913–7.
11. Karami H, Arbab AH, Hosseini SJ, et al. Impacted upper-ureteral calculi >1 cm: blind access and totally tubeless percutaneous antegrade removal or retrograde approach? J Endourol 2006;20(9):616–9.
12. Maheshwari PN, Oswal AT, Andankar M, et al. Is antegrade ureteroscopy better than retrograde ureteroscopy for impacted large upper ureteral calculi? J Endourol 1999;13(6):441–4.
13. Kumar V, Ahlawat R, Banjeree GK, et al. Percutaneous ureterolitholapaxy: the best bet to clear large bulk impacted upper ureteral calculi. Arch Esp Urol 1996;49(1):86–91.
14. Juan YS, Shen JT, Li CC, et al. Comparison of percutaneous nephrolithotomy and ureteroscopic lithotripsy in the management of impacted, large, proximal ureteral stones. Kaohsiung J Med Sci 2008;24(4):204–9.
15. Mendez Probst CE, Denstedt JD, Razvi H. Preoperative indications for percutaneous nephrolithotripsy in 2009. J Endourol 2009;23(10):1557–61.
16. Kacker R, Meeks JJ, Zhao L, et al. Decreased stone-free rates after percutaneous nephrolithotomy for high calcium phosphate composition kidney stones. J Urol 2008;180(3):958–60 [discussion: 960].
17. Tracy CR, Gupta A, Pearle MS, et al. Calcium phosphate content does not affect stone-free rate after percutaneous nephrolithotomy. J Urol 2012;187(1):169–72.
18. Joseph P, Mandal AK, Singh SK, et al. Computerized tomography attenuation value of renal calculus: can

it predict successful fragmentation of the calculus by extracorporeal shock wave lithotripsy? A preliminary study. J Urol 2002;167(5):1968–71.

19. Perks AE, Schuler TD, Lee J, et al. Stone attenuation and skin-to-stone distance on computed tomography predicts for stone fragmentation by shock wave lithotripsy. Urology 2008;72(4):765–9.
20. El-Nahas AR, El-Assmy AM, Mansour O, et al. A prospective multivariate analysis of factors predicting stone disintegration by extracorporeal shock wave lithotripsy: the value of high-resolution noncontrast computed tomography. Eur Urol 2007;51(6):1688–93 [discussion: 1693–4].
21. Gupta NP, Ansari MS, Kesarvani P, et al. Role of computed tomography with no contrast medium enhancement in predicting the outcome of extracorporeal shock wave lithotripsy for urinary calculi. BJU Int 2005;95(9):1285–8.
22. Pareek G, Hedican SP, Lee FT Jr, et al. Shock wave lithotripsy success determined by skin-to-stone distance on computed tomography. Urology 2005;66(5):941–4.
23. Pearle MS, Nakada SY, Womack JS, et al. Outcomes of contemporary percutaneous nephrostolithotomy in morbidly obese patients. J Urol 1998;160(3 Pt 1):669–73.
24. Bagrodia A, Gupta A, Raman JD, et al. Impact of body mass index on cost and clinical outcomes after percutaneous nephrostolithotomy. Urology 2008;72(4):756–60.
25. Grasso M, Nord R, Bagley DH. Prone split leg and flank roll positioning: simultaneous antegrade and retrograde access to the upper urinary tract. J Endourol 1993;7(4):307–10.
26. Ray AA, Chung DG, Honey RJ. Percutaneous nephrolithotomy in the prone and prone-flexed positions: anatomic considerations. J Endourol 2009;23(10):1607–14.
27. Honey RJ, Wiesenthal JD, Ghiculete D, et al. Comparison of supracostal versus infracostal percutaneous nephrolithotomy using the novel prone-flexed patient position. J Endourol 2011;25(6):947–54.
28. Valdivia Uria JG, Lachares Santamaria E, Villarroya Rodriguez S, et al. Percutaneous nephrolithotomy: simplified technique (preliminary report). Arch Esp Urol 1987;40(3):177–80 [in Spanish].
29. Valdivia Uria JG, Valle Gerhold J, Lopez Lopez JA, et al. Technique and complications of percutaneous nephroscopy: experience with 557 patients in the supine position. J Urol 1998;160(6 Pt 1):1975–8.
30. Steele D, Marshall V. Percutaneous nephrolithotomy in the supine position: a neglected approach? J Endourol 2007;21(12):1433–7.
31. Manohar T, Jain P, Desai M. Supine percutaneous nephrolithotomy: effective approach to high-risk and morbidly obese patients. J Endourol 2007;21(1):44–9.
32. Neto EA, Mitre AI, Gomes CM, et al. Percutaneous nephrolithotripsy with the patient in a modified supine position. J Urol 2007;178(1):165–8 [discussion: 168].
33. Ng MT, Sun WH, Cheng CW, et al. Supine position is safe and effective for percutaneous nephrolithotomy. J Endourol 2004;18(5):469–74.
34. Rana AM, Bhojwani JP, Junejo NN, et al. Tubeless PCNL with patient in supine position: procedure for all seasons?—with comprehensive technique. Urology 2008;71(4):581–5.
35. Scoffone CM, Cracco CM, Cossu M, et al. Endoscopic combined intrarenal surgery in Galdakao-modified supine Valdivia position: a new standard for percutaneous nephrolithotomy? Eur Urol 2008;54(6):1393–403.
36. Liu L, Zheng S, Xu Y, et al. Systematic review and meta-analysis of percutaneous nephrolithotomy for patients in the supine versus prone position. J Endourol 2010;24(12):1941–6.
37. Wu P, Wang L, Wang K. Supine versus prone position in percutaneous nephrolithotomy for kidney calculi: a meta-analysis. Int Urol Nephrol 2011;43(1):67–77.
38. Arrabal-Polo MA, Arrabal-Martin M, Saz T, et al. Emergency percutaneous nephrostomy in supine-oblique position without cushion. Urol Res 2011;39(6):521–2.
39. Xu KW, Huang J, Guo ZH, et al. Percutaneous nephrolithotomy in semisupine position: a modified approach for renal calculus. Urol Res 2011;39(6):467–75.
40. El-Husseiny T, Moraitis K, Maan Z, et al. Percutaneous endourologic procedures in high-risk patients in the lateral decubitus position under regional anesthesia. J Endourol 2009;23(10):1603–6.
41. Lezrek M, Ammani A, Bazine K, et al. The split-leg modified lateral position for percutaneous renal surgery and optimal retrograde access to the upper urinary tract. Urology 2011;78(1):217–20.
42. Jang WS, Choi KH, Yang SC, et al. The learning curve for flank percutaneous nephrolithotomy for kidney calculi: a single surgeon's experience. Korean J Urol 2011;52(4):284–8.
43. Karami H, Rezaei A, Mohammadhosseini M, et al. Ultrasonography-guided percutaneous nephrolithotomy in the flank position versus fluoroscopy-guided percutaneous nephrolithotomy in the prone position: a comparative study. J Endourol 2010;24(8):1357–61.
44. Bird VG, Fallon B, Winfield HN. Practice patterns in the treatment of large renal stones. J Endourol 2003;17(6):355–63.
45. Watterson JD, Soon S, Jana K. Access related complications during percutaneous

nephrolithotomy: urology versus radiology at a single academic institution. J Urol 2006;176(1):142–5.
46. El-Assmy AM, Shokeir AA, Mohsen T, et al. Renal access by urologist or radiologist for percutaneous nephrolithotomy—is it still an issue? J Urol 2007; 178(3 Pt 1):916–20 [discussion: 920].
47. Lashley DB, Fuchs EF. Urologist-acquired renal access for percutaneous renal surgery. Urology 1998;51(6):927–31.
48. Tomaszewski JJ, Ortiz TD, Gayed BA, et al. Renal access by urologist or radiologist during percutaneous nephrolithotomy. J Endourol 2010;24(11): 1733–7.
49. Kumari G, Kumar P, Wadhwa P, et al. Radiation exposure to the patient and operating room personnel during percutaneous nephrolithotomy. Int Urol Nephrol 2006;38(2):207–10.
50. Park S, Pearle MS. Imaging for percutaneous renal access and management of renal calculi. Urol Clin North Am 2006;33(3):353–64.
51. McAleer SJ, Loughlin KR. Nephrolithiasis and pregnancy. Curr Opin Urol 2004;14(2):123–7.
52. Evans HJ, Wollin TA. The management of urinary calculi in pregnancy. Curr Opin Urol 2001;11(4): 379–84.
53. Kavoussi LR, Albala DM, Basler JW, et al. Percutaneous management of urolithiasis during pregnancy. J Urol 1992;148(3 Pt 2):1069–71.
54. Francesca F, Felipetto R, Mosca F, et al. Percutaneous nephrolithotomy of transplanted kidney. J Endourol 2002;16(4):225–7.
55. Lu HF, Shekarriz B, Stoller ML. Donor-gifted allograft urolithiasis: early percutaneous management. Urology 2002;59(1):25–7.
56. Basiri A, Ziaee AM, Kianian HR, et al. Ultrasonographic versus fluoroscopic access for percutaneous nephrolithotomy: a randomized clinical trial. J Endourol 2008;22(2):281–4.
57. Basiri A, Ziaee SA, Nasseh H, et al. Totally ultrasonography-guided percutaneous nephrolithotomy in the flank position. J Endourol 2008; 22(7):1453–7.
58. Hosseini MM, Hassanpour A, Farzan R, et al. Ultrasonography-guided percutaneous nephrolithotomy. J Endourol 2009;23(4):603–7.
59. Karami H, Arbab AH, Rezaei A, et al. Percutaneous nephrolithotomy with ultrasonography-guided renal access in the lateral decubitus flank position. J Endourol 2009;23(1):33–5.
60. Agarwal M, Agrawal MS, Jaiswal A, et al. Safety and efficacy of ultrasonography as an adjunct to fluoroscopy for renal access in percutaneous nephrolithotomy (PCNL). BJU Int 2011;108(8): 1346–9.
61. Hagspiel KD, Kandarpa K, Silverman SG. Interactive MR-guided percutaneous nephrostomy. J Magn Reson Imaging 1998;8(6):1319–22.
62. Kariniemi J, Sequeiros RB, Ojala R, et al. MRI-guided percutaneous nephrostomy: a feasibility study. Eur Radiol 2009;19(5):1296–301.
63. Matlaga BR, Shah OD, Zagoria RJ, et al. Computerized tomography guided access for percutaneous nephrostolithotomy. J Urol 2003;170(1):45–7.
64. Lawson RK, Murphy JB, Taylor AJ, et al. Retrograde method for percutaneous access to kidney. Urology 1983;22(6):580–2.
65. Hunter PT, Hawkins IF, Finlayson B, et al. Hawkins-Hunter retrograde transcutaneous nephrostomy: a new technique. Urology 1983;22(6):583–7.
66. Kawahara T, Ito H, Terao H, et al. Ureteroscopy assisted retrograde nephrostomy: a new technique for percutaneous nephrolithotomy (PCNL). BJU Int 2012;110(4):588–90.
67. Grasso M, Lang G, Taylor FC. Flexible ureteroscopically assisted percutaneous renal access. Tech Urol 1995;1(1):39–43.
68. Kidd CF, Conlin MJ. Ureteroscopically assisted percutaneous renal access. Urology 2003;61(6):1244–5.
69. Khan F, Borin JF, Pearle MS, et al. Endoscopically guided percutaneous renal access: "seeing is believing". J Endourol 2006;20(7):451–5 [discussion: 455].
70. Yamaguchi A, Skolarikos A, Buchholz NP, et al. Operating times and bleeding complications in percutaneous nephrolithotomy: a comparison of tract dilation methods in 5,537 patients in the Clinical Research Office of the Endourological Society Percutaneous Nephrolithotomy Global Study. J Endourol 2011;25(6):933–9.
71. Helal M, Black T, Lockhart J, et al. The Hickman peel-away sheath: alternative for pediatric percutaneous nephrolithotomy. J Endourol 1997;11(3):171–2.
72. Jackman SV, Docimo SG, Cadeddu JA, et al. The "mini-perc" technique: a less invasive alternative to percutaneous nephrolithotomy. World J Urol 1998;16(6):371–4.
73. Knoll T, Wezel F, Michel MS, et al. Do patients benefit from miniaturized tubeless percutaneous nephrolithotomy? A comparative prospective study. J Endourol 2010;24(7):1075–9.
74. Cheng F, Yu W, Zhang X, et al. Minimally invasive tract in percutaneous nephrolithotomy for renal stones. J Endourol 2010;24(10):1579–82.
75. Mishra S, Sharma R, Garg C, et al. Prospective comparative study of miniperc and standard PNL for treatment of 1 to 2 cm size renal stone. BJU Int 2011;108(6):896–9 [discussion: 899–900].
76. Bader MJ, Gratzke C, Seitz M, et al. The "all-seeing needle": initial results of an optical puncture system confirming access in percutaneous nephrolithotomy. Eur Urol 2011;59(6):1054–9.
77. Desai MR, Sharma R, Mishra S, et al. Single-step percutaneous nephrolithotomy (microperc): the initial clinical report. J Urol 2011;186(1):140–5.

78. Netto NR Jr, Ikonomidis J, Ikari O, et al. Comparative study of percutaneous access for staghorn calculi. Urology 2005;65(4):659–62 [discussion: 662–3].
79. Kukreja R, Desai M, Patel S, et al. Factors affecting blood loss during percutaneous nephrolithotomy: prospective study. J Endourol 2004; 18(8):715–22.
80. Wong C, Leveillee RJ. Single upper-pole percutaneous access for treatment of > or = 5-cm complex branched staghorn calculi: is shockwave lithotripsy necessary? J Endourol 2002;16(7):477–81.
81. Landman J, Venkatesh R, Lee DI, et al. Combined percutaneous and retrograde approach to staghorn calculi with application of the ureteral access sheath to facilitate percutaneous nephrolithotomy. J Urol 2003;169(1):64–7.
82. Marguet CG, Springhart WP, Tan YH, et al. Simultaneous combined use of flexible ureteroscopy and percutaneous nephrolithotomy to reduce the number of access tracts in the management of complex renal calculi. BJU Int 2005;96(7): 1097–100.
83. Miller NL, Matlaga BR, Lingeman JE. Techniques for fluoroscopic percutaneous renal access. J Urol 2007;178(1):15–23.
84. Alken P, Hutschenreiter G, Gunther R. Percutaneous kidney stone removal. Eur Urol 1982;8(5):304–11.
85. Davidoff R, Bellman GC. Influence of technique of percutaneous tract creation on incidence of renal hemorrhage. J Urol 1997;157(4):1229–31.
86. Safak M, Gogus C, Soygur T. Nephrostomy tract dilation using a balloon dilator in percutaneous renal surgery: experience with 95 cases and comparison with the fascial dilator system. Urol Int 2003;71(4):382–4.
87. Gonen M, Istanbulluoglu OM, Cicek T, et al. Balloon dilatation versus Amplatz dilatation for nephrostomy tract dilatation. J Endourol 2008;22(5):901–4.
88. Joel AB, Rubenstein JN, Hsieh MH, et al. Failed percutaneous balloon dilation for renal access: incidence and risk factors. Urology 2005;66(1): 29–32.
89. Hendlin K, Monga M. Radial dilation of nephrostomy balloons: a comparative analysis. Int Braz J Urol 2008;34(5):546–52 [discussion: 552–4].
90. Pathak AS, Bellman GC. One-step percutaneous nephrolithotomy sheath versus standard two-step technique. Urology 2005;66(5):953–7.
91. Marberger M. Disintegration of renal and ureteral calculi with ultrasound. Urol Clin North Am 1983; 10(4):729–42.
92. Teh CL, Zhong P, Preminger GM. Laboratory and clinical assessment of pneumatically driven intracorporeal lithotripsy. J Endourol 1998;12(2):163–9.
93. Kuo RL, Paterson RF, Siqueira TM Jr, et al. In vitro assessment of lithoclast ultra intracorporeal lithotripter. J Endourol 2004;18(2):153–6.
94. Kim SC, Matlaga BR, Tinmouth WW, et al. In vitro assessment of a novel dual probe ultrasonic intracorporeal lithotriptor. J Urol 2007;177(4):1363–5.
95. Pietrow PK, Auge BK, Zhong P, et al. Clinical efficacy of a combination pneumatic and ultrasonic lithotrite. J Urol 2003;169(4):1247–9.
96. Krambeck AE, Miller NL, Humphreys MR, et al. Randomized controlled, multicentre clinical trial comparing a dual-probe ultrasonic lithotrite with a single-probe lithotrite for percutaneous nephrolithotomy. BJU Int 2011;107(5):824–8.
97. Maheshwari PN, Andankar MG, Bansal M. Nephrostomy tube after percutaneous nephrolithotomy: large-bore or pigtail catheter? J Endourol 2000; 14(9):735–7 [discussion :737–8].
98. Pietrow PK, Auge BK, Lallas CD, et al. Pain after percutaneous nephrolithotomy: impact of nephrostomy tube size. J Endourol 2003;17(6):411–4.
99. Wickham JE, Miller RA, Kellett MJ, et al. Percutaneous nephrolithotomy: one stage or two? Br J Urol 1984;56(6):582–5.
100. Winfield HN, Weyman P, Clayman RV. Percutaneous nephrostolithotomy: complications of premature nephrostomy tube removal. J Urol 1986; 136(1):77–9.
101. Bellman GC, Davidoff R, Candela J, et al. Tubeless percutaneous renal surgery. J Urol 1997;157(5): 1578–82.
102. Desai MR, Kukreja RA, Desai MM, et al. A prospective randomized comparison of type of nephrostomy drainage following percutaneous nephrostolithotomy: large bore versus small bore versus tubeless. J Urol 2004;172(2):565–7.
103. Marcovich R, Jacobson AI, Singh J, et al. No panacea for drainage after percutaneous nephrolithotomy. J Endourol 2004;18(8):743–7.
104. Aghamir SM, Hosseini SR, Gooran S. Totally tubeless percutaneous nephrolithotomy. J Endourol 2004;18(7):647–8.
105. Gupta V, Sadasukhi TC, Sharma KK, et al. Tubeless and stentless percutaneous nephrolithotomy. BJU Int 2005;95(6):905–6.
106. Crook TJ, Lockyer CR, Keoghane SR, et al. Totally tubeless percutaneous nephrolithotomy. J Endourol 2008;22(2):267–71.
107. Zilberman DE, Lipkin ME, de la Rosette JJ, et al. Tubeless percutaneous nephrolithotomy–the new standard of care? J Urol 2010;184(4):1261–6.
108. Yuan H, Zheng S, Liu L, et al. The efficacy and safety of tubeless percutaneous nephrolithotomy: a systematic review and meta-analysis. Urol Res 2011;39(5):401–10.
109. Wang J, Zhao C, Zhang C, et al. Tubeless vs standard percutaneous nephrolithotomy: a meta-analysis. BJU Int 2012;109(6):918–24.
110. Pearle MS, Watamull LM, Mullican MA. Sensitivity of noncontrast helical computerized tomography and

plain film radiography compared to flexible nephroscopy for detecting residual fragments after percutaneous nephrostolithotomy. J Urol 1999;162(1):23–6.

111. Portis AJ, Laliberte MA, Drake S, et al. Intraoperative fragment detection during percutaneous nephrolithotomy: evaluation of high magnification rotational fluoroscopy combined with aggressive nephroscopy. J Urol 2006;175(1):162–5 [discussion: 165–6].

112. Portis AJ, Laliberte MA, Holtz C, et al. Confident intraoperative decision making during percutaneous nephrolithotomy: does this patient need a second look? Urology 2008;71(2):218–22.

113. Raman JD, Bagrodia A, Gupta A, et al. Natural history of residual fragments following percutaneous nephrostolithotomy. J Urol 2009;181(3):1163–8.

114. Raman JD, Bagrodia A, Bensalah K, et al. Residual fragments after percutaneous nephrolithotomy: cost comparison of immediate second look flexible nephroscopy versus expectant management. J Urol 2010;183(1):188–93.

115. Ogan K, Corwin TS, Smith T, et al. Sensitivity of chest fluoroscopy compared with chest CT and chest radiography for diagnosing hydropneumothorax in association with percutaneous nephrostolithotomy. Urology 2003;62(6):988–92.

116. Bjurlin MA, O'Grady T, Kim R, et al. Is routine postoperative chest radiography needed after percutaneous nephrolithotomy? Urology 2012; 79(4):791–5.

117. Denstedt JD, Clayman RV, Picus DD. Comparison of endoscopic and radiological residual fragment rate following percutaneous nephrolithotripsy. J Urol 1991;145(4):703–5.

118. Roy OP, Angle JF, Jenkins AD, et al. Cone beam computed tomography for percutaneous nephrolithotomy: Initial evaluation of a new technology. J Endourol 2012;26(7):814–8.

The Emerging Role of Robotics and Laparoscopy in Stone Disease

Mitchell R. Humphreys, MD

KEYWORDS

• Laparoscopy • Robot-assisted surgery • Ureterolithotomy • Pyelolithotomy • Urolithiasis • Calculi

KEY POINTS

- The prevalence of open surgical procedures has decreased dramatically with the advent of minimally invasive and endourologic procedures in the United States and world wide.
- When endourologic procedures fail, laparoscopic or robot-assisted techniques offer patients significant benefits over open surgery.
- In certain clinical circumstances such as abnormal anatomy, the need for concomitant reconstruction efforts, the unavailability of endoscopic equipment or experience, robotic or laparoscopic approaches may be considered as initial treatment options for patients.

INTRODUCTION

The surgical management for urolithiasis has undergone a dramatic clinical evolution during the past 3 decades. Advances in endoscopic equipment and procedures have relegated the practice of open stone surgery nearly to one of historical interest. The defining developments of percutaneous nephrolithotomy (PNL), ureteroscopy (URS), extracorporeal shock-wave lithotripsy (SWL), laparoscopy, and robot-assisted surgery have diminished the role of open surgery in the modern day urologist's armamentarium. The European Association of Urologists (EAU) and American Urologic Association (AUA) have released guidelines that attempt to define the roles of various surgical procedures and techniques in the spectrum of surgical stone intervention. The in-depth rationale, benefits, and morbidities associated specifically with laparoscopic and robot-assisted approaches have yet to be fully adjudicated as urologists become more facile with these procedures. The following report will discuss the historical changes from open to minimally invasive treatment options and review the literature and indications of laparoscopic and robot-assisted approaches for the management of urolithiasis.

HISTORICAL PERSPECTIVE

Urolithiasis has plagued mankind since before recorded history; in 1901 a stone was extracted from an Egyptian mummy dating to 4800 BC.[1] During Hippocrates' era, specific surgical interventions, although crude by modern standards, were described to relieve the symptoms of stone disease.[2] The reports of successful stone surgery were rare in the subsequent millennia, with most procedures resulting in death and significant morbidities. In 1879, Heinke described the first pyelotomy incision with subsequent stone extraction.[2] During the next several decades, because of the complications associated with early attempts of nephrolithotomy, pyelolithotomy became standard therapy with the adjuvanted use of blood coagulum, fibrin and fibrinogen, or cryoprecipitate to assist with the removal of calyceal stones and

There are no financial relationships to disclose as it pertains to this article.
Department of Urology, Mayo Clinic, 5777 East Mayo Boulevard, Phoenix, AZ 85054, USA
E-mail address: Humphreys.mitchell@mayo.edu

Urol Clin N Am 40 (2013) 115–128
http://dx.doi.org/10.1016/j.ucl.2012.09.005

fragments.[3,4] Smith and Boyce then described the first anatrophic nephrolithotomy for staghorn calculi in 1968, which redefined the approach to large complex kidney stones.[5] This was predicated by the technical description by Josef Hyrtl (1882) and Max Brödel (1902) of the avascular plane of the kidney that allowed bloodless access to the renal collecting system.[6]

The recognition of ureteral calculi and their particular surgical management mirrored that of nephrolithiasis. Thomas Emmet of New York published his account in 1879 of 3 women with distally impacted ureteral stones that were treated by open ureterolithotomy, including one through a transvaginal approach.[7] Then, in 1910, Gibson described the extraperitoneal approach to the distal ureter that remained in practice during the next century.[7]

The role of open surgical consideration has given way to a collection of techniques and technology that have minimized the subsequent mortality and morbidity for most patients requiring stone surgery. Arthur Smith labeled the new frontier of minimally invasive surgical management: endourology, or the closed controlled manipulation within the urinary tract.[8] This shift in the treatment paradigm was established by several important developments that will only be briefly described in the context of the relevant surgical evolution. Fernström and Johansson described the first percutaneous removal of a kidney stone in 1976,[9] which was preceded by the initial description of percutaneous nephrostomy tube placement for hydronephrosis in 1955.[10] The subsequent development of an intracorporeal lithotripter in 1977[11] permitted PNL to become the mainstay of intervention for large renal stones. In a survey of disease codes, the annual use of PNL in the United Stated increased from 1.2 per 100,000 to 2.5 per 100,000 between 1988 and 2002.[12] Other surgical means of accessing the kidney and ureter for stone disease involved the development of retrograde approaches via URS.

URS was initially developed in the late 1970s to diagnosis and treat conditions of the distal ureter.[13] The introduction of rigid, semirigid, and flexible URS has allowed the usefulness of URS to increase dramatically during the past several decades.[14] This is predominantly a result of the vast technological advances made for URS stone management including miniaturization, new instruments, and lasers, in addition to the improved endoscopic skills of the urologist.

Further diminishing the role of open surgery was the development of SWL, first described by Chaussy and colleagues[15] in 1980 and approved by the US Food and Drug Administration in 1984. It has become the most commonly used therapeutic intervention for patients with upper tract stones.[16] The advantages of SWL include high patient tolerance because of the infrequent need for invasive surgical procedures and minimal morbidity.

The emergence of these technologies and procedures were followed by the development of minimally invasive surgery such as laparoscopy. Clayman and colleagues[17] reported the first transperitoneal laparoscopic nephrectomy in 1991, drawing attention to the capabilities of such a novel technique. Laparoscopy became an alternative to open surgery with decreased complications, less morbidity, and high stone-free rates and fostered the imagination of innovators to push the surgical envelope even further. The advanced engineering capabilities and desire to pursue remote surgery by the military gave rise to the modern day da Vinci Surgical System (Intuitive Surgical Inc, Sunnyvale, CA).[18] During the past, decade the US health care system has seen an explosion of robot-assisted surgical procedures. In June 2010, Jin and colleagues[19] randomly surveyed 400 US hospital Web sites and found that 41% of all hospitals described robotic surgery and statements of clinical superiority were made on 86% of these Web sites. The exponential growth of robot-assisted laparoscopic techniques has provided a critical enabling technology to the surgical armamentarium, making laparoscopy possible for those not proficient in 2-dimensional spatial relationships or lacking the dexterity for precise laparoscopic maneuvers.

PATIENT CONSIDERATIONS

The prevalence of open surgical procedures has decreased significantly with the advent of minimally invasive and endourologic procedures. In the United States in 2000, only 2% of Medicare patients were treated with open surgery when they required a stone operation.[20] Internationally, when alternative equipment and expertise are available, open surgery is done in only 1% to 5.4% of all patients requiring stone surgery.[20–27] Even in developing countries, the prevalence of open surgery has decreased from 26% to 3.5% of patients requiring stone surgery.[28,29] As such, even though the prevalence of open surgery has collapsed, there remain certain clinical scenarios when it may be indicated (**Table 1**). The maturity of laparoscopic proficiency, equipment, and robotic experience has shown the ability to duplicate nearly any open surgical procedure.[26] The advent of robot-assisted and laparoscopic approaches, when the resources and expertise

Table 1
Clinical conditions when laparoscopic or robot-assisted surgery may be offered

Organ	Procedure	Indication
Kidney	Pyelolithotomy	Failure of endourologic management
		Extremely large calculi with unfavorable collecting system anatomy
		Need for concomitant procedure (UPJ repair)
	Nephrolithotomy	Complex staghorn calculi
		Unfavorable collecting system anatomy (infundubuliar stenosis)
		Ectopic or malrotated kidney making other access difficult or impossible
		Calyceal diverticulum with stones (particularly when located anteriorly with thin overlying parenchyma)
	Nephrectomy	Polar nephrectomy with nonfunctional portion associated with calculi
		Nonfunctioning renal unit with significant stone burden
Ureter	Ureterolithotomy	Large impacted stone
		Failure or unavailability of endourologic procedure
		Large stones in megaureter
Bladder	Cystolithotomy	Large stone(s) in a urinary diversion
		Concomitant bladder diverticulectomy with stone removal

are available, have surpassed open surgery as the preferred approach for difficult or complex cases.

Endoscopic techniques can be difficult, especially in morbidly obese individuals, when fluoroscopy may have insufficient penetration to allow adequate visualization or if the patient's weight exceeds the limits of the fluoroscopy table. If percutaneous instrumentation is not long enough to provide sufficient access to the collecting system or if the patient cannot tolerate the prone position, certain approaches to the stone cannot be safely accomplished, thereby supporting the role for laparoscopic or robot-assisted management. Also, patients with skeletal abnormalities that preclude adequate imaging or positioning are candidates for alternative options. Occasionally, patients desire a treatment that gives them the highest potential to be 100% stone free after a single procedure that URS, SWL and PNL treatments cannot guarantee. Compared with the open surgical equivalent, laparoscopic and robot-assisted laparoscopic procedures tend to require less analgesia, are associated with shorter hospital stays and less convalescence, and have improved cosmetic results.[30–38]

APPROACHES FOR URETERAL STONES

The advent of flexible active deflection and semirigid ureteroscopes, digital image resolution, advances in lithotripsy devices such as the holmium:yttrium-aluminum-garnet laser, and the introduction of SWL has simplified the means and improved the outcomes for most patients requiring stone surgery while minimizing risks. The bevy of accompanying ureteroscopic instrumentation including nitinol baskets, ureteral access sheaths, retropulsion devices, and stents have further decreased the role of open surgical approaches. Matlaga recently evaluated the contemporary practice patterns of the surgical management of urinary calculi based on surgical logs reported to the American Board of Urology (ABU) as part of certification requirements and noted that recently trained urologists tended to embrace endoscopic treatment modalities such as URS, whereas SWL was used more often by earlier trained urologists.[39] The combined EAU/AUA guideline recommendation on the management of ureteral calculi recognizes the value and importance of these approaches by indicating either SWL or URS as the preferred first-line intervention.[40] However, open surgery has not been completely eradicated and, by extension, laparoscopic and robotic approaches offer a preferred method of stone eradication for complex cases. The EAU/AUA panel continued to suggest that laparoscopic or open stone removal may be considered in rare cases when SWL, URS, and percutaneous antegrade URS fail or are unlikely to succeed.[40]

The earliest report of laparoscopic ureterolithotomy was by Wickham in 1979 via a retroperitoneal approach.[41] The role of laparoscopy was limited with only sporadic case reports until in 1992 and 1993, when technology and skills provided a foundation for broader adoption.[42,43] The popularity also increased in developing countries where access to endourologic facilities is limited and the expense of disposable medical supplies made endourologic procedures cost prohibitive.[44] **Table 2** summarizes the largest reported

Table 2
Descriptive statistics and functional results of selected laparoscopic ureterolithotomy cases (≥30 patients)

Reference No.	No. of Procedures	TP/RP	Mean Stone Size, mm	Mean Operating Room Time, min	Mean Hospital Stay, d	Stricture, %	Conversions, %[a]	Stone-Free Rate, %[b]	Urine Leak, %	Stent, %	Closure of Ureterotomy, %
45	50	TP	22.4	127.8	5.8	-	4	90	16	-	100
54	33	-	34	85	3.4	-	0	100	-	-	-
47	126	RP	13.6	88	2.8	-	2.4	97.6	2.4	100	100
55	32	RP	18.1	118	5.9	3.1	3.1	93.8	-	100	100
30	55	RP	21	108.8	3.3	5.2	18	82	Yes	64	100
56	31	RP	2.2	67	2.4	-	-	-	6.5	No	100
48	75	RP 69/TP 6	25	45	3.0	No	1.3	98.7	8	97.3	100
53	30	RP	19	121.3	-	No	3.3	96.7	3.4	3.3	100
57	50	RP	17	97	6.8	No	8	92	20	-	-
49	40	RP	22.5	92.5	6.0	-	5	100	2.5	100	100
58	74	RP 66/TP 8	18	58.7	6.4	1.4	5.4	94.6	1.4	86.5	13.5
51	101	RP 100/TP 1	16	79	3.5	4	-	92	19.8	-	-

Abbreviation: TP/RP, transperitoneal/retroperitoneal.
[a] Most common cause of conversion was reported as stone migration into the kidney.
[b] Stone-free rate is reported according to author's imaging test of choice at last follow-up.

laparoscopic ureterolithotomy trials in the literature. One of the few prospective randomized trials comparing laparoscopic surgery to URS or PNL for upper ureteral stones of 1 cm or larger enrolled 150 patients. The stone-free rate at discharge was highest in the laparoscopic group (88%), followed by the PNL (64%) and URS (56%) groups. Operative times were 127.8 ± 41.8, 93.6 ± 28.9, and 42.7 ± 2.4 minutes in the laparoscopic, PNL, and URS groups, respectively, whereas the requirement for a secondary procedure was 10%, 14%, and 22%, respectively. Two conversions to open surgery occurred in the laparoscopic group because of a dropped stone in the abdomen and an inability to localize the ureteral stone.[45] This trial shows that despite endourologic management, laparoscopic surgery may offer better single-episode stone clearance with the least need for additional procedures. Another recent prospective randomized trial supported these finding when they compared SWL, URS, and laparoscopy in 48 patients with stones greater than 1 cm (mean, 14.7 mm). They showed that laparoscopy again was associated with a higher success rate with fewer required surgical procedures than the other interventions.[46] The success rate was 35.7% for SWL, 62.5% for semirigid URS, and 93.3% for laparoscopic ureterolithotomy. One patient in the laparoscopic group required open conversion and another required a secondary PNL.[46] Although laparoscopic management may not be a first-line treatment option, it remains a valuable tool in the therapeutic algorithm.

There is debate as to the ideal approach to the ureter: retroperitoneal or transperitoneal. Qadri and associates retrospectively reported their 10-year experience with retroperitoneal laparoscopic ureterolithotomy (RLU). They had 126 patients with large or impacted ureteral stones 86 (68.25%), 28 with failed URS (22.23%), and 12 with unsuccessful SWL (9.52%). Their mean operative time was 88 minutes, and surgery was successful in 97.6% of cases with a mean hospitalization of 2.8 days and no major complications. They concluded that RLU has the ability to render a patient stone free after 1 procedure even in salvage situations.[47] Furthermore, they advocate retroperitoneoscopy to alleviate the need for bowel mobilization, retraction, the risk of inadvertent injury, and postoperative ileus. They also suggest that abdominal adhesions, shoulder pain caused by the pneumoperitoneum, and potential contamination of the abdomen with urine or blood would be avoided via the retroperitoneal approach. However, the retroperitoneum offers its own set of challenges such as the unfamiliar surgical anatomy and landmarks in the setting of a restricted working space and the potential loss of visualization because of inadvertent peritoneotomy. Additionally, retroperitoneal access is limited by its ability to deal with upper or mid ureteral stones because exposure of the lower ureter is difficult, if not impossible.[48,49] Transperitoneal access has been promoted to surmount these limitations and is generally more acceptable by urologists because of the familiar landmarks and a larger working space facilitating intracorporeal suturing. Bovie and colleagues[50] compared transperitoneal to retroperitoneal access for laparoscopic ureterolithotomy in 35 consecutive patients. They found that the transperitoneal approach resulted in a shorter time to access and identify the ureter (14 vs 24 minutes), ureterotomy closure (16 vs 28 minutes), and total operative time (75 vs 102 minutes). The increased retroperitoneal operative time was attributed to accidental entry into the peritoneal cavity causing a loss of pneumoretroperitoneum. There were no conversions and no transfusions required. They concluded that for surgeons learning laparoscopy, the transperitoneal approach is better, but for those with demonstrated expertise, the approach should be left to the discretion of the surgeon.

The need to close the ureter or provide drainage has not reached consensus in the literature. Gaur and colleagues[51] reported that operative time for RLU was 66 minutes compared with 92 minutes if the ureterotomy was closed. They noted a prolonged postoperative urine leak in 19.8% (20/101) of patients in whom the ureter was not stented. However, of these patients, that 70% (14/20) also did not have the ureterotomy closed confounds the true impact of stenting on the risk of urine leak. They concluded that because 6 of these patients did have the ureterotomy closed, perhaps in cases of chronically inflamed, edematous, and friable ureters or after prolonged stone impaction or infection, the ureter should only be stented and left open.[51] Keeley and associates described the Edinburgh experience in which 9 patients underwent a salvage transperitoneal approach for failed URS (6 patients), SWL (2 patients), or both (1 patient), 5 primarily for a large ureteral stone (mean, 27.2 mm). The average operative time was 105 minutes with a 100% success rate and no need for open conversion. Only 5 patients had their ureterotomy closed and 2 subsequently developed strictures versus none of the 9 in the unclosed ureteral group. Only 1 patient with neither a stent nor ureterotomy closure developed a urine leak requiring prolong drainage.[52] They surmised that as long as a drain is maintained, even in the peritoneal cavity, the ureter can be left open if a stent is also provided.

Kijvikai and Patcharatrakul[53] instead preferred to suture the ureter and not provide a stent in their patients and noted a 3.4% incidence of urine leak and no development of strictures. The decision on how to manage the ureter seems to be one of surgeon preference; however, it would make sense to duplicate what is done in open surgery to prevent potential complications and morbidities for patients by at least closing the ureterotomy and providing drainage to the renal unit when appropriate.

The risks associated with laparoscopic or robot-assisted ureterolithotomy deserve consideration. The most common risk is that of urine leak (0%–20%) followed by stricture formation (1.4%–5.2%).[30,45–49,51,53–58] Ureteral strictures can develop independent of the surgical approach and may occur in up to 24% of patients after prolonged stone impaction.[59] However, several authors suggest keeping the length of the ureterotomy as short as possible to allow removal of the stone and using a cold knife instead of diathermy to create the ureterotomy.[45,53,60] Visualization may be improved with the use of thermal energy for hemostasis at the increased risk of stricture development. Bellman and Smith also suggested that the ureterotomy be made in a longitudinal manner to prevent disruption of the ureteral blood supply.[61] Visualization and vascular concerns are not the most cited reasons for open conversion; most series indicate the grounds for conversion was the inability to locate the stone or that it migrated into the kidney during the procedure. To prevent stone migration, placing some compressive device proximally on the ureter, such as a laparoscopic Babcock clamp or vessel loop, will prevent stone movement and provide an additional fixation point for the ureter during ureterotomy. The ability to locate large stones is apparent via visual cues, but for smaller impacted ureteral stones with associated inflammation or edema, this may represent a difficult aspect of the operation. It is possible to use laparoscopic ultrasonic probes to locate the stone or, alternatively, to place an open-ended ureteral catheter to the level of the stone to facilitate fluoroscopic imaging and subsequent stenting. If an open-ended catheter is placed, then a wire can be passed through the catheter with gentle manipulations to identify the corresponding section of ureteral obstruction. Gaur and colleagues[51] had a large series of more than 100 patients followed for 10 years and noted the following early in their laparoscopic experience: failure to locate the ureter via RLU (>30 minutes in 30/100 cases with eventual success in 24 of these), severe retroperitoneal fibrosis making progress impossible (3/100), and one accidental ureteral avulsion (1/100). The complications and rate of conversion decreased in time as one would expect with the maturity of the techniques and the accumulation of experience.

Any new technique or surgical procedure requires translation and adoption by the urologic community. The hurdles of this endeavor regarding how best to teach a procedure while ensuring the best possible outcomes for patients is always a challenge. The EAU has suggested that to acquire the dexterity and proficiency in laparoscopy, 50 cases are required to significantly decrease the complication rate.[62] Fan and associates compared their first 20 RLU cases to their next 20 cases and were able to demonstrate a decrease in their operative time from 120 to 65 minutes.[49] Additionally, they had 2 cases requiring open conversion and a complication rate of 15% in their first 20 procedures compared with zero in their last 20. The arduous pursuit of obtaining the needed laparoscopic proficiency to maintain optimal patient outcomes is difficult for most surgeons. However, this is perhaps one of the clear advantages that robot-assisted laparoscopic surgery can provide. The wristed instruments and 3-dimensional vision allow greater dexterity for the surgeon in a more ergonomic situation. This can facilitate the successful transition from open to laparoscopic surgery and can flatten the learning curve.

APPROACHES FOR KIDNEY STONES

The particular techniques of laparoscopic or robot-assisted management of nephrolithiasis can be placed into one of several broad classifications of technique: pyelolithotomy, nephrolithotomy, or combined procedures (concomitant ureteropelvic junction [UPJ] repair, calyceal diverticula ablation, or partial nephrectomy). The data associated with each type of procedure will be described next.

Laparoscopic/Robot-Assisted Pyelolithotomy

Laparoscopic pyelolithotomy was introduced by Gaur and associates in 1994 with the initial description of a retroperitoneal approach in 5 patients with stones not amenable to either SWL or PNL.[44] Multiple reports since that time have documented either a retroperitoneal or transperitoneal approach with stone-free rates ranging from 71% to 100% and conversion to open surgery from zero to 27%.[33,35] Most series tend to prefer the retroperitoneal approach because of the decreased risk of peritoneal contamination and because a posterior approach to the renal pelvis can be extended into a superior infundibulotomy without risk or limitation of the renal vasculature. Note in most cases the renal hilar vascular anatomy overlies the anterior surface of the renal pelvis, obstructing access to the upper calyceal system. **Table 3** provides a summary of these studies. Sinha and Sharma reported their results of retroperitoneal laparoscopy for 1.6- to 2.5-cm solitary renal pelvic stones that would have been susceptible to endourologic treatment had such facilities been available. They did not close the pyelotomy in 14 of the initial patients, 2 of whom experienced a prolonged urine leak, whereas in the 6 subsequent patients, with a closed pyelotomy, no leak occurred.[63] Meria and colleagues[64] compared 16 patients undergoing transperitoneal laparoscopic pyelolithotomy with 16 patients undergoing PNL for renal pelvic stones greater than 2 cm. Because the stone-free rates were similar (88% vs 82%), and the laparoscopic group had longer operative times and a 12% risk of developing a urine leak, and 2 patients required open conversion, they concluded that PNL should be the primary treatment of uncomplicated large pelvic stones. However, in anomalous kidneys this may not be as clearly indicated. Tunc and colleagues[65] examined 150 patients with 57 duplicated, 45 horseshoe, 30 malrotated, 14 pelvic, and 4 crossed fused ectopic kidneys treated with SWL (Siemens Lithostar Plus; Siemens, Erlanger, Germany). The overall stone-free rate was only 68% with the corresponding kidney-specific stone-free rates of 80.7%, 66.7%, 56.7%, 57.2%, and 25%, respectively. Braz and colleagues[66] have reported an improved 81% stone-free rate for bulky stone disease at 3 months following ureteroscopic treatment, but still 62% of patients required ancillary procedures. Laparoscopic pyelotomy has been advocated because of avoidance of nephron damage and decreased risk of bleeding that may complicate PNL.[67] This may be especially important for patients who already have impaired renal function and require a procedure to give them the best chance of eradication of the stone in a single procedure. The prohibitive factor has generally been the acceptance and implementation of laparoscopic reconstructive techniques.

The limitation of the skills needed to be able to effectively suture intracorporeally with laparoscopy has always been a barrier to widespread adoption. However, robot-assisted surgery is the great equalizer providing a translation of open suturing technique to the laparoscopic environment with 3-dimensional visualization, magnification, and tremor dampening. Badani and associates published their series of 13 patients who underwent robot-assisted extended pyelolithotomy for mostly partial and 1 complete staghorn calculi with a mean stone size of 4.2 cm in 2006.[68] All procedures were transperitoneal with no open conversions, transfusions, or urine leaks. Two of these patients required lower pole nephrotomies to render them stone free, which all patients were except for 1 who had a complete staghorn calculus. Their mean operative time was 158 minutes (range, 90–257 minutes) with a mean console time of 108 minutes (range, 60–193 minutes). The only difficulty was in extending the pyelotomy to the upper pole because of hindrance of the renal vasculature, but they thought that the wristed instrumentation gave them a distinct advantage compared with pure laparoscopic approaches.[68] In 2010, Hemal and colleagues[69] described their experience with 50 robot-assisted cases in the management of urolithiasis: 36 stone extractions with reconstructive procedures, 8 pyelolithotomies, 4 nephrectomies, and 2 nephroureterectomies. They reported complete clearance of stones in 93.1% of cases, 1 open conversion because of nonlocalization of the stone, and 1 postoperative case of prolonged hematuria resolving after selective angioembolization. Based on their extensive laparoscopic and robot-assisted surgical experience, they thought that the control, dexterity, and precision of the robot-assisted approach were superior and provided a significant advantage in reconstructive efforts.[69]

One of the main concerns with robot-assisted surgery is the associated equipment, maintenance, and expense. Link and colleagues[70] developed a model of mathematical cost showing that robot-assisted pyeloplasty is 2.7 times more expensive than the laparoscopic counterpart. In contrast, an earlier report by be Gettman and colleagues[71] described only a 1.7-fold increase in cost of the robotic approach and much longer operative times for the laparoscopic (235 minutes) versus the robotic (140 minutes) technique. The expense is considerable regardless whether it is 1.7- or 2.5-fold higher than laparoscopy, but it is reasonable to expect the impact of depreciation to be mitigated at high-volume robot-assisted surgery centers.

Laparoscopic/Robot-Assisted Nephrolithotomy

The feasibility of performing laparoscopic anatrophic nephrolithotomy was first demonstrated by Kaouk and colleagues[72] in 2003. In a porcine survival study, after first creating chronic radiolucent staghorn calculi (maturation for 2 weeks), the renal hilum was controlled with a laparoscopic

Table 3
Descriptive statistics and functional results of selected laparoscopic or robot-assisted nephrolithiasis cases

Reference No.	No. of Procedures	Procedure	TP/RP	Mean Stone Size, mm	Mean Operating Room Time, min	Mean Hospital Stay, d	Stricture, %	Conversions, %	Stone-Free Rate, %[a]	Urine Leak, %	Stent, %	Closure of Incision, %
63	20	LAP	RP	16–25	80.2	3.6	0	20	100	10	-	30
64	16	LAP	TP	>20	129	6.5	-	12	88	12	-	-
93	56	LAP	RP	27.5	81	4.0	-	3.6	96	-	100	100
68	13	RAP	TP	42	158	-	-	0	92.3	0	100	100
69	8[b]	RAP	TP	35	106	2.7	-	12.5	93.1	0	100	100
94	5[c]	RAP	TP	38.4	315	3.8	-	20	75	0	100	100
95	11	LAN	TP	52	139	-	-	0	90.9	27.3	-	100[d]
74	5	LAN	TP	53	170	5.4	-	0	60	0	0	100
75	15	LPS	TP	5.8	174	1.6	-	0	80	0	100	100
76	19	LPS	TP	-	276	3.4	-	0	90	-	100	100
78	8	RPS	TP	2–35 mm[e]	275.8	1.1	-	0	100	-	100	100
79	13	RPS	TP	-	235.9	2.0	-	0	95.7	-	100	100
36	5	LCD	RP	-	133.8	1.5	-	0	100	0	100	-
86	3	LPN	TP	-	360	10.6	-	33	67	33	0	0
91	9	NAL	TP	29	176	3.7	-	0	100	0	100	100

Abbreviations: LAP, laparoscopic pyelolithotomy; RAP, robot-assisted pyelolithotomy; LAN, laparoscopic anatrophic nephrolithotomy; LPS, laparoscopic pyeloplasty with removal of stone; RPS, robot-assisted pyeloplasty and stone removal; LCD, laparoscopic calyceal diverticulectomy; LPN, laparoscopic partial nephrectomy for stones; NAL, nephroscopy-assisted laparoscopic pyelolithotomy; TP/RP, transperitoneal/retroperitoneal.

[a] Stone-free rate is reported according to author's imaging test of choice at last follow-up.
[b] One of these cases was a robotic ureterolithotomy.
[c] Note all patients were adolescents with a mean age of 16.6 years, 4 with staghorn cystine stones, and 1 with concomitant UPJ repair.
[d] Collecting system and renal parenchyma were closed with a single layer of 3-0 polyglactin suture.
[e] No mean stone size reported, only range of stone sizes.

Satinsky clamp, allowing successful completion of the laparoscopic anatrophic nephrolithotomy in all animals, closing the renorrhaphy in 2 layers.[72] The mean operative time was 125 minutes and warm ischemia time was 30 minutes, indicating this to be a reasonable and feasible approach. This was first successfully reported in humans by Deger and colleagues[73] in 2004. Simforoosh and colleagues[74] reported 5 cases of transperitoneal laparoscopic anatrophic nephrolithotomy, clamping only the renal artery with a laparoscopic bulldog clamp. The mean stone size was 53 mm (range, 45–65 mm), warm ischemia time was 32 minutes (range, 29–35 minutes), and operative time was 170 minutes (range, 120–225 minutes). No transfusions were needed, and the only 2 patients who were not stone free at initial procedure were stone free after subsequent treatment with SWL. Additionally, even though they closed the renal parenchyma and collecting system in 1 layer, the authors had no patient develop infundibular stenosis on subsequent radiographic evaluation.[74] The authors thought that this approached showed promise but that additional study was needed before widespread adoption.

Laparoscopic/Robot-Assisted Approaches for Urolithiasis and Concomitant Procedures

In centers of established experience in advanced reconstructive laparoscopy, the goal of stone clearance and correction of malformations in a single procedure combines surgical efficacy with minimally invasive surgery. This has most commonly been reported in situations of UPJ repair with concomitant management of renal calculi, from both a laparoscopic and a robot-assisted approach.

UPJ obstruction is an independent risk factor for the subsequent development of nephrolithiasis. Traditionally, PNL with simultaneous percutaneous endopyelotomy has been the preferred minimally invasive treatment option. However, investigators at Cleveland Clinic reviewed their series of laparoscopic pyeloplasties (117 patients) and found that 15 patients (12.8%) also underwent concomitant ipsilateral stone treatment of 1 to 21 stones per patient with a mean size of 5.8 mm.[75] They performed transperitoneal repair in 86.7% of patients and removed the stones after dismembering the UPJ and extending the pyelotomy in an average of 174 minutes. They were successful in 80% of patients with no complications or need for conversion to open surgery.[75] Confirming the excellent results, Ramakumar and colleagues[76] reported a 90% stone-free rate in 19 patients who underwent transperitoneal laparoscopic pyelolithotomy and pyeloplasty. Srivastava and colleagues[77] treated 20 patients with laparoscopic UPJ repair and pyelolithotomy with only a 75% stone clearance rate, but after 3 patients underwent SWL and 2 underwent PNL, all were stone free at 6 months and diuretic renography was improved in 90% of patients (the other 10% had symptomatic improvement). Atug and coworkers reported the first robot-assisted experience; they performed 55 robot-assisted transperitoneal pyeloplasties in which 8 patients also had kidney stones. The number of stones ranged from 1 to more than 30 with a size of 2 to 35 mm in diameter, and they were able to achieve a 100% stone-free rate. The requirement for the management of stones at time of surgery resulted in a mean 61.7 minutes longer of operative time with no postoperative complications and a hospital stay of 1.1 days.[78] Mufarrij and colleagues[79] also retrospectively examined their series of robot-assisted pyeloplasties in 140 patients and found similar excellent stone-free and functional results. They noted that 13 required concomitant stone extraction, with 95.7% of all patients showing resolution of their obstruction and only a 7.1% major and 2.9% minor complication rate. The combined efficiency of a single procedure to clear the stone burden while correcting anatomic obstruction provides a clear indication for laparoscopic or robot-assisted techniques.

The approach to symptomatic calyceal diverticula with stones offers an additional indication for laparoscopic or robot-assisted procedures. Although the occurrences of diverticula are relatively rare, 0.2% to 0.5% of the US population, alternative management options to endourologic procedures require consideration.[80] This is especially true for anterior located diverticula when percutaneous access is difficult or impossible and previous endourologic management has failed. Gluckman and associates performed the first laparoscopic unroofing and fulguration of a calyceal diverticulum in 1993.[80] Miller and colleagues[36] reported their outcomes in 5 patients who underwent retroperitoneal laparoscopic management without the need for open conversion. Mean operative time was 133.8 minutes and the mean hospital stay was only 36 hours. They used various techniques of calyceal localization as none were apparent based on laparoscopic inspection of the renal surface. In 1 patient, retrograde indigo carmine was injected identifying blue discoloration resulting from the thin overlying renal parenchyma, which was unsuccessful in the subsequent patient who required intraoperative fluoroscopy to guide the nephrotomy incision. In the other cases, intraoperative laparoscopic ultrasound was used to direct the surgeon to the appropriate site. The use of intraoperative B-mode scanning and Doppler sonography[81,82] may be the most reproducible and reliable method of definitively identifying the avascular areas in the renal parenchyma close to the stone or dilated calices. This calyceal localization technique also allows removal of large staghorn stones by multiple small radial nephrotomies, without risking significant loss of kidney function. Most calyceal diverticula are ablated or fulgurated, but others report the use of laparoscopic figure-of-8 suture closure of the diverticulum neck,[36] closure with perirenal fat,[83] and even injection of gelatin-resorcinol-formaldehyde-glutaraldehyde glue.[84] These studies indicate the safety of laparoscopy or robotic procedures as an alternative or adjunct to endourologic procedures.

Laparoscopic nephrectomy and partial nephrectomy for stone disease are equivalent to their oncologic counterparts in terms of success and benefit to the patient. The first laparoscopic partial nephrectomy for a stone-bearing hydrocalyx (a rare situation) was reported by Winfield and colleagues[85] in 1992. They subsequently updated their experience with success in 4 of 5 similar patients.[86] Although reports in the literature about robot-assisted partial nephrectomy for stone disease are scarce, the benefits that this platform affords make it well suited for translation of laparoscopic skills to such an endeavor.

COMBINED LAPAROSCOPIC AND ENDOUROLOGIC PROCEDURES

Occasionally, rare and complex cases require more than one treatment modality to achieve the greatest level of success for the patient. Laparoscopic and robot-assisted techniques can be and are often combined with endourologic procedures for those individuals with complicated stone disease and underlying urinary abnormalities, usually for assistance in retrieving fragments.[87] Eshghi and associates reported the first use of laparoscopic guided percutaneous removal of a staghorn calculus in a pelvic kidney in 1985.[88] Such an approach allows safe retraction of overlying structures and percutaneous access in a controlled fashion under direct vision, reducing the risk of complications compared with radiographic assisted endourologic approaches. Exploitation of this technique has also been reported for patients with stones in ectopic pelvic renal units and in horseshoe kidneys with aberrant vasculature.[32,89] In addition, laparoscopic and robot techniques facilitate antegrade stent placement while also allowing suture closure of the nephrotomy or pyelotomy tract to prevent bleeding and urine leakage.

In most cases of endourologic assistance, nephroscopes or ureteroscopes are used to visualize different portions of the renal collecting system to allow surgeons to break up and remove stone fragments in an effort to eradicate all stones in one procedure. For example, Nadu and colleagues[90] described using a flexible nephroscope passed through a 10-mm port during laparoscopic pyeloplasty to perform laser lithotripsy and stone retrieval in 10 patients. Salvadó and colleagues[91] performed cystoscopic assisted laparoscopic pyelolithotomy to remove all stone fragments in 9 patients with a mean stone size of 20 mm, mean operative time of 176 minutes, and mean hospital stay of 3.7 days. The additional irrigation posed no problems or complications for the patients. Endoscopic measures are often necessary to retrieve small fragments because fluoroscopic images through an insufflated abdomen can be challenging to interpret and identify residual fragments. The operating room constraints with laparoscopic and/or robotic equipment coupled with patient positioning and the bulk of a c-arm make the addition of fluoroscopy a challenge. The relatively small mobile endoscopy towers can be arranged to allow stone management in a complementary fashion when needed. Nadu and colleagues[90] also described a technique to help identify calyceal diverticula during laparoscopy by creating access to the renal pelvis and guiding the nephroscope into the area of infundibular stricture for obstructed hydrocalyx or the diverticula neck to guide the nephrotomy as a "cut to the light" procedure. They performed this in 2 patients and lost 2 small stones.

The fate of lost stones during laparoscopic and robot-assisted procedures deserves some consideration. During endoscopic procedures, the urinary system is a closed system, so the "wandering stone" or fragment becomes a localization issue and a minor nuisance. At open surgery, exploration and recovery of stones are easily accomplished, which generally is not the case for laparoscopy. One of the major reasons cited for the need for open conversion is to identify lost stones.[45] Although specific reports of the consequences of retained or lost stone fragments during laparoscopy or robot-assisted surgery are scarce, it is possible to draw some important lessons from the general surgery literature. In a description of lost gallstones during laparoscopic cholecystectomy, several adverse events have been reported: intraperitoneal and abdominal wall abscess formation, fistula, and prolonged fever.[92] It should be the aim of urologic stone procedures to maintain the principles of the open or endourologic equivalent. Lost stone fragments represent all the potential of a retained foreign object. This requires the laparoscopic or robot-assisted surgeon to take great care in ensuring all stones are removed or at least only retained in the closed urinary system if unable to treat.

SUMMARY

The surgical approach to most cases of urolithiasis is defined by endourogic techniques and technology including SWL, PNL, or URS. However, despite the numerous advantages and advances in endourology, open surgical approaches cannot be entirely replaced. Laparoscopic and robot-assisted urological surgery is increasingly replacing open surgery as a result of accumulated surgical experience. The need for open surgical management is shrinking, especially when equivalent outcomes can be achieved with minimally invasive techniques such as laparoscopy and robot-assisted surgery. The implementation and use of these approaches, when available, have further relegated the role of open surgery to that of historical interest as the benefits to patients become more apparent. Laparoscopic and robot-assisted stone surgery is not meant to compete with endourologic procedures but instead complement them and offer the patients the best possible outcomes with the lowest risks and morbidity. The skills, technology, and costs currently available limit the current adoption of these approaches, but the number of reports extolling the relative benefits is growing. The techniques will continue to have a role in the urologist's armamentarium for the modern surgical approach for urolithiasis.

REFERENCES

1. Eknoyan G. History of urolithiasis. Clin Rev Bone Miner Metab 2004;2(3):177–85.
2. Wershub LP. Urology, from antiquity to the 20th century. St Louis (MO): WH Green; 1970.
3. Marshall S. Coagulum pyelolithotomy. Urol Clin North Am 1983;10:659–64.
4. Fischer CP, Sonda LP, Diokno AC. Use of cryoprecipitate coagulum in extracting renal calculi. Urology 1980;15:6–13.
5. Smith MJ, Boyce WH. Anatrophic nephrotomy and plastic calyrhaphy. J Urol 1968;99:521–7.
6. Schultheiss D, Engel RM, Crosby RW, et al. Max Brödel (1870-1941) and medical illustration in urology. J Urol 2000;164:1137–42.
7. Ballenger EG, Frontz WA, Hamer HG, et al. History of urology. Prepared under the auspices of the American Urological Association. Baltimore (MD): Williams & Wilkins; 1933.
8. Smith AD, Lange PH, Fraley EE. Applications of percutaneous nephrostomy: new challenges and opportunities in endo-urology. J Urol 1979; 121(3):382.
9. Fernström I, Johansson B. Percutaneous pyelolithotomy: a new extraction technique. Scand J Urol Nephrol 1976;10:157–9.
10. Goodwin WE, Casey WC, Woolfe W. Percutaneous trocar (needle) nephrostomy in hydronephrosis. JAMA 1955;157:891–4.
11. Kurth K, Hohenfellner R, Altwein JE. Ultrasound lithopaxy of a staghorn calculus. J Urol 1977;117: 242–3.
12. Morris DS, Wei JT, Taub DA, et al. Temporal trends in the use of percutaneous nephrolithotomy. J Urol 2006;175:1731–6.
13. Lyon ES, Kyker JS, Schoenberg HW. Transurethral ureteroscopy in women: a ready addition to the urological armamentarium. J Urol 1978;119(1): 35–6.
14. Krameck AE, Murat FJ, Gettman MT, et al. The evolution of ureteroscopy: a modern single-institution series. Mayo Clin Proc 2006;81(4):468–73.
15. Chaussy C, Brendel W, Schmiedt E. Extracorporeal induced destruction of kidney stones by shock waves. Lancet 1980;2(8207):1265–8.
16. Pearle MS, Calhoun EA, Curhan GC. Urologic Diseases in America Project: urolithiasis. J Urol 2005;173:848–57.
17. Clayman RV, Kavoussi L, Soper N, et al. Laparoscopic nephrectomy: initial case report. J Urol 1991;146:278–82.
18. Satava RM. Robotic surgery: from past to future – a personal journey. Surg Clin North Am 2003;83(6): 1491–500.
19. Jin LX, Ibrahim AM, Newman NA, et al. Robotic surgery claims on United States hospital websites. J Heatlhc Qual 2011;33(6):48–52.
20. Kerbl K, Rehman J, Landman J, et al. Current management of urolithiasis: progress or regress? J Endourol 2002;16:281–8.
21. Assimos DG, Boyce WH, Harrison LH, et al. The role of open surgery since extracorporeal shock wave lithotripsy. J Urol 1989;142:263–7.
22. Segura JW. Current surgical approaches to nephrolithiasis. Endocrinol Metab Clin North Am 1990;19: 912–25.
23. Bichler KH, Lahme S, Strohmaier WL. Indications for open stone removal of urinary calculi. Urol Int 1997; 59:102–8.
24. Rocco F, Casu M, Carmingnani L, et al. Long-term results of intrarenal surgery for branched calculi: is surgery still valid? BJU Int 1998;81:796–800.
25. Paik ML, Wainstein MA, Spirnak JP, et al. Current indications for open stone surgery in the

treatment of renal and ureteral calculi. J Urol 1998;159:374–9.
26. Matlaga BR, Assimos DG. Changing indications of open stone surgery. Urology 2002;59:490–4.
27. Alivizatos G, Skolarikos A. Is there still a role for open surgery in the management of renal stones? Curr Opin Urol 2006;16:106–11.
28. Honeck P, Wendt-Nordahl G, Krombach P, et al. Does open stone surgery still play a role in the treatment of urolithiasis? Data of a primary urolithiasis center. J Endourol 2009;23(7):1209–12.
29. Paik ML, Resnick MI. Is there a role for open stone surgery? Urol Clin North Am 2000;27(2): 323–31.
30. Goel A, Hemal AK. Upper and mid-ureteric stones: a prospective unrandomized comparison of retroperitoneoscopic and open ureterolithotomy. BJU Int 2001;88:679–82.
31. Hruza M, Schulze M, Teber D, et al. Laparoscopic techniques for removal of renal and ureteral calculi. J Endourol 2009;23(10):1713–8.
32. Mousavi-Bahar SH, Amir-Zargar MA, Gholamrezaie HR. Laparoscopic assisted percutaneous nephrolithotomy in ectopic pelvic kidneys. Int J Urol 2008;15(3): 276–8.
33. Nambirajan T, Jeschke S, Albqami N, et al. Role of laparoscopy in management of renal stones: single-center experience and review of literature. J Endourol 2005;19(3):353–9.
34. Ramakumar S, Segura JW. Laparoscopic surgery for renal urolithiasis: pyelolithotomy, caliceal diverticulectomy, and treatment of stones in a pelvic kidney. J Endourol 2000;14(10):829–32.
35. Hemal AK, Goel A, Kumar M, et al. Evaluation of laparoscopic retroperitoneal surgery in urinary stone disease. J Endourol 2001;15(7):701–5.
36. Miller SD, Ng CS, Streem SB, et al. Laparoscopic management of a calyceal diverticular calculi. J Urol 2002;167(3):1248–52.
37. Troxel SA, Low RK, Das S. Extraperitoneal laparoscopy-assisted percutaneous nephrolithotomy in a left pelvic kidney. J Endourol 2002;16(9):655–7.
38. Gaur DD, Trivedi S, Prabhudesai MR, et al. Retroperitoneal laparoscopic pyelolithotomy for staghorn stones. J Laparoendosc Adv Surg Tech A 2002; 12(4):299–303.
39. Matlaga BR. Contemporary surgical management of upper urinary tract calculi. J Urol 2009;181: 2152–6.
40. Preminger GM, Tiselium HG, Assimos DG, et al. 2007 guideline for the management of ureteral calculi. J Urol 2007;178:2418–34.
41. Wickham JE. The surgical treatment of renal lithiasis. In: Wickham JE, editor. Urinary calculous disease. Edinburgh (Scotland): Churchill Livingstone; 1979.
42. Raboy A, Ferzli GS, Ioffreda R, et al. Laparoscopic ureterolithotomy. Urology 1992;39(3):323–5.
43. Wuernschimmel E, Lipsky H. Laparoscopic treatment of upper ureteral stone. J Laproendosc Surg 1993;3(3):301–7.
44. Gaur DD, Agarwal DK, Purohit KC. Retroperitoneal laparoscopic pyelolithotomy. J Urol 1994; 151:927–9.
45. Basiri A, Simforoosh N, Ziaee A, et al. Retrograde, antegrade, and laparoscopic approaches for the management of large, proximal ureteral stones: a randomized clinical trial. J Endourol 2008;22(12): 2677–80.
46. Lopes Neto AC, Korkes F, Silva JL 2nd, et al. Prospective randomized study of treatment of large proximal ureteral stones: extracorporeal shock wave lithotripsy versus ureterolithotripsy versus laparoscopy. J Urol 2012;187(1):164–8.
47. Farooq Qadri SJ, Kahn N, Kahn M. Retroperitoneal laparoscopic ureterolithotomy – a single centre 10 year experience. Int J Surg 2011;9(2):160–4.
48. Flasko T, Holman E, Kovacs G, et al. Laparoscopic ureterolithotomy: the method of choice in selected cases. J Laparoendosc Adv Surg Tech A 2005; 15(2):149–52.
49. Fan T, Xian P, Yang L, et al. Experience and learning curve of retroperitoneal laparoscopic ureterolithotomy for upper ureteral calculi. J Endourol 2009;23(11):1867–70.
50. Bove P, Micali S, Miano R, et al. Laparoscopic ureterolithotomy: a comparison between the transperitoneal and the retroperitoneal approach during the learning curve. J Endourol 2009;23(6):953–7.
51. Gaur DD, Trivedi S, Prabhudesai MR, et al. Laparoscopic ureterolithotomy: technical considerations and long-term follow-up. BJU Int 2002;89(4):339–43.
52. Keeley FX, Gialas I, Pillai M, et al. Laparoscopic ureterolithotomy: the Edinburgh experience. BJU Int 1999;84:765–9.
53. Kijvikai K, Patcharatrakul S. Laparoscopic ureterolithotomy: its role and some controversial technical considerations. Int J Urol 2006;13(3):206–10.
54. Leonardo C, Simone G, Rocco P, et al. Laparoscopic ureterolithotomy: minimally invasive second line treatment. Int Urol Nephrol 2011;43(3):651–4.
55. Ko YH, Kang SG, Park JY, et al. Laparoscopic ureterolithotomy as a primary modality for large proximal ureteral calculi: comparison to rigid ureteroscopic pneumatic lithotripsy. J Laparoendosc Adv Surg Tech A 2011;21(1):7–13.
56. Hemal AK, Goel A, Goel R. Minimally invasive retroperitoneoscopic ureterolithotomy. J Urol 2003;169: 480–2.
57. Derouiche A, Belhaj K, Garbouj N, et al. Retroperitoneal laparoscopy for hte management of lumbar ureter stones. Prog Urol 2008;18(5):281–7.
58. El-Moula MG, Abdallah A, El-Anany F, et al. Laparoscopic ureterolithotomy: our experience with 74 cases. Int J Urol 2008;15(7):593–7.

59. Roberts WW, Cadeddu JA, Micali S. Ureteral stricture formation after removal of impacted calculi. J Urol 1998;159(3):723–6.
60. Nouira Y, Kallel Y, Binous MY, et al. Laparoscopic retroperitoneal ureterolithotomy: initial experience and review of literature. J Endourol 2004;18(6): 557–61.
61. Bellman GC, Smith AD. Special considerations in the technique of laparoscopic ureterolithotomy. J Urol 1992;151(1):146–9.
62. EAU guidelines on laparoscopy 2002. Available at: www.uroweb.org. Accessed July 10, 2012.
63. Sinha R, Sharma N. Retroperitoneal laparoscopic management of urolithiasis. J Laparoendosc Adv Surg Tech A 1997;7(2):95–8.
64. Meria P, Milcent S, Desgrandchamps F, et al. Management of pelvic stones larger than 20 mm: laparoscopic transperitoneal pyelolithotomy or percutaneous nephrolithotomy? Urol Int 2005;75(4): 322–6.
65. Tunc L, Tokgoz H, Tan MO, et al. Stones in anomalous kidneys: results of treatment by shock wave lithotripsy in 150 patients. Int J Urol 2004;11(10): 831–6.
66. Braz Y, Ramon J, Winkler H. Ureterorenoscopy and holmium laser lithotripsy for large renal stone burden: a reasonable alternative to percutaneous nephrolithotomy. Eur Urol 2005;Suppl 4(3):264.
67. Micali S, Pini G, Sighinolfi MC, et al. Laparoscopic simultaneous treatment of peripelvic renal cysts and stones: case series. J Endourol 2009;23(11): 1851–6.
68. Badani KK, Hemal AK, Fumo M, et al. Robotic extended pyelolithotomy for treatment of renal calculi: a feasibility study. World J Urol 2006;24: 198–201.
69. Hemal AK, Nayyar R, Gupta NP, et al. Experience with robotic assisted laparoscopic surgery in upper tract urolithiasis. Can J Urol 2010;17(4):5299–305.
70. Link RE, Bhayani SB, Kavoussi LR. A prospective comparison of robotic and laparoscopic pyeloplasty. Ann Surg 2006;243(4):486–91.
71. Gettman MT, Peschel R, Neururer R, et al. A comparison of laparoscopic pyeloplasty performed with the da Vinci robotic system versus standard laparoscopic techniques: initial clinical results. Eur Urol 2002;42:453–7.
72. Kaouk JH, Gill IS, Desai MM, et al. Laparoscopic anatrophic nephrolithotomy: feasibility study in a chronic porcine model. J Urol 2003;169(2):691–6.
73. Deger S, Tuellmann M, Schoenberger B, et al. Laparoscopic anatrophic nephrolithotomy. Scand J Urol Nephrol 2004;38:263–5.
74. Simforoosh N, Aminsharifi A, Tabibi A, et al. Laparoscopic anatrophic nephrolithotomy for managing large staghorn calculi. BJU Int 2008;101(10): 1293–6.
75. Stein RJ, Turna B, Nguyen MM, et al. Laparoscopic pyeloplasty with concomitant pyelolithotomy: technique and outcomes. J Endourol 2008;22(6): 1251–5.
76. Ramakumar S, Lancini V, Chan DY, et al. Laparoscopic pyeloplasty with concomitant pyelolithotomy. J Urol 2002;167:1378–80.
77. Srivastava A, Singh P, Gupta M, et al. Laparoscopic pyeloplasty with concomitant pyelolithotomy – is it an effective mode of treatment? Urol Int 2008;80: 306–9.
78. Atug F, Castle EP, Burgess SV, et al. Concomitant management of renal calculi and pelvi-ureteric junction obstruction with robotic laparoscopic surgery. BJU Int 2005;96:1365–8.
79. Mufarrij PW, Woods M, Shah OD, et al. Robotic dismembered pyeloplasty: a 6-year multi-institutional experience. J Urol 2008;180(4):1391–6.
80. Gluckman GR, Stroller M, Irby P. Laparoscopic pyelocaliceal diverticular ablation. J Endourol 1993;7(4): 315–7.
81. Thüroff JW, Frohneberg D, Riedmiller R, et al. Localization of segmental arteries in renal surgery by Doppler sonography. J Urol 1982;127(5):863–6.
82. Alken P, Thüroff JW, Riedmiller H, et al. Doppler sonography and B-mode ultrasound scanning in renal stone surgery. Urology 1984;23(5): 455–60.
83. Harewood LM, Agarwal D, Lindsay S, et al. Extraperitoneal laparoscopic caliceal diverticulectomy. J Endourol 1996;10:425–30.
84. Hoznek A, Herard A, Oqiez N, et al. Symptomatic caliceal diverticula treated with extraperitoneal laparoscopic marsupialization fulguration and gelatine resorcinol formaldehyde glue obliteration. J Urol 1998;160:352–5.
85. Winfield HN, Donovan JF, Godet AS, et al. Laparoscopic partial nephrectomy: initial case report for benign disease. J Endourol 1993;7:521–6.
86. Winfield HN, Donovan JF, Lund GO, et al. Laparoscopic nephrectomy: initial experience and comparison to the open surgical approach. J Urol 1995;153: 1409–14.
87. Saussine C, Lechevallier E, Traxer O. Urolithiasis and laparoscopy. Treatment of renal stones in special anatomical and functional conditions. Prog Urol 2008;18:948–51.
88. Eshghi AM, Roth JA, Smith AD. Percutaneous transperitoneal approach to a pelvic kidney for endourological removal of staghorn calculus. J Urol 1985; 134:525.
89. Tahmaz L, Ozgok Y, Zor M, et al. Laparoscopy-assisted tubeless percutaneous nephrolithotomy in previously operated ectopic pelvic kidney with fragmented J-J stent. Urol Res 2009;37:257–60.
90. Nadu A, Schatloff O, Morag R, et al. Laparoscopic surgery for renal stones: is it indicated in the

modern endourology era? Int Braz J Urol 2009; 35(1):9–18.

91. Salvadó JA, Guzman S, Trucco CA, et al. Laparoscopic pyelolithotomy: optimizing surgical technique. J Endourol 2009;23(4):575–8.

92. Memon MA, Deeik RK, Maffi TR, et al. The outcome of unretrieved gallstones in the peritoneal cavity during laparoscopic cholecystectomy. A prospective analysis. Surg Endosc 1999;13:848–57.

93. Chander J, Suryavanshi M, Lal P, et al. Retroperitoneal pyelolithotomy for management of renal calculi. J Soc Laparoendosc Surg 2005;9(1):97–101.

94. Lee RS, Passerotti CC, Cendron M, et al. Early results of robot assisted laparoscopic lithotomy in adolescents. J Urol 2007;177:2306–10.

95. Zhou L, Xuan Q, Wu B, et al. Retroperitoneal laparoscopic anatrophic nephrolithotomy for large staghorn calculi. Int J Urol 2011;18(2):126–30.

Cost-effectiveness Treatment Strategies for Stone Disease for the Practicing Urologist

Elias S. Hyams, MD[a], Brian R. Matlaga, MD, MPH[b,*]

KEYWORDS

• Kidney stones • Nephrolithiasis • Cost-effectiveness

KEY POINTS

- Kidney stones have been rising in prevalence in the United States and worldwide, and represent a significant cost burden based on direct and indirect treatment costs.
- Cost-effectiveness research in this area may enable improvements in treatment efficiency that can benefit patients, providers, and the health care system.
- There has been limited research in the cost-effectiveness of surgical interventions for stone disease, despite the diverse treatment approaches that are available.
- Medical expulsive therapy has been shown to improve rates of stone passage for ureteral stones, and there is evidence that this practice should be liberalized from the standpoints of clinical and cost-effectiveness.
- Although conservative treatment following a primary stone event seems to be cost-effective, the economic impact of medical therapy for recurrent stone formers requires clarification despite its clinical efficacy.

INTRODUCTION

The prevalence of kidney stones has steadily risen in recent decades, with upward of 8% of the United States' population presently being affected.[1] The economic burden of kidney stone treatment is substantial, with annual estimates up to $5 billion including direct and indirect costs.[2,3] Unfortunately, despite this considerable cost burden, there has been limited investigation of the cost-effectiveness of treatment approaches to stone disease. Indeed, efforts to maximize the ratio of benefit to cost are needed to ensure that health care costs are controlled, and to enable practitioners to maintain control of their treatment options. Treatment of stone disease is a ripe area for cost-effectiveness research, given the diverse technologies that are available, as well as variable practice patterns for both medical and surgical treatment.[4] Impediments to cost-effectiveness research in the urological community in general, and for kidney stone treatment in particular, have included the complexity of these analyses, which require consideration of direct and indirect costs; difficulty accessing actual cost data; the need for long-term follow-up of patients susceptible to disease recurrence; institutional, regional and global variations in cost structures; and limitations of clinical research itself that does not provide clarity regarding comparative effectiveness.[5] This article reviews existing data regarding cost and efficacy of surgical and medical interventions for stone disease to guide the individual provider in

Conflict of interest: None.
Funding source: None.
[a] Division of Urology, Dartmouth-Hitchcock Medical Center, 1 Medical Center Drive, Lebanon, NH 03756, USA;
[b] Brady Urological Institute, Johns Hopkins Hospital, 600 North Wolfe Street, Park 221, Baltimore, MD 21287, USA
* Corresponding author.
E-mail address: bmatlag1@jhmi.edu

Urol Clin N Am 40 (2013) 129–133
http://dx.doi.org/10.1016/j.ucl.2012.09.010

his or her clinical decision-making, and identifies areas in which further research is needed to clarify which strategies are cost-effective.

TREATMENT OF KIDNEY STONES

Medical Expulsive Therapy

Because most kidney stones are treated conservatively, medical expulsive therapy (MET) has been a useful tool to expedite stone passage.[6] However, MET does incur a direct medication cost and, potentially, an "opportunity cost." If surgical treatment is delayed in a case where the stone does not pass, additional care is rendered and there is additional lost time from work. The question of cost-effectiveness of MET was explored by Bensalah and colleagues[7] in a decision analysis. These investigators found that MET was cost-effective for distal ureteral stones even when making "worst case" assumptions of a low cost of treatment (ie, ureteroscopy), a small benefit of MET, and/or low rates of spontaneous passage. Other studies have suggested that MET may be cost-effective for mid- or proximal ureteral stones because even a small increase in the likelihood of spontaneous passage enables a cost advantage.[8] This evidence argues for liberal use of MET; however, clinical judgment is needed to ensure that larger and more proximal stones have a lower threshold to proceed with surgical intervention. Further research is needed in the cost-effectiveness of MET versus prompt surgical treatment of stones of various sizes in different anatomic positions.

Surgical Management

Shockwave lithotripsy

Shockwave lithotripsy (SWL) has historically been the most common treatment method for small renal and ureteral stones.[4,9] Selecting patients who are more likely to succeed with SWL may improve the clinical and cost-effectiveness of this treatment. Favorable characteristics include smaller stones, lower Hounsfield units (<1000), shorter skin-to-stone distance (<10 cm), and, in the case of lower pole stones, favorable lower pole anatomy, including infundibulopelvic angle and length.[10,11] Also, evidence demonstrates that slowing SWL rate significantly improves treatment efficiency and reduces the cost of SWL by 50%.[12] Although extra time is required for the treatment, there is higher treatment success and less need for auxiliary treatment.

Ureteroscopy

Use of endoscopy has become more common in recently trained urologists.[4] Although the literature comparing ureteroscopy with SWL has been limited,[5] studies demonstrate a clinical advantage of ureteroscopy for distal ureteral stones, with a lack of rigorous evidence to definitively compare outcomes for stones in other locations. Studies of economic outcomes of ureteroscopy versus SWL have found that, despite the heterogeneity and limited quality of the evidence, ureteroscopy may be cost-effective compared with SWL.[13]

Flexible ureteroscopy, in particular, has enabled access to all renal calyces and direct visualization and removal of stones by a retrograde approach. Options for treatment include active extraction of fragments, typically with a ureteral access sheath, or a "dusting" technique with stent placement enabling small fragments to pass spontaneously over time. There is no consensus on the optimal technique, and studies regarding the comparative effectiveness of these approaches are ongoing. Future studies of the cost-effectiveness of these approaches will need to include short-term costs (eg, operating room time, supplies) and long-term costs (eg, future stone events and/or interventions).

Although flexible ureteroscopy is effective for small-to-medium size stones, the cost of the instruments, as well as maintenance, can be substantial. Furthermore, after one repair, the risk of requiring additional maintenance increases significantly, such that it may be cost advantageous to replace a damaged scope rather than repair it repeatedly.[14] There are important techniques for maximizing the longevity of flexible ureteroscopes; these are likely to benefit both the provider and health system in reducing costs and ensuring functional equipment. These include displacing lower pole stones to more accessible calyces to prevent excessive torque, ensuring that the Holmium laser fiber is not advanced through a curved scope, and taking care not to fire the laser in the channel. Also, use of nitinol devices, smaller caliber laser fibers (ie, 200 μgm), and use of a ureteral access sheath for larger stone burdens may minimize strain on the scope.[15] Careful supervision and education of trainees is needed to ensure these lessons are inculcated and the equipment is preserved. Finally, it may be that having the urology staff process and clean ureteroscopes themselves may reduce processing-related damages and save costs compared with central processing.[14,16]

An area of investigation has been the cost-effectiveness of prestenting patients undergoing ureteroscopy. Chu and colleagues[17] retrospectively studied 104 patients with upper tract (primarily ureteral) stones with a wide range of stone sizes (0.3–4 cm; median 1 cm).[17] The investigators found that prestenting significantly reduced the total costs (direct and indirect) for treatment of patients with stones greater than 1 cm, even when assuming a cost of prestenting up to 6.2 times the current cost. A limitation of this study was use of reimbursement data, instead of actual cost data. Nonetheless, there seemed to be a cost advantage for prestenting patients with larger stone burdens undergoing ureteroscopy. Additional research is needed to better delineate the cost-effectiveness of endoscopic treatments for larger stone burdens, in terms of timing of stent placement, the use of staged procedures, and comparison with alternative approaches such as percutaneous surgery.

Percutaneous nephrolithotomy

Percutaneous nephrolithotomy (PCNL) remains the standard of care for treatment of large (>2 cm) and/or complex renal calculi.[18,19] In addition to superior stone clearance for larger burdens, there is evidence that PCNL is cost-effective for these patients.[20] Although PCNL does incur higher costs in the short-term based on an inpatient hospitalization and higher disposable costs, superior stone eradication leads to a long-term cost advantage.[13,20]

Certain investigators have examined ways to further improve the cost-effectiveness of PCNL. Investigating predictors of cost of this procedure, Bagrodia and colleagues[21] found that only stone burden independently predicted cost, and the main impact of large stone size related to the use of second-look flexible nephroscopy (SLFN). Follow-up study of the cost-effectiveness of SLFN was performed by Raman and colleagues,[22] who reported that this procedure was cost advantageous for residual fragments greater than 4 mm but not for those less than or equal to 4 mm, based on future risk of stone events requiring treatment. The investigators discussed how their cost benefit analysis was dramatically influenced by assumptions regarding likelihood of stone events, the need for surgical treatment, and surgical costs.

There is also some evidence that increased surgical experience enables more efficient and effective treatment of PCNL. Hyams and colleagues[23] reported a lower rate of 30-day mortality and ICU hospitalization for high-volume providers in a Maryland state database. Also, increased surgical experience has been associated with decreased operative time, which may have cost implications.[24] This may also reflect the experience of the operating room staff because troubleshooting instrumentation for PCNL and overall efficiency can be improved with experienced personnel. Finally, operating and fluoroscopy time have been showed to decrease up to 60 cases within a learning curve.[25] These data suggest that referral for treatment of PCNL to higher volume providers and/or institutions may be cost advantageous, though additional research in this area is needed.

The cost-effectiveness of PCNL has been compared with ureteroscopy for treatment of larger renal stones. Hyams and Shah[26] recently demonstrated lower cost associated with ureteroscopy for 2 to 3 cm stones versus PCNL in a retrospective analysis with medium term follow-up. Higher cost for PCNL was based primarily on a high rate of second-stage treatment with PCNL, though there was superior stone clearance in this group of patients. The investigators framed a tradeoff in cost and stone-free rate, with the caveat that long-term follow-up was needed to assess the need for future interventions in patients with small residual fragments. The investigators concluded that, although PCNL was the standard of care, the cost-profile and clinical outcomes of ureteroscopy made it a reasonable option for patients with contraindications to or preference against percutaneous surgery.

In patients with bilateral large stone burdens, it is not clear whether simultaneous or staged PCNL is cost-advantageous. There has been one study in this area by Bagrodia and colleagues,[27] who reported that synchronous bilateral PCNL decreased cumulative operative room time, length of stay, and cost, and thus was advantageous to patients and third-party payers. The investigators noted that physician reimbursement was significantly less compared with staged procedures, providing a disincentive to perform this procedure. This is an important point because a reimbursement scheme can influence practice patterns and provide a disincentive to render care that might be a cost-effective approach overall.

Finally, tubeless PCNL has become increasingly popular to decrease the morbidity and hasten the recovery from PCNL without conceding patient safety. Literature has demonstrated improvements in hospital stay, postoperative analgesic use, and urinary leakage, as well as in operative time.[28,29] Although tubeless procedures may be cost-effective in properly selected patients, investigation in this area is needed because these patients frequently have ureteral stents placed and may have subsequent retrograde procedures and/or SWL.

Prevention of Kidney Stones

Primary prevention

Primary prevention of stone disease has been considered in populations that may be at increased risk based on geography (ie, warmer climates), familial or medical risk factors, genetic testing, or changes in environment (eg, military deployment).[8,30] Lotan and Pearle[31] investigated the cost-effectiveness of primary prevention strategies using a decision-analysis model. They found that primary prevention of stones may be cost-effective depending on assumptions of cost, risk, and efficacy. Specifically, an intervention would be cost-effective if the incidence of disease was at least 1%, cost did not exceed $20 per person per year, and the strategy was at least 50% effective at stone prevention. Thus, these interventions may be worthwhile in certain populations, depending on risk, because there are low-cost interventions, such as education regarding water consumption, which can be considered.[31] Indeed, Lotan and colleagues[30] reported a cost model in which increased water intake would theoretically be cost-effective for a national payer system for prevention of stone disease.

Secondary prevention

First-time stone formers generally are counseled on conservative treatment measures, including dietary manipulations, to decrease risk of recurrence. These inexpensive interventions include increased water intake[32] and dietary changes that have been shown to modulate stone risk.[33,34] For recurrent stone formers, conservative treatment is generally insufficient because of the high rate of recurrence.[35] Medical therapy is considered in these patients and has been shown to reduce risk of recurrence in certain patients.[36,37] Importantly, however, these medications have side effects, inconvenience, and cost that can affect patient compliance.[8,20,38] Although older studies found that screening and treating stone patients with medical therapy lowered costs,[39,40] these studies did not necessarily account for the benefit of conservative treatment alone, the costs of metabolic evaluation, and that not all recurrent stones necessitate treatment.[41] Nonetheless, more recent studies have concluded that medical treatment in known stone formers is likely to be cost-effective depending on assumptions regarding effectiveness, cost of therapy, and rate of stone recurrence.[2]

Lotan and colleagues[35] investigated the cost-effectiveness of conservative therapy versus drug treatment for first-time versus recurrent stone formers. In a decision-analysis model, they concluded that conservative treatment was cost-effective for first-time stone formers, whereas the higher cost of drug treatment strategies was justified for recurrent stone formers. Lotan and colleagues[41] also performed an international comparison of cost-effectiveness of medical management strategies for recurrent stone disease. Contrastingly, they found that dietary treatment was the most cost-effective approach because of the relatively low cost of surgery (which was required infrequently) compared with medication (which was required daily). Empiric and directed medical therapy were more effective at controlling stone disease; however, they were not cost-effective because of the low likelihood of surgical intervention and the relatively low cost of surgery. This was true except in the United Kingdom where medication costs were sufficiently low so that empiric therapy was more cost-effective than conservative therapy. Thus, improving cost-effectiveness of medical therapy requires additional research to reduce costs of medical therapy, improve compliance, identify patients who are most likely to benefit, and to improve the efficacy of medical management itself.[8]

SUMMARY

Kidney stone disease is rising in global prevalence, and the cost burden of this condition is substantial. Although cost-effectiveness considerations are typically made by policymakers, individual practitioners have become increasingly involved in these discussions so that they may affect the rising costs of care and assert control of treatment options. Although progress is being made, there are essential areas in which additional investigation is required.

REFERENCES

1. Scales CD Jr, Smith AC, Hanley JM, et al. Prevalence of kidney stones in the United States. Eur Urol 2012;62:160–5.
2. Saigal CS, Joyce G, Timilsina AR. Direct and indirect costs of nephrolithiasis in an employed population: opportunity for disease management? Kidney Int 2005;68:1808–14.
3. Pearle MS, Calhoun EA, Curhan GC. Urologic Diseases in America project: urolithiasis. J Urol 2005;173:848–57.
4. Matlaga BR, American Board of Urology. Contemporary surgical management of upper urinary tract calculi. J Urol 2009;181:2152–6.
5. Matlaga BR, Jansen JP, Meckley LM, et al. Treatment of ureteral and renal stones: a systematic review and meta-analysis of randomized, controlled trials. J Urol 2012;188:130–7.
6. Hollingsworth JM, Rogers MA, Kaufman SR, et al. Medical therapy to facilitate urinar stone passage: a meta-analysis. Lancet 2006;368:1171–9.
7. Bensalah K, Pearle M, Lotan Y. Cost-effectiveness and medical explusive therapy using alpha-blockers for

the treatment of distal ureteral stones. Eur Urol 2008; 53:411–9.
8. Lotan Y. Economics and cost of care of stone disease. Adv Chronic Kidney Dis 2009;16(1):5–10.
9. Bandi G, Best SL, Nakada SY. Current practice patterns in the management of upper urinary tract calculi in the north central United States. J Endourol 2008;22:631–6.
10. Raman JD, Pearle MS. Management options for lower pole renal calculi. Curr Opin Urol 2008;18:214–9.
11. Pearle MS. Shock-wave lithotripsy for renal calculi. N Engl J Med 2012;367(1):50–7.
12. Koo V, Beattie I, Young M. Improved cost-effectiveness and efficiency with a slower shock-wave delivery rate. BJU Int 2009;105:692–6.
13. Matlaga BR, Jansen JP, Meckley LM, et al. Economic outcomes of treatment for ureteral and renal stones: a systematic literature review. J Urol 2012;188:449–54.
14. Carey RI, Gomez CS, Maurici G, et al. Frequency of ureteroscope damage seen at a tertiary care center. J Urol 2006;176:607–10.
15. Pietrow PK, Auge BK, Delvecchio FC, et al. Techniques to maximize flexible ureteroscope longevity. Urology 2002;60(5):784–8.
16. Semins MJ, George S, Allaf ME, et al. Ureteroscope cleaning and sterilization by the urology operating room team: the effect on repair costs. J Endourol 2009;23(6):903–5.
17. Chu L, Farris CA, Corcoran AT, et al. Preoperative stent placement decreases cost of ureteroscopy. Urology 2011;78:309–13.
18. Preminger GM, Assimos DG, Lingeman JE, et al. Chapter 1: AUA guideline on management of staghorn calculi: diagnosis and treatment recommendations. J Urol 2005;173(6):1991–2000.
19. Kim SC, Kuo RL, Lingeman JE. Percutaneous nephrolithotomy: an update. Curr Opin Urol 2003;13(3): 235–41.
20. Lotan Y, Pearle MS. Economics of stone management. Urol Clin North Am 2007;34(3):443–53.
21. Bagrodia A, Gupta A, Raman JD, et al. Predictors of cost and clinical outcomes of percutaneous nephrostolithotomy. J Urol 2009;182:586–90.
22. Raman JD, Bagrodia A, Bensalah K, et al. Residual fragments after percutaneous nephrolithotomy: cost comparison of immediate second look flexible nephroscopy versus expectant management. J Urol 2010;183:188–93.
23. Hyams ES, Mullins JK, Pierorazio PM, et al. Impact of surgeon and hospital volume on short term outcomes of percutaneous nephrolithotomy. J Urol 2012;187(Suppl 4):e687.
24. Akman T, Binbay M, Akcay M, et al. Variables that influence operative time during percutaneous nephrolithotomy: an analysis of 1897 cases. J Endourol 2011;25(8):1269–73.
25. Tanriverdi O, Boylu U, Kendirci M, et al. The learning curve in the training of percutaneous nephrolithotomy. Eur Urol 2007;52(1):206–11.
26. Hyams ES, Shah O. Percutaneous nephrostolithotomy versus flexible ureteroscopy/Holmium laser lithotripsy: cost and outcome analysis. J Urol 2009; 182(3):1012–7.
27. Bagrodia A, Raman JD, Bensalah K, et al. Synchronous bilateral percutaneous nephrostolithotomy: analysis of clinical outcomes, cost and surgeon reimbursement. J Urol 2009;181:149–53.
28. Yuan H, Zheng S, Liu L, et al. The efficacy and safety of tubeless percutaneous nephrolithotomy: a systematic review and meta-analysis. Urol Res 2011;39:401–10.
29. Akman T, Binbay M, Yuruk E, et al. Tubeless procedure is most important factor in reducing length of hospitalization after percutaneous nephrolithotomy: results of univariable and multivariable models. Urology 2011;77:299–304.
30. Lotan Y, Jimenez IB, Lenoir-Wijnkoop I, et al. Primary prevention of nephrolithiasis is cost-effective for a national healthcare system. BJU Int 2012. [Epub ahead of print].
31. Lotan Y, Pearle MS. Cost-effectiveness of primary prevention strategies for nephrolithiasis. J Urol 2011;186:550–5.
32. Borghi L, Meschi T, Amato F, et al. Urinary volume, water and recurrences in idiopathic calcium nephrolithiasis: a 5-year randomized prospective study. J Urol 1996;155(3):839–43.
33. Borghi L, Schianchi T, Meschi T, et al. Comparison of two diets for the prevention of recurrent stones in idiopathic hypercalciuria. N Engl J Med 2002;346:77–84.
34. Taylor EN, Fung TT, Curhan GC. DASH-style diet associates with reduced risk for kidney stones. J Am Soc Nephrol 2009;20:2253–9.
35. Lotan Y, Cadeddu JA, Roerhborn CG, et al. Cost-effectiveness of medical management strategies for nephrolithiasis. J Urol 2004;172(6 Pt 1):2275–81.
36. Mardis HK, Parks JH, Muller G, et al. Outcome of metabolic evaluation and medical treatment for calcium nephrolithiasis in a private urological practice. J Urol 2004;171(1):85–8.
37. Pearle MS, Roehrborn CG, Pak CY. Meta-analysis of randomized trials for medical prevention of calcium oxalate nephrolithiasis. J Endourol 1999;13:679–85.
38. Robertson WG. Is prevention of stone recurrence financially worthwhile? Urol Res 2006;34:157–61.
39. Parks JH, Coe FL. The financial effects of kidney stone prevention. Kidney Int 1996;50:1706–12.
40. Fine JK, Pak CY, Prèminger GM, et al. Effect of medical management and residual fragments on recurrent stone formation following shock wave lithotripsy. J Urol 1995;153(1):27–32.
41. Lotan Y, Cadeddu JA, Pearle MS. International comparison of cost effectiveness of medical management strategies for nephrolithiasis. Urol Res 2005;33:223–30.

http://dx.doi.org/10.1016/j.uc
0094-0143/12/$ – see front

Impact of Stone Disease

Chronic Kidney Disease and Quality of Life

Ganesh Kartha, MD[a], Juan C. Calle, MD[b,*], Giovanni Scala Marchini, MD[a], Manoj Monga, MD[a]

KEYWORDS

• Nephrolithiasis • Quality of life • Renal function • Chronic kidney disease

KEY POINTS

- Kidney stone disease can impact renal function - with the greatest risk being related to infection stones and patients with significant comorbidities including obesity, hypertension and diabetes.
- Kidney stone disease can have a significant impact on psychological distress and quality of life.
- Vigilance is warranted to permit early detection and intervention for renal insufficiency, psychological disorders, and diminished quality of life in chronic stone formers.

INTRODUCTION

Urolithiasis is a disease with rising prevalence in the United States.[1] With a growing burden, a better understanding of the disease process and methods for prevention and treatment are being widely researched. Over the years, there has been a great leap in technology for minimally invasive management of urinary stones. The era of open pyelolithotomy has passed and currently there are much less invasive treatments, such as percutaneous nephrolithotomy (PCNL), ureteroscopy (URS), and shockwave lithotripsy (SWL). Nonetheless, recurrent stone formation is still a major issue among patients with urolithiasis.[2] The propensity for recurrence, necessity of lifestyle change, and frequent interventions associated with urinary stone disease may significantly affect both the risk for development of chronic kidney disease (CKD) and the quality of life (QOL) of patients burdened with this disease.

Nephrolithiasis is a worldwide health problem responsible for significant economic cost to society and serious effects on QOL, affecting both men and women with a lifetime prevalence of 13% and 7%, respectively.[3] Over the past few decades, it has been shown that stone disease incidence and prevalence is steadily increasing, a trend which has been attributed to changes in diet and lifestyle. Moreover, it may be related to the increasing prevalence of obesity and diabetes mellitus, which have also been linked to kidney stone formation. Lastly, environmental changes, namely global warming, may play a role.[4–6] In contrast, other reports suggest that the prevalence of nephrolithiasis is stable or even decreasing in the last decade in specific parts of the globe.[7] Incidence rates peak in both male and female around the fourth decade. In terms of race and ethnicity, prevalence and incidence of nephrolithiasis seem to be highest in white individuals, followed by Hispanics, blacks, and Asian natives. However, the rates for black Americans seem to have increased specifically at older ages.[7]

The risk of recurrence after a first kidney stone episode is controversial. In the beginning of the nineteenth century, Lamson[8] reported a wide range for nephrolithiasis recurrence rate, from 10% to 48 %. Recent uncontrolled studies show similar figures (30%–50%) within the first 5 years

[a] Department of Urology, Glickman Urological & Kidney Institute, The Cleveland Clinic, 9500 Euclid Avenue, Cleveland, OH 44120, USA; [b] Department of Nephrology, Glickman Urological & Kidney Institute, The Cleveland Clinic, 9500 Euclid Avenue, Cleveland, OH 44120, USA
* Corresponding author.
E-mail address: juancallecano@yahoo.com

Urol Clin N Am 40 (2013) 135–147
http://dx.doi.org/10.1016/j.ucl.2012.09.004

of the first stone-related event.[9] If the follow-up period is extended to 25 years, virtually all patients are expected to have some sort of stone recurrence, corroborating the complex and heterogeneous natural history of nephrolithiasis.[10,11] However, recent data from randomized, controlled trials suggest significantly lower rates, ranging from 2% to 5% per year. Furthermore, the risk of recurrence seems to increase with each new stone formed.[12]

Certain special patient groups may be at higher risk for impact of disease on CKD and QOL. Though the overall incidence of nephrolithiasis in renal transplant recipients is quite low (0.4%–1%), the effects can be devastating if left unattended.[13–15] Over the past few years, interest has renewed in the impact of bariatric surgery on calcium oxalate stone disease and oxalate nephropathy. Jejunoileal bypass surgery was abandoned in the 1990s due to major complications including nephrolithiasis and renal failure in as many as 37% of patients.[16,17] Similar concerns are arising with newer gastric bypass procedures.[18–20] Primary hyperoxaluria often presents with symptomatic urolithiasis earlier in life when compared with the general population and have higher chances of progressing to renal failure due to their disease.[21,22] Struvite stones, also known as triple phosphate, magnesium ammonium phosphate, or infection stones harbor a higher risk of sepsis, renal dysfunction, and death than other stone compositions.[23,24]

Finally, cystine stones are caused by an autosomal disorder transmitted in either a recessive or a dominant manner with incomplete penetrance due to mutations that include missense, nonsense, splicing defects, frameshift, deletions, and insertions of a single amino acid residue, and large rearrangements.[25] Although cystinuria accounts for only 1% to 2% of all urolithiasis in adults, it is more common in children, accounting for almost 8% of renal stones in the pediatric population. Commonly, the disease manifests in the second and third decades of life and carries a higher risk of CKD.[26,27]

Renal colic or nephrolithiasis related events account for more than 1 to 2 million emergency room visits per year, ensuing in an expensive burden to the health care system. If the number of days lost at work is considered, the scenario is even worse. Saigal and colleagues[28] retrospectively calculated the direct cost of stone disease based on data from a privately insured, employed population in the United States and found it to be more than 4.5 billion dollars in 1 year. After summing up conservative estimates for indirect costs, such as workdays lost due to the disease, the amount increased to more than 5.3 billion dollars.

This article focuses on the hidden costs of nephrolithiasis: namely the impact it has on kidney function and CKD, and the QOL of patients who suffer from recurrent bouts of debilitating pain.

Nephrolithiasis and CKD

CKD is a major public health problem and affects 13% of the adult population.[29] CKD can be classified into five categories according to their estimated glomerular filtration rate (eGFR) (in milliliters/minute/1.73 m^2) with or without renal damage for greater than or equal to 3 months. The categories, or stages, have an eGFR of (1) $\geq$90, (2) 60–89, (3) 30–59, (4) 15–29, and (5) <15 (ml/min/1.73 m^2).

With more than $23 billion spent by Medicare in 2009 in the United States for patients on any type of renal replacement therapy or renal transplantation, significant efforts have been made to prevent and treat possible causes of CKD.[30,31] According to the United States Renal Data System (USRDS), the prevalence of CKD has remained relatively stable over the last decade, despite the use of different formulas to calculate kidney function. In contrast, data extracted from Medicare claims for CKD demonstrate a clear increase from 3.3% in 1998 to 8.5% in 2009. Similarly, the 2005 to 2008 analysis of the National Health and Nutrition Examination Survey (NHANES) reports that the prevalence of CKD has increased to 15.1% and an incidence rate for end stage renal disease (ESRD) of 355 new cases per million population in 2009.[30]

Although nephrolithiasis is rarely identified as a prominent risk factor for either CKD or ESRD, there are many studies that associate stone disease with varying degrees of renal insufficiency.[32,33] The cause of renal insufficiency in patients with nephrolithiasis is multifactorial and includes renal obstruction, recurrent urinary tract infection (UTI), repeated surgical interventions, and coexisting medical disease.[34–40] Early recognition of CKD and management of its underlying factors could help prevent several adverse effects and decrease the risk of morbidity and mortality associated with this disease, including long-term renal replacement therapy and transplantation, as well as social and psychological distress. Patients with CKD represent 0.8% to 17.5% of those presenting with urinary stone disease.[34,35] CKD remains an uncommon event among stone formers and nephrolithiasis-related CKD accounts for only a small percentage (usually lower than

3%) of patients for whom renal replacement therapy is necessary.[36]

It has been assumed that CKD will develop in 3 of 100,000 stone formers annually.[40] In a cohort of 171 subjects with severe idiopathic calcium stone disease, Marangella and colleagues[35] reported that 18% had mild renal insufficiency, with a mean GFR of 67 mL/min/1.73 m^2 at referral; but there was no significant decline during a mean follow-up of nearly 3.5 years. Similarly, of the 3266 subjects with nephrolithiasis reported by Worcester and colleagues,[41] CKD did not develop in any of them and there was no significant decline in creatinine clearances on long-term follow-up. On the other hand, the same investigators reported that renal function decreased with age in stone formers at a higher pace than in non–stone formers.

In the general population, lower eGFR has been observed in overweight or obese patients and also in stone formers with hypertension (HTN).[42,43] Gillen and colleagues[42] used NHANES III of the US population to compare eGFR between the 6% who reported a history of kidney stones and the rest who did not report a history of kidney stones. Among individuals who were overweight or obese, a history of kidney stones was associated with an eGFR that was 3.4 mL/min/1.73 m^2 lower after multivariate adjustment. A similar association in normal-weight individuals was not evident. Vupputuri and colleagues[43] demonstrated that subjects who had CKD (identified by diagnostic codes) and elevated serum creatinine (SCr) levels were 1.9 times more likely to report a history of kidney stones on telephone interview when compared with matched community control subjects. Interestingly, the association was strongest in individuals without HTN and in individuals who were identified by CKD diagnostic codes for interstitial nephritis or diabetic nephropathy. Because cases were identified via hospital record review, they may have had more undiagnosed comorbidities than did control subjects. Population-based prospective cohort studies with active follow-up to determine the risk for CKD among stone formers are lacking. In a population-based historical cohort evaluation, Rule and colleagues[44] compared subjects with diagnostic codes and/or elevated SCr levels (or eGFR <60 mL/min/1.73 m^2) sustained for at least 3 months with a matched control group. With a mean follow-up of 8.6 years, the risk for clinical diagnosis of CKD was 50% to 67% higher, risk for a sustained elevated SCr was 26% to 46% higher, and risk for a sustained reduced eGFR was 22% to 42% higher in the stone group. These increased risks were independent of any comorbidities associated with CKD.

Although kidney stones may be associated with future CKD, paradoxically, there is reason to believe that CKD is protective against formation of kidney stones. As GFR declines, it is followed by a fall in urine calcium excretion, an important risk factor for stone formation.[45] Indeed, evidence suggests that stone recurrence rates may be lower in stone formers with a reduced GFR.[35] Ironically, if kidney stones lead to CKD, the risk for stone recurrence may decrease, leading to an underrecognition of the contribution of kidney stones to the development of ESRD. It is important to distinguish stone formers in whom stones are the primary cause of ESRD from those in whom they are only a contributing risk factor. Jungers and colleagues[40] specifically investigated ESRD cases that had been attributed to kidney stones by reviewing the case histories of 1391 consecutive subjects with ESRD in France. Forty-five (3.2%) had ESRD attributed primarily or exclusively to kidney stones, with a significant proportion being attributed to struvite stones (42%). Tosetto and colleagues[46] identified a history of kidney stones in only 3.2% of 1901 subjects who had ESRD and were on hemodialysis, two-thirds of whom (2.1%) had ESRD attributed to the kidney stones. The USRDS reports kidney stones to be the primary cause of ESRD in only 0.2% (908 or 546,878) of all-incident subjects from 2004 to 2008.[47] Nevertheless, their findings took in consideration the ESRD Medical Evidence form (CMS 2728) and not a comprehensive chart review.

In a case-control study, Stankus and colleagues[48] surveyed 300 black subjects with hemodialysis for a history of kidney stones and compared findings with the 5341 black individuals who participated in NHANES III. The likelihood of self-reported past kidney stones was higher for patients with ESRD than for the population control subjects (8% vs 3%, respectively). Of the 25 subjects with ESRD and a history of kidney stones, only five had a stone episode within 5 years of starting dialysis and only two had ESRD that was primarily attributed to the stone disease. Hippisley-Cox and Coupland[49] reported an increased risk for ESRD with women (hazard ratio of 2.1), but not men, stone formers in a cohort study. In contrast, though the Olmsted County study demonstrated significant links between CKD and stone disease, there was no statistical impact on the development of ESRD or mortality.[44]

STONE TREATMENT AND CKD

Gupta and colleagues[33] reported that 75.8% of subjects with urinary stone disease and CKD had undergone multiple surgical procedures for stone treatment. These subjects also frequently had several coexisting comorbidities (diabetes, HTN, anemia and/or bleeding disorders), some of which could either lead to the development of CKD or be a manifestation of the disease. The coexistence of medical conditions associated with CKD may increase operative risk, the incidence of postoperative complications, and ultimately affect outcomes. This complex interplay between stone disease, medical comorbidities, and surgical interventions make it difficult to attribute specific risk for the development of CKD.

Jungers and colleagues[40] found that 40% of stone formers who developed ESRD had a solitary functioning kidney before developing ESRD. Although nephrolithiasis is rarely identified as a prominent risk factor for either CKD or ESRD, there are many studies that associate them with stone disease. Worcester and colleagues[41] evaluated the cause of a solitary functioning kidney among 115 stone formers. The most common culprits reported were large stone burden (29%), infection (23%), and ureteral obstruction (21%). Surgical procedures were responsible for only 8% of the solitary kidneys in this group.

The evolution of minimally invasive procedures for nephrolithiasis has been scrutinized for impact on renal function. Typically an eGFR of 60 has been used as a threshold to identify iatrogenic changes in renal function after intervention.[50,51]

SWL

SWL is widely used to treat proximal ureteral calculi less than 1 cm and renal stones less than 2 cm in diameter.[52–54] In animal models, SWL has been shown to induce parenchymal injury, which increases with the number of shocks, level of energy, and also with smaller kidneys. Furthermore, SWL is associated with an acute reduction in GFR and renal blood flow due to vasoconstriction.[55,56] Evaluation of "shocked" kidneys with magnetic resonance imaging, contrast urogram, and nuclear scintigraphy revealed that 74% of patients had abnormal findings after SWL consistent with a renal contusion. However, a long-term effect of SWL on kidney function has not been definitively demonstrated. Eassa and colleagues[57] found no change in eGFR or in the relative differential renal function of the treated kidney using nuclear scintigraphy at approximately 4 years of follow-up. Even longer follow-up studies suggest that the risk for an elevated SCr level is not increased with SWL compared with PCNL or conservative management.[58] HTN has been described as a possible long-term complication of SWL in some[59–61] but not all[57,62,63] trials. A recent population-based study did not find an increased risk, suggesting that this complication rarely affects stone formers following SWL.[64] Pretreatment with low-energy shockwaves followed by a ramp-up protocol in energy seems to be protective against renal injury.[65] Recently, el-Assmy and colleagues[66] retrospectively evaluated the long-term effects of SWL in subjects with solitary kidneys with a mean follow-up of 3.8 years and found no significant difference in SCr, systolic and diastolic blood pressure, new onset HTN, calculated GFR, and kidney morphology before and after treatment.

SWL success is dependent of several factors. Stone-free rate (SFR) is influenced by stone size,[67–70] location,[71–74] symptom duration previous to the procedure,[71–74] presence of ureteral stent,[67,68] gender,[70] stone density (Hounsfield Units), skin-to-stone distance, and stone composition.[70,75] The influence of renal function on success rates after SWL, however, is debatable. Lee and colleagues[76] reported a significantly lower SFR of 57% for subjects with preoperative SCr between 2.0 and 2.9 mg/dL compared with 66% if SCr was less than 2.0 mg/dL ($P<.05$). Hung and colleagues[70] reported that subjects with proximal ureteral calculi had SFR of only 50% if they had underlying CKD, compared with 93% for subjects with an eGFR greater than 60 mL/min/1.73 m^2. On multivariate logistic regression analysis, factors negatively affecting SFR were gender (females), eGFR less than 60 mL/min/1.73 m^2, and stone width greater than 7 mm. Conversely, other studies have failed to find an association between SWL outcomes and preoperative impaired renal function.[77,78]

PCNL

There have been some attempts to identify predictors of prognosis and outcomes for patients with CKD who have upper urinary tract calculi.[79,80] Paryani and Ather[79] retrospectively reviewed 500 subjects with urolithiasis (40% with complete or partial staghorn calculi) and reported that in the 12% with baseline renal insufficiency, most had improvements in function independent of relief of obstruction. Singh and colleagues[80] prospectively followed 70 subjects with CKD (mean preoperative SCr of 4.76 mg/dL) who underwent PCNL for staghorn or calyceal stones. They reported an average decrease in SCr of 1.53 mg/dL (32%) and an average functional improvement by renal dynamic scans of 20% 9 months postoperative.

Agrawal and colleagues[81] published their experience with PCNL in 78 subjects with calculous nephropathy and advanced renal failure. An improvement in renal function was seen in most (82%) subjects, whereas in 11 subjects it remained unaltered or deteriorated. Nevertheless, in their study baseline renal function evaluation was performed at presentation, instead of after placing a percutaneous nephrostomy tube or treating any UTI to rule out an overlying component of acute renal failure. They reported parenchymal thickness greater than or equal to 7 mm, clear urine in the collecting system, absence of urosepsis, and recent onset azotemia were predictors of renal recovery. Kukreja and colleagues[82] reviewed the impact of PCNL on renal function in 84 CKD subjects with renal stones. Subjects with acute rise in creatinine due to obstruction or infection were excluded from the study, but SCr, instead of eGFR, was used to evaluate renal function. They reported an overall improvement in renal function in 33 subjects (39%), stable function in 24 (29%), and decreased function in 27 (32%) with a mean follow-up of 2.2 years. Factors predicting deterioration in renal function were proteinuria greater than 300 mg/d, atrophic cortex less than 5 mm, recurrent UTI, stone burden greater than 1500 mm^2, time elapsed after PCNL surgery less than 15 years, and finally pediatric age group. In a retrospective study by Canes and colleagues,[83] the impact of PCNL on renal function was evaluated in 81 subjects with a solitary kidney. Mean eGFR increased from 44.9 mL/min/1.73 m^2 preoperatively to 51.5 mL/min/1.73 m^2 1 year after intervention. In another large series, Bilen and colleagues[51] evaluated 185 subjects with eGFR less than 60 mL/min/1.73 m^2 undergoing PCNL and found the mean preoperative eGFR significantly increased from 42.4 to 48.4 mL/min/1.73 m^2 at three months follow-up. None of the subjects required dialysis during that relatively shorter follow-up. They also found that nearly all subjects with stage 5 CKD had some benefit from surgery, whereas half of stage 4 subjects and only 25% of stage 3 subjects improved. Renal function improvement was the greatest in stage 5 and the least in stage 2 subjects. They hypothesized that the impact of the calculi itself in a severely compromised kidney is greater than the impact of PCNL and the opposite is probably true for moderately affected kidneys in which the harm of PCNL may be more significant, particularly if associated with UTI.

Kurien and colleagues[84] studied 91 adult subjects with SCr greater than 1.5 mg/dL who underwent PCNL. Most subjects had stage 3 or 4 CKD and most showed improvement or stabilization in renal function after PCNL. Postoperative complications and peak eGFR were the main factors predicting deterioration of kidney function during follow-up. Similarly, Akman and colleagues[85] followed 177 subjects who underwent PCNL and had preoperative GFR less than 60 mL/min/1.73 m^2 for at least 1 year and found a significant improvement in eGFR after a mean 43-month follow-up.

Another important factor that has been proposed to affect renal function in patients with CKD is the number of tracts. Animal studies have shown that PCNL tracts were associated with minimal scar tissue and no significant morphologic or functional alterations.[86,87] Handa and colleagues[86] also evaluated the impact of multiple-tract PCNL in pigs and found no significant difference in renal function loss compared with single-tract PCNL. Human studies revealed that renal damage from nephrostomy tracts is minimal based on nuclear renography and has no effect on systemic renal function.[88,89] Akman and colleagues[85] series compared 142 subjects treated with one access to 35 subjects with multiple-tract PCNL and found similar renal function among them, even when considering CKD subjects.

SFR after PCNL for patients with CKD depend on imaging modality to define it and timing of the examination itself. Bilen and colleagues[51] reported complete stone-free status on postoperative radiograph of 81.1% in subjects with CKD undergoing PCNL. Clinically significant residual stones (>5 mm) were present in 21 renal units (10.7%) and insignificant residual fragments were seen in the remaining 16 (8.1%). Overall, 5 renal units underwent adjuvant SWL, 10 had second-look PCNL, and 5 underwent ureteroscopy. Kurien and colleagues[84] defined complete clearance as nonvisualization of residual fragments on radiograph and ultrasonography at 1 month after PCNL. Stone-free status was achieved in 98 renal units (83.7%) with a mean of 1.3 stages per renal unit. SWL as an auxiliary procedure was required for clearance of residual stones in 2.5%. Akman and colleagues[85] reported SFR at postoperative month 3 of 80.2% (142 out of 177). Definition was based on radiograph, ultrasound, and/or CT. Stone recurred during long-term follow-up in 25.3% of these subjects.

PCNL remains the primary modality for treating complex stones in patients with CKD. However, it is not without complications and the most common are hypothermia, bleeding, metabolic acidosis, serum electrolytes disturbances, urosepsis, and rarely death.[90,91] Overall PCNL complication rate is 13% to 35% and bleeding remains the leading problem.[81–85] Anemia and underlying platelet dysfunction in patients with CKD may play an important role in the high rate of transfusion. Bilen and colleagues[51] reported that 38% of CKD subjects had anemia preoperatively and that blood transfusion rates were as high as 36%. Kurien and colleagues[84] and Akman and colleagues[85] had a lower, but still significant, transfusion rate of 20.5% and 9.6%, respectively. Efforts to reduce hemorrhagic complications include ultrasound-guided access, balloon-tract dilatation, optimization of operating time, and staging procedures in cases of large stone burden.[92]

Despite prophylactic antibiotics, urosepsis remains a major concern, even in patients with CKD who have sterile preoperative urine cultures. Because of the inhibition of cell-mediated immunity and humoral defense mechanisms, sepsis may easily develop in patients with CKD. Agrawal and colleagues[81] reported septic complications in eight of the 78 subjects, out of whom three died (3.8%) despite intensive care. Bilen and colleagues[51] reported septic shock in three subjects, regardless of appropriate antibiotic treatment. Only one subject survived and the overall mortality rate was 1.1%. Kurien and colleagues[84] reported UTI, defined as culture proven or prolonged febrile episodes, in nine subjects (7.7%) of their series. There were two postoperative deaths and one related septic shock. In the series of Akman and colleagues,[85] urosepsis was detected in five subjects (2.8%) who were successfully treated with intravenous broad-spectrum antibiotics. No deaths occurred. Steps used in attempts to avoid postoperative infection include adequate preoperative collecting system drainage and preemptive administration of broad-spectrum antibiotics. During the procedure, the use of a large caliber Amplatz sheath to maintain low intrarenal pressure may decrease the incidence of bacteremia in patients with infected stones.[93,94] Importantly, complete stone clearance is essential to remove all foci of infection. Furthermore, adequate postoperative drainage through a nephrostomy tube or a ureteral stent may reduce bacterial load in the pelvicalyceal system, decreasing the chance of bacteremia.[95,96] Efforts should also be spent to reduce hospital-acquired infections.

NEPHROLITHIASIS AND QOL

Overview

There are very few studies in regard to urolithiasis that investigate the impact of the disease process, treatment (both medical and surgical) and implementation of lifestyle modifications on the QOL of patients. Most studies look at SFR as an endpoint for effective management. Looking at the nature of the disease, a patient often is diagnosed with urolithiasis due to the onset of debilitating flank pain. Intervention may or may not be indicated. The patients are often asked to change their diet or begin medications to lower stone recurrence rates. All of these associations, in addition to the high recurrence rates, can have a significant impact on the QOL of a patient.

Stone formers have been shown to have more stressful life events. There have even been links to renal colic and symptoms of anxiety and depression. Furthermore, interventions for urolithiasis can also have an effect on QOL. Ureteral stents, PCNL, URS, and SWL all have their own associated side effects and complications that can affect outcomes in regard to patient well-being beyond SFR.

The following is a comprehensive look at the literature and compilation of a review of the effects of urolithiasis on patient QOL. Associations between stone disease and stress and/or psychiatric disorders and how interventions (surgical and medical) may affect patient QOL are discussed.

Stress, Depression, and QOL in Patients with Urolithiasis

Negative emotional and psychological effects of chronic disease can be seen in stone formers. Like other chronic diseases, there have been associations between urolithiasis and stress, depression, and further psychological disorders. Stress is a psychological term related to the perception of one's mental and physical well-being. It is not clear whether stress is a cause or an effect of a given condition or situation. Either way, patients experience a change in their perception of their own well-being and sometimes have physiologic reactions to these stressors. It is well known that chronic diseases are associated with increased stress levels.

When compared with the general population, recurrent stone formers and those with other chronic diseases have higher stress levels. In stone formers, increased stress has been associated with presence of symptoms.[97] It has been shown in case control studies that stressful life events were significantly greater in patients with recurrent painful renal colic.[98] When comparing validated stress questionnaires, Miyaoka and colleagues[97] have shown increased stress levels in those with the presence of symptoms but no significant difference in stress between recurrent stone formers and nonrecurrent stone formers. One might infer from this data that acute exacerbations of chronic illness cause increased stress levels, and the presence of symptoms (ie, renal colic) is the true stressor independent of chronicity of disease.

Najem and colleagues[99] have shown an increase in incidence of symptomatic stone disease in subjects who have preceding stressful life events. The notion of stress causing renal calculi has been proposed, but difficult to prove. Onset of stress can easily be determined from good history taking and the timing of stressful life events such as loss of employment, death of a loved one, or other traumatic event. However, it is difficult to determine the onset of calculi formation in relation to the timing of the stressor. Because all stones must start from a nidus and are initially asymptomatic, it proves difficult to determine if stone formation precedes the stressor (ie, the effect model of stress) or if the stressor actually predates the calculi formation (ie, the cause model of stress).[97,99]

Depression has also been linked to chronic diseases, and it is no surprise that there is a higher prevalence of reported depression in patients with urolithiasis. In the United States, depression has a lifetime prevalence of 16.5%.[100] Diagnosis of depression is defined by the *Diagnostic and Statistical Manual of Mental Disorders* (*DSM*) *IV* criteria. Patients must exhibit depressed mood and/or decreased functionality in addition to five or more of the following: weight loss or weight gain, insomnia, psychomotor agitation or retardation, fatigue, feelings of worthlessness, decreased ability to think or concentrate, or recurrent thought of death or suicidal ideation.[100]

A key characteristic for clinically diagnosed depression is that the *DSM IV* criteria cannot be caused by an underlying medical condition.[101] When assessing chronic diseases like urolithiasis, it is important to determine if the *DSM IV* criteria are caused by associated symptoms of stone disease. When looking at increased depression rates in chronic diseases, such as chronic obstructive pulmonary disease, asthma, diabetes, and congestive heart failure, one can postulate that the depressive symptoms exist during and well after acute exacerbations of the underlying chronic disease. However, there have not been many studies looking at clinically diagnosed depression and urolithiasis. Angell and colleagues[102] reported a correlation between depression and urolithiasis; however, this study used a depression symptom questionnaire and did not clinically diagnose depression as defined by the *DSM IV*. Patients with a stone episode within the past year and those requiring greater than one emergency room visit had a "significant level of physiologic distress" according to their scores on the depression questionnaire. A study from Taiwan reported that subjects with newly diagnosed urinary calculi are 1.75 times more likely to be diagnosed with depressive disorder within 1 year than controls.[103] Diniz and colleagues[104] have shown a significant linear correlation between symptoms of depression and the number of recurrent renal colic episodes. As shown in other illnesses with pain exacerbations, there is a reciprocal correlation between pain and depressive symptoms. For example, individuals with chronic lower back pain are more likely to have depressive symptoms after 2 years, and patients with baseline depressive symptoms are more likely to experience debilitating lower back pain exacerbations.[105]

Researchers have started to look at overall QOL in regard to patients with chronic urolithiasis. Instead of looking at stress and depression as individual symptoms, QOL questionnaires can encompass a variety of symptoms and give investigators a better understanding of how chronic urolithiasis affects patients' perception of their own mental and physical well-being. There have been many studies looking at urolithiasis and health-related QOL outcomes. Similar to stress and depressive symptom studies, QOL investigations assess patient well-being in relation to renal colic symptoms, chronicity of disease, and urolithiasis interventions. QOL studies may provide better insight (compared with stress and depressive studies) into how recurrent stone formers perceive their own health and may potentially influence management and treatment outcomes with overall patient well-being taken into consideration.

QOL is usually determined via a questionnaire or survey. Based on scores, the QOL of patients with urolithiasis can be compared with the general population. The most commonly used QOL questionnaire for urolithiasis in the literature is the SF-36 (Short Form-36) health survey, a validated 36 item general health and well-being questionnaire split into domains encompassing physical, social, and emotional health. In total there are eight domains: physical functioning, role limitations due to physical health, bodily pain, general health, vitality, social functioning, role-emotional. and mental health.

Similar to increased stress and depression symptoms, patients with recurrent symptomatic urolithiasis have a decreased QOL. In case control studies, subjects with recurrent painful renal colic have a substantially impaired QOL.[106] Patients with a stone episode less than 1 month before surveying also have lower QOL scores; however, as seen with stress and depression indices, people with remote stone episodes have comparable QOL scores to those of the general public.[107] Within groups of patients with urolithiasis, patients with comorbid conditions such as obesity, HTN, and diabetes tend to have worse QOL scores than their associated counterparts.[107,108] Female stone formers also tend to have a lower QOL compared with their male counterparts.[108] Universal among studies comparing stone formers' QOL with the general population show that all domains are not uniformly lower in stone formers. Penniston and Nakada[108] found statistically significant differences in stone formers in the bodily pain and general health domains only. Bensalah and colleagues[107] found lower scores in five of eight domains (physical functioning, role-physical. general health, role-emotional. and social functioning) in their stone formers compared with the US general population. Bryant and colleagues[109] found decreased QOL scores in six of eight domains (physical function, role physical. bodily pain, general health, vitality, and social function) in their stone former population. They reported lower QOL in patients with recent stone events, greater than one emergency room visit, and in those with greater than two surgical procedures.

Discrepancies in QOL scores between populations of stone formers at different institutions are evident when reviewing the literature. Donnally and colleagues[110] looked at these discrepancies by questioning the validity of the SF-36 QOL questionnaire in subjects with urolithiasis. When comparing QOL after a recent stone event to those 18 months later with no recurrence, there were no differences in QOL scores. One would anticipate that an improvement in disease and an absence of symptomatic recurrence would show an improvement in QOL scores. By definition, in order for a QOL questionnaire to be validated for a specific disease, there must be improvements in scores when there are improvements in the disease on follow-up survey.

Importantly, 20 of the 36 questions in the SF-36 questionnaire are specific to events within the last 4 weeks. This could be why recent symptomatic stone events correlate to significantly lower QOL scores. Score and domain discrepancies in the QOL questionnaire between populations of recurrent stone formers at different institutions can in part be attributed to the natural progression of recurrent stone formation and the timing bias seen in the SF-36 questionnaire.

Management of Urolithiasis and QOL

In addition to QOL evaluation for urolithiasis and its associated symptoms, it is also important to evaluate QOL in regard to management of urinary stone disease. Urolithiasis has multiple treatment modalities. Over the years, treatment of kidney stones has become less invasive and there has been broader adoption of medical management and dietary modifications to prevent recurrence. Historically, endpoints of clinical studies have been SFR, which are defined by nonstandardized postmanagement imaging. Patients are counseled on which intervention and/or management strategy would achieve optimal SFR. QOL is not usually addressed with the proper attention.

The European Association of Urology (EAU) and American Urological Association (AUA) have established treatment guidelines for urolithiasis based mainly on stone size, location, and density (EAU/AUA Guidelines, 2005–2008). Most of these recommendations were tailored based on trials' SFR and even within guidelines there are still some areas of uncertainty, including management of asymptomatic renal stones, lower pole calculi, and small ureteral calculi. Urologists may propose multiple surgical interventions as options to their patients if a definitive treatment modality has not yet been proved superior. Overall, there are few clinical trials prospectively comparing different surgical management options for urolithiasis with QOL incorporated as an endpoint.

Keeley and Assimos[111] and Keeley and colleagues[112] showed that, in subjects with asymptomatic renal calculi, SWL had a reduced need for surgical intervention after a 2-year follow-up compared with observation. However, there was no difference in QOL or SFR between the two groups. When reviewing the literature on lower pole calculi, SFR are higher in subjects receiving PCNL and URS compared with SWL.[111–114] Clinically, SWL is not as effective for lower pole calculi but, when looking at QOL outcomes, patients who underwent SWL compared with URS had fewer complications, required less pain relief, and were more likely to choose SWL again.[111,113] According to Albala and colleagues,[114] when compared with PCNL for lower pole calculi, SWL had similar SF-36 scores, indicating no difference in QOL outcomes. Again, the PCNL group had a higher SFR, but had more complications. When comparing PCNL to URS for lower pole stones, higher SFR and a reduced need for secondary procedures were seen in the PCNL group, but a similar QOL score was found among cohorts. Even though the PCNL group had more complications, when questioned, more subjects would prefer PCNL again in comparison to URS for management of their lower pole calculi.[111] When looking at ureteral calculi, URS achieves higher SFRs and a reduced need for repeat intervention when compared with SWL.[115] However, URS is associated with a higher complication rate and increased hospital stay, both of which can affect QOL outcomes.

In addition to the above-mentioned controversies, disagreement also persists concerning ureteral stenting for stone disease. With regard to SFR, stenting versus not stenting for URS is similar.[116] Ureteral stenting in combination with SWL or URS may be required but is not without drawbacks that should be addressed during patient counseling. Most individuals will experience one or more known side effects: irritative voiding symptoms, pain, incontinence, and/or hematuria. Joshi and colleagues[117,118] looked at QOL issues in subjects with ureteral stenting and the SF-36 questionnaire was shown to be neither specific nor sensitive in these studies. The investigators developed disease-specific QOL questionnaires, which incorporated general health scores and the described stent-associated symptoms, as well as sexual health complications. It was determined by using these validated disease-specific questionnaires that ureteral stenting is associated with significant morbidity and reduced QOL in 80% of patients with stents. These results strongly reinforce the need for QOL measures to be considered when determining management of urolithiasis. Based on the studies of Joshi and colleagues,[117,118] it becomes clear that a critical evaluation of indications for ureteral stenting after uncomplicated urolithiasis procedures is required to identify those patients who will benefit from temporary diversion.

Strong efforts have been made in the basic science and clinical research arenas to better understand the pathophysiology of stone disease and to prevent recurrent stone disease. Nevertheless, half of patients have repeated stone episodes after their initial event regardless of initial intervention.[119,120] Evidence shows that increasing fluid intake can greatly reduce the risk of repeat stone formation, regardless of the type of calculi. Meta-analysis through systematic review of randomized controlled trials by Fink and colleagues[121] established the efficacy of fluid intake modification by showing that high water intake lowered the long-term risk of nephrolithiasis recurrence by 60%. The efficacy of dietary modification is less understood, but low animal protein diets, and decreased sodium and oxalate intake have been shown to decrease stone recurrence rates.[120–122] As more is understood about metabolic abnormalities in recurrent stone formers, targeted medical therapy is being investigated to reduce repeat stone episodes. Potassium citrate can reduce stone formation rates by greater than 90% in patients with hypocitraturia.[123]

Despite the abundant data supporting dietary modifications and long-term medication use for reducing stone recurrence, to the authors knowledge there are no evaluations correlating dietary modifications and long-term medications to patient QOL in stone formers. Both increased fluid intake and chronic medication use can have compliance issues and dramatically affect ones QOL. For example, some patients' daily lives may not be very accommodating to the frequent restroom breaks which are associated with increased fluid intake, including health professionals, teachers, and truck drivers. Furthermore, it may be unfair to compare chronic medication use in other diseases that may lead to life-threatening sequelae (eg, diabetes, HTN) with the need for chronic medication for stone formers. Each medication has specific side-effect profiles to consider that may affect QOL and compliance. To address this, new formularies, such as Urocit-K 15, are being developed to allow increased dosing flexibility, improved compliance, and better tolerability.[120] Drug companies and physicians should continue to strive for improved treatment regimens that emphasize patient compliance and tolerability in hopes that this improves QOL.

SUMMARY

Although stone research has lead to evolution in the understanding of stone pathophysiology, revolution in approaches to stone prevention, and innovation in surgical management of calculi, the next step is a critical assessment of the impact of these advancements on patients' QOL and CKD. Physicians should strive to treat the disease and the patient, with an eye on optimizing patient well-being. For a generally non–life-threatening disease such as urolithiasis, QOL outcomes and impact on renal function must be taken into consideration.

Initial studies using the SF-36 questionnaire have been promising in determining patients' perception of their own well-being in regards to stone disease management. However, the evident discrepancies in SF-36 results among different populations at various institutions warrant critique of this generalized questionnaire. Validated urolithiasis-specific QOL questionnaires are needed. By combining a stone-specific questionnaire with the SF-36, some investigators were able to better correlate certain stone specific variables with lower QOL scores.[109] With a validated urolithiasis QOL questionnaire, appropriate interventions and proper management to prevent recurrence can be evaluated beyond the objective scope of stone-free and reduced recurrence rates. Validated questionnaires, such as the SHIM (sexual health inventory for men) score and AUA-SS (American Urological Association Symptom Score), have been used in the management and treatment of other urologic diseases, such as erectile dysfunction and lower urinary tract pathologic states, and it is time for the same caliber of validated questionnaire for the treatment and management of stone disease.

REFERENCES

1. Lotan Y. Economics and cost of care of stone disease. Adv Chronic Kidney Dis 2009;16(1):5–10.
2. Pearle MS, Calhoun EA, Curhan GC. Urologic diseases in America project: urolithiasis. J Urol 2005;173(3):848–57.
3. Stamatelou KK, Francis ME, Jones CA, et al. Time trends in reported prevalence of kidney stones in the United States: 1976–1994. Kidney Int 2003; 63(5):1817–23.
4. Lieske JC, Peña de la Vega LS, Slezak JM, et al. Renal stone epidemiology in Rochester, Minnesota: an update. Kidney Int 2006;69(4):760–4.
5. Taylor EN, Stampfer MJ, Curhan GC. Obesity, weight gain, and the risk of kidney stones. JAMA 2005;293:455–62.
6. Taylor EN, Stampfer MJ, Curhan GC. Diabetes mellitus and the risk of nephrolithiasis. Kidney Int 2005; 68(3):1230–5.
7. Romero V, Akpinar H, Assimos DG. Kidney stones: a global picture of prevalence, incidence, and associated risk factors. Rev Urol 2010;12(2–3):e86–96.
8. Lamson OF. Recurrent nephrolithiasis. Ann Surg 1920;71(1):16–21.
9. Hall PM. Nephrolithiasis: treatment, causes, and prevention. Cleve Clin J Med 2009;76(10):583–91.
10. Coe FL, Keck J, Norton ER. The natural history of calcium urolithiasis. JAMA 1977;238(14):1519–23.
11. Williams RE. Long-term survey of 538 patients with upper urinary tract stone. Br J Urol 1963;35:416–37.
12. Borghi L, Schianchi T, Meschi T, et al. Comparison of two diets for the prevention of recurrent stones in idiopathic hypercalciuria. N Engl J Med 2002;346: 77–84.
13. Poullain J, Devevey JM, Mousson C, et al. Management of lithiasis of kidney transplant. Prog Urol 2010;20(2):138–43.
14. Challacombe B, Dasgupta P, Tiptaft R, et al. Multimodal management of urolithiasis in renal transplantation. BJU Int 2005;96(3):385–9.
15. Stravodimos KG, Adamis S, Tyritzis S, et al. Renal transplant lithiasis: analysis of our series and review of the literature. J Endourol 2012;26(1):38–44.
16. Griffen WO Jr, Bivins BA, Bell RM. The decline and fall of the jejunoileal bypass. Surg Gynecol Obstet 1983;157(4):301–8.
17. Requarth JA, Burchard KW, Colacchio TA, et al. Long-term morbidity following jejunoileal bypass. The continuing potential need for surgical reversal. Arch Surg 1995;130(3):318–25.
18. Sinha MK, Collazo-Clavell ML, Rule A, et al. Hyperoxaluric nephrolithiasis is a complication of Roux-en-Y gastric bypass surgery. Kidney Int 2007; 72(1):100–7.
19. Lieske JC, Kumar R, Collazo-Clavell ML. Nephrolithiasis after bariatric surgery for obesity. Semin Nephrol 2008;28(2):163–73.
20. Durrani O, Morrisroe S, Jackman S, et al. Analysis of stone disease in morbidly obese patients undergoing gastric bypass surgery. J Endourol 2006; 20(10):749–52.
21. Milliner DS, Wilson DM, Smith LH. Phenotypic expression of primary hyperoxaluria: comparative features of types I and II. Kidney Int 2001;59(1):31–6.
22. Harambat J, Fargue S, Bacchetta J, et al. Primary hyperoxaluria. Int J Nephrol 2011;2011:864580.
23. Griffith DP. Struvite stones. Kidney Int 1978;13(5): 372–82.
24. Rodman JS. Struvite stones. Nephron 1999; 81(Suppl 1):50–9.
25. Font-Llitjós M, Jiménez-Vidal M, Bisceglia L, et al. New insights into cystinuria: 40 new mutations, genotype-phenotype correlation, and digenic inheritance causing partial phenotype. J Med Genet 2005;42(1):58–68.
26. Milliner DS. Cystinuria. Endocrinol Metab Clin North Am 1990;19(4):889–907.
27. Shekarriz B, Stoller ML. Cystinuria and other noncalcareous calculi. Endocrinol Metab Clin North Am 2002;31:951–77.
28. Saigal CS, Joyce G, Timilsina AR. Direct and indirect costs of nephrolithiasis in an employed population: opportunity for disease management? Kidney Int 2005;68(4):1808–14.
29. Coresh J, Selvin E, Stevens LA, et al. Prevalence of chronic kidney disease in the United States. JAMA 2007;298:2038–47.
30. United States renal data system. 2011 annual data report. Available at: http://www.usrds.org/adr.aspx. Accessed October 15, 2012.
31. Couser WG, Riella MC, Joint International Society of Nephrology, International Federation of Kidney Foundations World Kidney Day 2011 Steering Committee. World Kidney Day 2011: protect your kidneys, save your heart. Clin J Am Soc Nephrol 2011;6(2):235–8.
32. Goel MC, Ahlawat R, Kumar M, et al. Chronic renal failure and nephrolithiasis in a solitary kidney: role of intervention. J Urol 1997;157:1574.
33. Gupta NP, Kochar GS, Wadhwa SN, et al. Management of patients renal and ureteric calculi presenting with chronic renal insufficiency. Br J Urol 1985; 57:130.
34. Gupta M, Bolton DM, Gupta PN, et al. Improved renal function following aggressive treatment of urolithiasis and concurrent mild to moderate renal insufficiency. J Urol 1994;152:1086.

35. Marangella M, Bruno M, Cosseddu D, et al. Prevalence of chronic renal insufficiency in the course of idiopathic recurrent calcium stone disease: risk factors and patterns of progression. Nephron 1990;54:302.
36. Gambaro G, D'Angelo A, Favaro S. Risk for renal failure in nephrolithiasis. Am J Kidney Dis 2001; 37:233.
37. Frymoyer PA, Scheinman SJ, Dunham PB, et al. X-linked recessive nephrolithiasis with renal failure. N Engl J Med 1991;325:681–6.
38. Leumann EP. Primary hyperoxaluria: an important cause of renal failure in infancy. Int J Pediatr Nephrol 1985;6:13–6.
39. Worcester EM, Coe FL, Evan AP, et al. Reduced renal function and benefits of treatment in cystinuria vs other forms of nephrolithiasis. BJU Int 2006;97:1285–90.
40. Jungers P, Joly D, Barbey F, et al. ESRD caused by nephrolithiasis: prevalence, mechanisms, and prevention. Am J Kidney Dis 2004;44:799–805.
41. Worcester E, Parks JH, Josephson MA, et al. Causes and consequences of kidney loss in patients with nephrolithiasis. Kidney Int 2003;64: 2204–13.
42. Gillen DL, Worcester EM, Coe FL. Decreased renal function among adults with a history of nephrolithiasis: a study of NHANES III. Kidney Int 2005; 67:685–90.
43. Vupputuri S, Soucie JM, McClellan W, et al. History of kidney stones as a possible risk factor for chronic kidney disease. Ann Epidemiol 2004;14: 222–8.
44. Rule AD, Bergstralh EJ, Melton LJ 3rd, et al. Kidney stones and the risk for chronic kidney disease. Clin J Am Soc Nephrol 2009;4:804–11.
45. Craver L, Marco MP, Martínez I, et al. Mineral metabolism parameters throughout chronic kidney disease stages 1–5: Achievement of K/DOQI target ranges. Nephrol Dial Transplant 2007;22: 1171–6.
46. Tosetto E, Graziotto R, Artifoni L, et al. Dent's disease and prevalence of renal stones in dialysis patients in Northeastern Italy. J Hum Genet 2006; 51:25–30.
47. Collins AJ, Foley RN, Herzog C, et al. US renal data system 2010 annual data report. Am J Kidney Dis 2001;57(Suppl 1):A8, e521–A8, e526.
48. Stankus N, Hammes M, Gillen D, et al. African American ESRD patients have a high pre-dialysis prevalence of kidney stones compared to NHANES III. Urol Res 2007;35:83–7.
49. Hippisley-Cox J, Coupland C. Predicting the risk of chronic kidney disease in men and women in England and Wales: prospective derivation and external validation of the QKidney scores. BMC Fam Pract 2010;11:49.
50. Levey AS, Bosch JP, Lewis JB, et al. A more accurate method to estimate glomerular filtration rate from serum creatinine: a new prediction equation. Modification of diet in renal disease study group. Ann Intern Med 1999;16:461–70.
51. Bilen CY, Inci K, Kocak B, et al. Impact of percutaneous nephrolithotomy on estimated glomerular filtration rate in patients with chronic kidney disease. J Endourol 2008;22:895–900.
52. Lotan Y, Pearle MS. Economics of stone management. Urol Clin North Am 2007;34:443–53.
53. Preminger GM, Tiselius HG, Assimos DG, et al. 2007 Guideline for the management of ureteral calculi. Eur Urol 2007;52:1610–31.
54. Preminger GM, Tiselius HG, Assimos DG, et al. 2007 guideline for the management of ureteral calculi. J Urol 2007;178:2418–34.
55. Willis LR, Evan AP, Connors BA, et al. Relationship between kidney size, renal injury, and renal impairment induced by shock wave lithotripsy. J Am Soc Nephrol 1999;10:1753–62.
56. Evan AP, Willis LR, Lingeman JE, et al. Renal trauma and the risk of long-term complications in shock wave lithotripsy. Nephron 1998;78:1–8.
57. Eassa WA, Sheir KZ, Gad HM, et al. Prospective study of the long-term effects of shock wave lithotripsy on renal function and blood pressure. J Urol 2008;179:964–8 [discussion: 968–9].
58. Krambeck AE, LeRoy AJ, Patterson DE, et al. Long-term outcomes of percutaneous nephrolithotomy compared to shock wave lithotripsy and conservative management. J Urol 2008;179:2233–7.
59. Krambeck AE, Gettman MT, Rohlinger AL, et al. Diabetes mellitus and hypertension associated with shock wave lithotripsy of renal and proximal ureteral stones at 19 years of followup. J Urol 2006;175:1742–7.
60. Janetschek G, Frauscher F, Knapp R, et al. New onset hypertension after extracorporeal shock wave lithotripsy. Age related incidence and prediction by intrarenal resistive index. J Urol 1997;158: 346–51.
61. Barbosa PV, Makhlouf AA, Thorner D, et al. Shock wave lithotripsy associated with greater prevalence of hypertension. Urology 2011;78(1):22–5.
62. Sato Y, Tanda H, Kato S, et al. Shock wave lithotripsy for renal stones is not associated with hypertension and diabetes mellitus. Urology 2008;71: 586–91 [discussion: 591–2].
63. Elves AW, Tilling K, Menezes P, et al. Early observations of the effect of extracorporeal shockwave lithotripsy on blood pressure: a prospective randomized control clinical trial. BJU Int 2000;85:611–5.
64. Krambeck AE, Rule AD, Li X, et al. Shock wave lithotripsy is not predictive of hypertension among community stone formers at long-term followup. J Urol 2011;185:164–9.

65. Willis LR, Evan AP, Connors BA, et al. Prevention of lithotripsy-induced renal injury by pretreating kidneys with low-energy shock waves. J Am Soc Nephrol 2006;17:663–73.
66. el-Assmy A, el-Nahas AR, Hekal IA, et al. Long-term effects of extracorporeal shock wave lithotripsy on renal function: our experience with 156 patients with solitary kidney. J Urol 2008;179(6):2229–32.
67. Abdel-Khalek M, Sheir K, Elsobky E, et al. Prognostic factors for extracorporeal shock-wave lithotripsy of ureteric stones—a multivariate analysis study. Scand J Urol Nephrol 2003;37:413–8.
68. Abdel-Khalek M, Sheir KZ, Mokhtar AA, et al. Prediction of success rate after extracorporeal shock-wave lithotripsy of renal stones—a multivariate analysis model. Scand J Urol Nephrol 2004;38:161–7.
69. Salman M, Al-Ansari AA, Talib RA, et al. Prediction of success of extracorporeal shock wave lithotripsy in the treatment of ureteric stones. Int Urol Nephrol 2007;39:85–9.
70. Hung SF, Chung SD, Wang SM, et al. Chronic kidney disease affects the stone-free rate after extracorporeal shock wave lithotripsy for proximal ureteric stones. BJU Int 2010;105(8):1162–7.
71. Seitz C, Fajkovic H, Remzi M, et al. Rapid extracorporeal shock wave lithotripsy treatment after a first colic episode correlates with accelerated ureteral stone clearance. Eur Urol 2006;49:1099–105.
72. Tombal B, Mawlawi H, Feyaerts A, et al. Prospective randomized evaluation of emergency extracorporeal shock wave lithotripsy (ESWL) on the short-time outcome of symptomatic ureteral stones. Eur Urol 2005;47:855–9.
73. Tligui M, El Khadime MR, Tchala K, et al. Emergency extracorporeal shock wave lithotripsy (ESWL) for obstructing ureteral stones. Eur Urol 2003;43:552–5.
74. Seitz C, Tanovic E, Kikic Z, et al. Rapid extracorporeal shock wave lithotripsy for proximal ureteral calculi in colic versus noncolic patients. Eur Urol 2007;52:1223–7.
75. Madaan S, Joyce AD. Limitations of extracorporeal shock wave lithotripsy. Curr Opin Urol 2007;17:109–13.
76. Lee C, Ugarte R, Best S, et al. Impact of renal function on efficacy of extracorporeal shockwave lithotripsy. J Endourol 2007;21:490–3.
77. Bhatia V, Biyani CS, al-Awadi K. Extracorporeal shockwave therapy for urolithiasis with renal insufficiency. Urol Int 1995;55:11–5.
78. Srivastava A, Sinha T, Karan SC, et al. Assessing the efficiency of extracorporeal shockwave lithotripsy for stones in renal units with impaired function: a prospective controlled study. Urol Res 2006;34:283–7.
79. Paryani JP, Ather MH. Improvement in serum creatinine following definite treatment of urolithiasis in patients with concurrent renal insufficiency. Scand J Urol Nephrol 2002;36:134–6.
80. Singh I, Gupta NP, Hemal AK, et al. Efficacy and outcome of surgical intervention in patients with nephrolithiasis and chronic renal failure. Int Urol Nephrol 2001;33:293–8.
81. Agrawal MS, Aron M, Asopa HS. Endourological renal salvage in patients with calculus nephropathy and advanced uraemia. BJU Int 1999;84:252–6.
82. Kukreja R, Desai M, Patel SH, et al. Nephrolithiasis associated with renal insufficiency: factors predicting outcome. J Endourol 2003;17:875–9.
83. Canes D, Hegarty NJ, Kamoi K, et al. Functional outcomes following percutaneous surgery in the solitary kidney. J Urol 2009;181:154.
84. Kurien A, Baishya R, Mishra S, et al. The impact of percutaneous nephrolithotomy in patients with chronic kidney disease. J Endourol 2009;23:1403.
85. Akman T, Binbay M, Aslan R, et al. Long-term outcomes of percutaneous nephrolithotomy in 177 patients with chronic kidney disease: a single center experience. J Urol 2012;187(1):173–7.
86. Handa RK, Willis LR, Connors BA, et al. Time-course for recovery of renal function after unilateral (single-tract) percutaneous access in the pig. J Endourol 2010;24:283.
87. Traxer O, Smith TG 3rd, Pearle MS, et al. Renal parenchymal injury after standard and mini percutaneous nephrostolithotomy. J Urol 2001;165:1693.
88. Unsal A, Koca G, Reşorlu B, et al. Effect of percutaneous nephrolithotomy and tract dilatation methods on renal function: assessment by quantitative single-photon emission computed tomography of technetium-99m dimercaptosuccinic acid uptake by the kidneys. J Endourol 2010;24:1497.
89. Moskovitz B, Halachmi S, Sopov V, et al. Effect of percutaneous nephrolithotripsy on renal function: assessment with quantitative SPECT of 99mTc-DMSA renal scintigraphy. J Endourol 2006;20:102.
90. Gopalakrishnan G, Prasad GS. Management of urolithiasis with chronic renal failure. Curr Opin Urol 2007;17:132–5.
91. Michel MS, Trojan L, Rassweiler JJ. Complications in percutaneous nephrolithotomy. Eur Urol 2007;51:899–906.
92. Kukreja R, Desai M, Patel S, et al. Factors affecting blood loss during percutaneous nephrolithotomy: prospective study. J Endourol 2004;18:715–22.
93. Troxel SA, Low RK. Renal intrapelvic pressure during percutaneous nephrolithotomy and its correlation with the development of postoperative fever. J Urol 2002;168:1348–51.
94. Zhong W, Zeng G, Wu K, et al. Does a smaller tract in percutaneous nephrolithotomy contribute to high

renal pelvic pressure and postoperative fever? J Endourol 2008;22:2147–51.
95. Joshi HB, Kumar PV, Timoney AG. Citric acid (solution R) irrigation in the treatment of refractory infection (struvite) stone disease: Is it useful? Eur Urol 2001;39:586–90.
96. Collins S, Ortiz J, Maruffo F, et al. Expediated struvite-stone dissolution using a high-flow low-pressure irrigation system. J Endourol 2007;21:1153–8.
97. Miyaoka R, Ortiz-Alvarado O, Kriedberg C, et al. Correlation between stress and kidney stone disease. J Endourol 2012;26(5):551–5.
98. Diniz DH, Schor N, Blay SL. Stressful life events and painful recurrent colic of renal lithiasis. J Urol 2006;176(6 Pt 1):2483–7 [discussion: 2487].
99. Najem GR, Seebode JJ, Samady AJ, et al. Stressful life events and risk of symptomatic kidney stones. Int J Epidemiol 1997;26(5):1017–23.
100. Kessler RC, Berglund P, Demler O. Lifetime prevalence and age-of-onset distributions of DSM-IV disorders in the National Comorbidity Survey Replication. Arch Gen Psychiatry 2005;62:593–602.
101. American Psychiatric Association. Diagnostic and statistical manual of mental disorders. Revised 4th edition. Washington, DC: Author; 2000.
102. Angell J, Bryant M, Tu H, et al. Association of depression and urolithiasis. Urology 2012;79(3):518–25.
103. Chung SD, Keller JJ, Lin HC. Increased risk of depressive disorder within 1 year after diagnosis with urinary calculi in Taiwan. Psychiatry Res 2012. [Epub ahead of print].
104. Diniz DH, Blay SL, Schor N. Anxiety and depression symptoms in recurrent painful renallithiasis colic. Braz J Med Biol Res 2007;40(7):949–55.
105. Meyer T, Cooper J, Raspe H. Disabling low back pain and depressive symptoms in the community-dwelling elderly: a prospective study. Spine 2007;32(21):2380–6.
106. Diniz DH, Blay SL, Schor N. Quality of life of patients with nephrolithiasis and recurrent painful renal colic. Nephron Clin Pract 2007;106(3):c91–7.
107. Bensalah K, Tuncel A, Gupta A, et al. Determinants of quality of life for patients with kidney stones. J Urol 2008;179(6):2238–43 [discussion: 2243].
108. Penniston KL, Nakada SY. Health related quality of life differs between male and female stone formers. J Urol 2007;178(6):2435–40 [discussion: 2440].
109. Bryant M, Angell J, Tu H, et al. Health related quality of life for stone formers. J Urol 2012;188(2):436–40.
110. Donnally CJ 3rd, Gupta A, Bensalah K, et al. Longitudinal evaluation of the SF-36 quality of life questionnaire in patients with kidney stones. Urol Res 2011;39(2):141–6.
111. Keeley FX Jr, Assimos DG. Clinical trials of the surgical management of urolithiasis: current status and future needs. Adv Chronic Kidney Dis 2009;16(1):65–9.
112. Keeley FX Jr, Tilling K, Elves A, et al. Preliminary results of a randomized controlled trial of prophylactic shock wave lithotripsy for small asymptomatic renal caliceal stones. BJU Int 2001;87(1):1–8.
113. Pearle MS, Lingeman JE, Leveillee R, et al. Prospective randomized trial comparing shock wave lithotripsy and ureteroscopy for lower pole caliceal calculi 1 cm or less. J Urol 2008;179(5 Suppl):S69–73.
114. Albala DM, Assimos DG, Clayman RV, et al. Lower pole I: a prospective randomized trial of extracorporeal shock wave lithotripsy and percutaneous nephrostolithotomy for lower pole nephrolithiasis-initial results. J Urol 2001;166(6):2072–80.
115. Aboumarzouk OM, Kata SG, Keeley FX, et al. Extracorporeal shock wave lithotripsy (ESWL) versus ureteroscopic management for ureteric calculi. Cochrane Database Syst Rev 2012;(5):CD006029.
116. Nabi G, Cook J, N'Dow J, et al. Outcomes of stenting after uncomplicated ureteroscopy: systematic review and meta-analysis. BMJ 2007;334(7593):572.
117. Joshi HB, Newns N, Stainthorpe A, et al. Ureteral stent symptom questionnaire: development and validation of a multidimensional quality of life measure. J Urol 2003;169(3):1060–4.
118. Joshi HB, Stainthorpe A, Keeley FX Jr, et al. Indwelling ureteralstents: evaluation of quality of life to aid outcome analysis. J Endourol 2001;15(2):151–4.
119. Raynal G, Petit J, Saint F. Which efficiency index for urinary stones treatment? Urol Res 2009;37(4):237–9.
120. Lipkin ME, Preminger GM. Demystifying the medical management of nephrolithiasis. Rev Urol 2011;13(1):34–8.
121. Fink HA, Akornor JW, Garimella PS, et al. Diet, fluid, or supplements for secondary prevention of nephrolithiasis: a systematic review and meta-analysis of randomized trials. Eur Urol 2009;56(1):72–80.
122. Ortiz-Alvarado O, Miyaoka R, Kriedberg C, et al. Impact of dietary counseling on urinary stone risk parameters in recurrent stone formers. J Endourol 2011;25(3):535–40.
123. Robinson MR, Leitao VA, Haleblian GE, et al. Impact of long-term potassium citrate therapy on urinary profiles and recurrent stone formation. J Urol 2009;181(3):1145–50.

Urol Clin N Am
http://dx.doi.org/10.1016/
0094-0143/13/$ – see front matter

Index

Note: Page numbers of article titles are in **boldface** type.

Urol Clin N Am 40 (2013) 149–154
http://dx.doi.org/10.1016/S0094-0143(12)00115-2
0094-0143/13/$ – see front matter

M

N

O

P

U

Printed and bound by CPI Group (UK) Ltd, Croydon, CR0 4YY

03/10/2024

01040347-0010